THE
Transformation

THE
Transformation

DISCOVERING WHOLENESS AND
HEALING AFTER TRAUMA

JAMES S. GORDON, MD

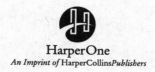

HarperOne
An Imprint of HarperCollinsPublishers

HarperOne

THE TRANSFORMATION. Copyright © 2019 by James S. Gordon. All rights reserved. Printed in the United States of America. No part of this book may be used or reproduced in any manner whatsoever without written permission except in the case of brief quotations embodied in critical articles and reviews. For information, address HarperCollins Publishers, 195 Broadway, New York, NY 10007.

HarperCollins books may be purchased for educational, business, or sales promotional use. For information, please email the Special Markets Department at SPsales@harpercollins.com.

FIRST EDITION

Designed by Lucy Albanese

Library of Congress Cataloging-in-Publication Data is available upon request.

ISBN 978-0-06-287071-1

19 20 21 22 23   LSC   10 9 8 7 6 5 4 3 2 1

For Gabriel Gordon-Berardi and Jamie Lord: I hold you in my heart
and
William Alfred, Robert Coles, Sharon Curtin, and Shyam Singha:
you lighted my path and warmed me on my way

Contents

Introduction

THERE ARE TWO common and dangerous misconceptions about psychological trauma.

The first is that trauma (the word is Greek and means "injury") comes only to some of us: combatants or civilians in a war, victims of natural disasters, survivors of rape and incest, children who've grown up in the most callous and sordid families.

The second is that trauma is an unmitigated disaster, causing permanent emotional crippling, requiring never-ending treatment, severely limiting the lives of those who've experienced it.

IN FACT, TRAUMA COMES, sooner or later, to all of us. In a recent government survey, 60 percent of US adults said that as children they had experienced significant abuse and/or neglect. Studies of adverse childhood experiences (ACEs) in the 1990s reported that more than a quarter of the middle-class, well-educated, and financially secure

Americans who were surveyed were as children "often or very often hit . . . so hard that [they] had marks or were injured."

Having a life-threatening illness, a long-term disability, or chronic pain is traumatic. So is caring for someone with these conditions.

Poverty is traumatizing, and so are racism and gender discrimination.

Loss of a loving relationship is deeply traumatizing. So is the loss of a job that gave our lives meaning and purpose.

And all of us, if we live long enough, will have to contend with the trauma of losing loved ones, and with old age, physical frailty, and death.

Trauma comes to all of us, and its consequences can be terrible. That's the truth and the bad news. The good news is that all of us can use tools of self-awareness and self-care to heal our trauma and, indeed, to become healthier and more whole than we've ever been. If we accept the pain that trauma inflicts, it can open our minds and bodies to healing change. If we relax with the chaos it brings, a new, more flexible, and more stable order can emerge. Our broken hearts can open with tender consideration and new love for others, as well as ourselves.

This is the timeless wisdom of the shamans, our planet's oldest indigenous healers, and also of our great religious and spiritual traditions: suffering is the soil in which wisdom and compassion grow; it is the school from which we graduate, committed to healing others' hurt. Recent scientific studies on post-traumatic growth yield similar conclusions.

This is what I know after fifty years of clinical work with traumatized people and from wrestling with and learning from the ordinary challenges and heartbreaking losses of my own long life. This is what I want to share with you, here, now, in *The Transformation*.

FIFTY YEARS AGO, as a resident in the emergency room of Jacobi, the Bronx's public hospital, I met Diana and began my trauma-healing work.

In medical school, I'd learned to enter the inner world of troubled children and older people struggling with life-threatening illness and also to listen to my own confusion and troubles. I reached out for help to Robert Coles, a young psychiatrist at the Harvard Health Services, who was working with the Black kids who were braving murderous mobs to integrate New Orleans schools. Bob helped me learn for myself the lessons that Freud had taught—how early childhood trauma of loss and forgotten abuse had made me more vulnerable to present loss. He also set an example of personal vulnerability and courageous commitment, sharing with me his own pain and loss and showing me I could make a healing difference in the larger world as well as with individual patients. And Bob helped me begin to know who I was, to appreciate my identity—an enduring sense of myself that has pulled me through troubled times.

While I was working as a student on medical and psychiatric wards, I was also welcoming other teachers who began to appear—in books as well as in my life.

Early on, there was *Man's Search for Meaning*, a slim memoir by Viktor Frankl, an Austrian Jewish psychiatrist whom the Nazis had confined in concentration camps. In Auschwitz, in the midst of the most inhumane abuse and unimaginable suffering, Frankl had found the meaning and purpose of his life. "Suffering ceases to be suffering," Frankl wrote, "at the moment it finds a meaning." He found his in appreciating, understanding, and having compassion for his fellow inmates and himself. He realized, even while his wife was being condemned to death in another camp, that "love is the ultimate good to which man can aspire." He learned to "say yes to life in spite of everything." Reading Frankl, admiring him, I knew I wanted to do the same.

HELPING DIANA HEAL called on everything Bob—and books, medical school, and my internship—had taught me and demanded a willingness to learn and take emotional chances I couldn't have imagined.

Diana arrived in the middle of the usual late-night chaos. She had a pixie face, chopped-off brown hair, and a compact body. She wore a pencil skirt and a Peter Pan blouse, and spoke in a wised-up Bronx way that mixed foul-mouthed street talk with offhand, spot-on psychological observation. Her medical chart was filled with dire diagnoses. Several psychiatrists had referred to a "borderline personality disorder," another, "multiple personalities"; one suggested she was "schizophrenic." She told me her current therapist was finishing his residency and that she was thinking of killing herself.

For the next two years, Diana and I met three or four times a week. I was her doctor, and she was my teacher. Every session was compelling, surprising, absorbing. I never knew who would appear in my office: a terrified eight-year-old; a snarling murderous version of her mother; a hip twenty-something; a helpless, thumb-sucking infant.

Diana's features seemed to change to fit the personality who was appearing. Her voice fell with whimpers and rose with screams and shouts. Sometimes she shrank into a corner and stared wildly, as if seeing her mother's ghost. Her severe trauma had apparently caused her self to fragment, to dissociate into different personalities that were unaware of one another. Freud's case histories were coming alive.

It became clear to me that Diana's diagnosis was far less important than the early, deep, and often repeated trauma that was responsible for her tortured ways. Over time I became aware of how childhood abuse shaped some of Diana's most disturbing and bewildering symptoms. "I am garbage. I stink," she growled at me one afternoon more than a year into our therapy, as enraged as she was ashamed. "My mother," she said between sobs and gasps, reliving it now, "used to force my head into the garbage. She told me that's where I belonged."

Sometimes I was stunned by Diana's rage—at my inattention

or the least hint of less than honest words. Sometimes I was flat-out frightened by what she was going through and of what she might do to hurt herself. And in between one or another kind of fear and all my effort to understand her and what she was teaching me about myself as a therapist and as a person, I felt my heart opening, maybe more than it ever had, my arms reaching to hold close the terrified child, the whole person, who lived inside this divided, troubled, brave young woman.

Slowly, slowly, Diana became aware that present challenges—her young children's needs, her husband's anger and sexual demands, my upcoming vacation—were evoking, "triggering," memories of the unmet needs, threatening rages, exploitation, and abandonment that had deformed her childhood.

As Diana shared and played out her past trauma with me, she seemed to grow taller, stand straighter. "I felt safe with you. There was a 'me' in there that was real," she told me years later. "I was drowning and you were warm and solid. I felt accepted, more full. Finally me."

As Diana felt safer, she became kinder and more generous to her kids. As her anxiety subsided, her "crazy" fears and rages began to quiet, and the light of her fine mind turned on.

Diana would have years more of demanding psychological work to do, but I could already feel the fragments of her being beginning to knit together. Healing, I was coming to understand, was possible even for the terribly traumatized.

Exploring Alternatives

My psychiatric residency was intense, focused. My ten years as a researcher at the National Institute of Mental Health (NIMH) were expansive and exploratory. I began by bringing what I learned from Diana and in the Bronx to runaway and homeless kids and their counselors, on the streets in Washington, DC, and nearby Prince George's County, and later, after I was selected to create a national program, to troubled kids and their families everywhere in America.

I now knew that all of us had suffered or would suffer trauma—hospitalized elders, obviously disturbed people like Diana, abused and confused homeless and runaway kids and their bewildered parents, as well as my colleagues, my teachers, and me. And I was coming to believe that all of us could recover from past trauma and meet future threats and blows with resiliency, even grace.

Still, I knew there were pieces missing from my trauma recovery program. I had to find ways to better understand the physical and spiritual as well as the mental, social, and emotional dimensions of our lives, ways to make them part of my healing work.

Many psychiatrists were now seeing emotional problems as brain disorders that demanded drug treatment. But this apparently rational biological approach seemed imprecise, inadequate, and even dangerous. Some people on psychiatric medication did feel better. Many, however, felt that taking the drugs defined them as sick, drug dependent, and incapable of acting to help themselves. Others were sure the meds blunted their emotions and stunted their creativity.

Studies were even then showing that antidepressant and antipsychotic drugs often disturbed digestion, put weight on those who took them, made their heads ache and their hands shake. And my own clinical experience was making it clear that the drugs were mostly treating symptoms, suppressing rather than resolving the trauma that caused so many of my patients' problems.

I wanted to find other answers: safe, nonpharmacological ways to promote a biological transformation that matched and enhanced the work I was doing with psychological healing.

The research I was reading on stress and stress-related illness was pointing in a new direction. I was learning that our biochemistry and physiology are affected by our thoughts and moods, where we live and whom we spend our time with. And I could feel it in myself. When I was hobbled by back pain, my mood plummeted. When I was frustrated and agitated, my back got in trouble.

Published studies were revealing that we could consciously use this mind-body connection to reverse emotional and physical damage. The research was telling us that forty minutes a day of silent meditation could lower blood pressure, quiet anxiety, improve mood, decrease pain, and enhance immunity and brain functioning. Like every doctor, I knew that Hippocrates, the father of Western medicine, had admonished us to "first do no harm." If meditation worked so well, with no downside, then it seemed to me that it should be the first line of treatment, and medication, with its damaging side effects, a last resort.

Expanding my trauma-healing work to include the spiritual was more challenging. Indigenous healers, I was learning, had been spiritual teachers as well as physicians; so, too, were the monks and nuns who, until the late Middle Ages, practiced medicine in the West. But concerns about ultimate meaning and purpose, questions about God, and mystical experiences of union with something beyond the human were ignored in modern medical practice or labeled "psychopathology." This seemed shortsighted. Ignorant.

I'd long ago sensed deep truth in biblical mysteries: Jacob wrestling with the angel, Moses's uncanny connection to God, the extraordinary wisdom, compassion, and sanity in Jesus's parables and injunctions—to let go of pride and material wealth, and to love one another, especially those who'd hurt us. More recently I'd been drawn to Buddhism's calm, clear-eyed acceptance of life's suffering. Still, these were stories to me, giving glimpses, ideals. I wanted to make them facts of my daily life and my psychiatric practice.

Then, in 1973, I met Shyam Singha, a man as fluent in the inspired poetry of the spirit as he was in the elegant prose of the mind-body connection and the worlds of non-Western, "alternative" medicine.

Shyam was a Kashmir-born, London-based osteopath, naturopath, acupuncturist, herbalist, and meditation master. He looked and moved like a big cat—sly, knowing, unpredictable—and spoke with offhand familiarity of yin and yang; heaven, earth, and man; and the five elements of Chinese medicine. When we cooked together, he created endless improbable combinations of meats and fruit, nuts and vegetables, herbs and spices in an infinite variety of dishes that delighted my digestion and left me energized and relaxed, satisfied and intrigued.

Shyam showed me the transformative power of intensely physical meditations that mixed Indian, Middle Eastern Sufi, Chinese, and Tibetan traditions with Western body-oriented psychotherapies like so many spices—fast, deep breathing followed by shouting and pounding; jumping up and down and landing on my heels; whirling; Shaking and Dancing; talking gibberish; and laughing at myself in a mirror. These "expressive meditations" relieved my physical and emotional tension, called up and released long-suppressed fear and anger, and opened the door to a sweet, easy connection to an ever-changing, always enlivening world.

AT NIMH IN the late 1970s, I helped create and provide the scientific basis for the new fields of holistic, integrative, and mind-body medicine. I coedited two books—comprehensive accounts of what we then knew of the benefits and limitations of these approaches: meditation, Biofeedback, nutrition, herbalism, homeopathy, musculoskeletal manipulation, environmental medicine, Ayurveda, and Chinese medicine. I chaired the Special Study on Alternative Mental Health Services for President Jimmy Carter.

What I was learning, from the research, with Shyam, and as a psychiatrist working with patients, was turning conventional wisdom on its head, showing me another way. Physical, emotional, and spiritual distress were inextricably connected. Natural, side-effect-free approaches to the cause, rather than the symptoms, of illness could reverse biological and psychological damage and enlarge and vastly improve our health, help us move through life's inevitable traumas, and find the awareness and acceptance, the love and compassion promised by all spiritual traditions.

I was tasting it in my food, feeling it in my body, seeing it in my life, reading it in the new research, and proving it in my practice. Leaving NIMH in 1982, I wondered how I could continue to help it happen—for me and everyone else.

Self-Care Is the True Primary Care

After nine years of private practice and writing, I found an answer: create a nonprofit organization. At The Center for Mind-Body Medicine (CMBM) we would live the principles and practices of what I was calling "The New Medicine." Our hopeful, immodest mission was to make self-care and the group support that enhanced it central to all health care, to the training of all health professionals and the education of our children, to create for ourselves "a healing community and a community of healers."

I started CMBM in 1991, with no money and no paid staff. Friends and colleagues, like Mary Lee Esty, a social worker and psychologist who had also studied with Shyam, volunteered their skills and enthusiasm.

Mary Lee and I and the others began to create a model that brought together the techniques and approaches we'd been exploring: slow, deep, Soft Belly breathing and mindfulness exercises; expressive meditations; Guided Imagery, Biofeedback, and yoga; experiments with words and Drawings, music and movement and food; healing Rituals from many traditions.

We learned together and taught what we were learning in small, supportive groups to some of the people in the DC area who we felt needed it most: inner-city Black and Hispanic kids, devastated and psychologically disabled by poverty, violence, abuse, and neglect; people with life-threatening and chronic illnesses, like cancer, HIV, heart disease, and depression; Washington professionals who were, as one congressman-patient observed to me, "too stressed out to deal with our stress"; my Georgetown medical students, whose fears threatened to constrict their future practice and crush their compassion; and the stream of refugees who had survived torture or their family members' executions and were now filling my private practice.

Within two years, Mary Lee and I, along with the first people we had taught, had organized a national training in mind-body medicine.

Teaching Thousands to Heal Millions

I loved the teaching that was the focus of our work at CMBM and the community of healers we were creating, and I was thoroughly enjoying the role to which President Bill Clinton soon appointed me: chairman of the advisory council to the National Institutes of Health's newly created Office of Alternative Medicine.

Still, some other need was growing in me. I wanted to know if our mind-body approach, which was beginning to work so well in hospitals, clinics, schools, and private practices in the US, could help the most troubled and traumatized people in some of the darkest places on our planet.

Family physician Susan Lord and I took that question and ourselves to Bosnia in 1997, just after the Dayton Peace Accords were signed. Four years of war had devastated Bosnia, leaving more than 200,000 killed; tens of thousands had been imprisoned in rape camps. Now, Bosnian men and women seemed to move with difficulty, often anesthetized with alcohol, through clouds of tobacco smoke. Depression, insomnia, alcoholism, and post-traumatic stress disorder were off the charts. Years of trauma had tripled the incidence of chronic physical illnesses, including heart disease, cancer, diabetes, and arthritis. Men who had never raised their hands in anger were beating their wives.

IN 1998, WHEN the war between the Kosovar rebels and the Serbian government began, Susan and I had to be there, to begin work before the horrors of war caused the kind of post-traumatic psychological catastrophe we were witnessing in Bosnia.

During the war, we taught meditation to the international soldiers who recovered the bodies of the dead, going unarmed and fearful between warring Kosovar guerrillas and Serbian paramilitaries. We heard trauma in the words of the mothers and children who had been bombed out of their homes, saw it in their drawings of burning buildings and dead and dismembered bodies, in eyes blanked by relived horror. As they breathed slowly and deeply with us, and shared their stories and their Drawings, we watched feeling come back into their faces, saw their shoulders relax, and heard their words of appreciation. It was becoming clear that our model of self-care and group support was well tailored to relieve trauma's symptoms, to make healing happen.

The war ended and in the next six years, my CMBM colleagues and I trained six hundred Kosovar psychiatrists, psychologists, nurses, counselors, and teachers. Mind-body medicine became an official part of the new nation's mental health system.

We worked intensively in the Suhareka region, where 80 percent of the homes had been destroyed and 20 percent of the kids in the New Life High School had lost one or both parents. Five years after the war was over, almost half of these normal-looking kids and many of the teachers still had the signs and symptoms of full-blown, disabling post-traumatic stress disorder (PTSD): they were anxious and agitated, had trouble focusing and sleeping; the kids fought with classmates and parents. Their nights were haunted by dreams of death and destruction—bullets exploding heads, hands reaching out of graves— and their days punctuated by flashbacks. They felt distant from family and friends, emotionally numb. The kids' grades had plummeted.

The New Life teachers who came to our trainings found relaxation and relief and a new way to help their students. We taught them to lead small Mind-Body Skills Groups (MBSGs) where the kids, feeling safe and understood, were able for the first time to cry for parents, brothers, and sisters who had been murdered, for the beatings and rapes they'd suffered. The teachers taught the kids to quiet their agitation, release the tension in their bodies, and imagine a more hopeful future for themselves and their families. Kids and teachers came to understand that trauma and its strange symptoms had come to all of them, and that they could learn together to deal with what had happened to them.

We published a pilot study on the MBSGs the teachers led, and then, in a major psychiatric journal, a randomized controlled trial (RCT), the gold standard of medical research. The RCT compared kids with PTSD who had been randomly assigned to a program of eleven weekly Mind-Body Skills Groups with others who were similar in age and gender, as well as diagnosis. It was the first published RCT of *any* intervention—drugs, psychotherapy, whatever—with war-traumatized kids. After eleven weeks, more than 80 percent of the teenagers who began our groups with the symptoms of PTSD no longer qualified for the diagnosis. The gains held at three months follow-up. Over two years, all one thousand kids in the school participated in these groups.

These studies and others since then, in the Gaza Strip and the US, have shown that our model is powerfully effective for relieving psychological trauma, decreasing anger, improving sleep and mood, and enhancing hope. The Kosovo studies also demonstrated that intelligent people of good will—rural high school teachers—could, with supervision by experienced clinicians, use our approach as skill-fully as any MD or PhD.

These were crucial findings. If you want to help an entire trau-matized population, you need to be able to rely on many people, not just the few available psychiatrists, psychologists, and clinical social workers. The findings are also very good news for all of you reading this book. Any of you, like the Suhareka teachers and kids, can learn and successfully use our approach.

IN THE TWENTY years since, my CMBM colleagues and I have led trainings in every part of the United States and traveled to sites of over-whelming violence, devastation, and poverty. Our now international faculty of 130 has trained more than six thousand clinicians, teachers, religious and community leaders, and peer counselors. And they in turn have shared our program with many hundreds of thousands of children and adults: people here in the US, just like those of you reading this book; survivors of wars in Bosnia, Kosovo, Macedonia, Israel, Gaza, Syria, and South Sudan; those who've lived through hurricanes in New Orleans, Houston, and New York, the earthquake in Haiti, the wildfires in California, and school shootings in Sandy Hook, Connecticut, Broward County, Florida, and Santa Fe, Texas. We've trained eight hundred clinicians and veteran peer counselors who work with active-duty US military, veterans, and their families and created programs for New York City firefighters and their families after 9/11.

In 2015, after several years of volunteering, we began to work in-tensively on the impoverished Pine Ridge Indian Reservation in South Dakota. Twenty kids had killed themselves in the year before we were invited to offer our training to teachers, counselors, and elders who combined it with traditional Lakota healing; in the three years since, there has been only one youth suicide.

The people our trainees work with seem so different from one another, but this is only apparent. The Gaza widow in the black, body-denying, face-obscuring burqa, and the stylish Silicon Valley executive whose recent divorce is calling up the grief and terror of childhood neglect are sisters in suffering. They are alike, too, in the way they use slow, deep breathing to quiet anxiety and agitation, feel freedom in exuberant Shaking and Dancing, and haltingly, then happily, learn to trust their intuition and look forward to their future.

The research we've continued to do—on traumatized and depressed children and adults, on stressed-out, often burnt-out medical students and professionals, and on vets with PTSD and chronic pain—can inform and comfort you. Published in medical and psychological journals, these studies reinforce the *yes* of our CMBM experience with definitive, visible, verifiable scientific evidence. What we're doing works.

This approach, which I've spent fifty years learning and using and developing, which works so well with so many different kinds of people, is the one I bring you in *The Transformation*.

AS YOU READ, I hope you'll feel me alongside you, holding you close and steady as you move through your pain and discover strengths you didn't know or had forgotten that you had.

I've written this book so you can take this healing journey on your own, in your own way and in your own time. And I also encourage you to share the journey with people who are dear to you, to use the tools and techniques with a spouse or partner, with friends, parents, or children.

Some of the people you'll meet in this book will resemble you in the specific problems they face and the traumas they've suffered, in their age and gender, occupation and ethnicity. Others will be different in many ways. They've all been my teachers, and they can be yours as well.

Sometimes this learning can and will be challenging. It's not pleasant or easy to feel long-suppressed pain or deal with present or anticipated threats. But it turns out to be such a relief to finally face our losses and fears, so satisfying to reverse the biological damage that trauma inflicts, to free ourselves from past suffering and present fear. And it turns out to be such a joy to share the lessons that are enriching our lives with others who want and need them.

I believe that in *The Transformation*, you, like the people you'll meet in this book, and like me, will discover hidden resources of physical and mental energy and hope, as well as the capacity to imagine and make use of perspectives and solutions that may have previously been unthinkable. You may also, as shamans and spiritual teachers have long taught, discover in the ruins of trauma the treasure of Meaning and Purpose, and a Love for others and yourself that will warm and brighten all the moments of your life.

1

An Invitation

WHEN SHE SITS with CBS *60 Minutes* correspondent Scott Pelley, nine-year-old Azhaar Jendia will be solemn and composed. Today, in the damp courtyard of a bleak school in Shuja'iyya, a Gaza neighborhood bombed into rubble in the 2014 war with Israel, she's crying. I'm sitting with Azhaar and a circle of seven other children. All of their fathers were killed in that war six months earlier. Fatma, a Palestinian teacher who has led a nine-session Mind-Body Skills Group for the children, is there, and so is Jamil, the psychologist who is the Gaza program director for The Center for Mind-Body Medicine.

I've been explaining, to the puzzlement of the kids (their looks ask why I would ever want to come to Gaza), that I'm an American psychiatrist and have been working in Gaza since 2002, before they were born. My multinational CMBM team and I have trained Jamil and Fatma and seven hundred other Gazan doctors, nurses, counselors, teachers, and activist women. And they in turn have led the small groups where these kids, and tens of thousands of other children and adults, have come to know that someone hears and cares—that hope and relief and healing from their terrible trauma are possible.

Azhaar's long, dark curls frame her face as she bends to point out the carefully crayoned details in two sets of Drawings: one she did at the beginning of her first MBSG, the other three weeks later, at the end of the ninth and last group. In between, Azhaar and the other kids have learned to use the self-care tools we teach. A little boy, Azhaar's younger brother, buries his head in her side as she begins to speak.

Azhaar points to the first Drawing in the first set, which is, in fact, a combination of the first two Drawings we usually do: participants are told to draw "Yourself" and "Yourself with your biggest problem." On the left-hand side of the page, stones are falling from the wall of her home, which is being bombed by the Israeli planes that fly above it. On the ground next to the house is a body drenched in red. "This is my father," Azhaar tells us. Nearby, side by side, are two more bloody bodies—her uncles—and not far away a fourth, "my aunt." The graves of Azhaar's father, her uncles, and her aunt are high on the page, above the Israeli planes, as if they had already ascended to heaven; the woman's grave is decorously separated from the men's. "These are Shuja'iyya martyrs," she tells us. In the lower right-hand corner is a tiny stick figure, its mouth turned down in sadness. "This is me," says Azhaar.

It's all there, as it often is with adults' as well as children's drawings. The terrible losses are so clear. The traumatized person is tiny, diminished, peripheral, barely surviving.

This first Drawing is painful. The second, a response to the request to draw "Yourself with your biggest problem solved," is excruciating. A grayish rectangle fills the page. "It's me in a grave," Azhaar explains. She looks like a medieval knight on a sarcophagus. "The solution to my problem," she announces, remembering her state of mind when she began our program, "is for me to be murdered by the Israelis. It's a good thing. I'll be with my father, whom I love. There is nothing for me in this life."

Our circle sits in stunned silence. I know well that when we've been traumatized, we may despair of change and recovery. Still, the terrible, firm finality of Azhaar's picture and words sits inside my belly like a rock.

"And here," Azhaar goes on, her smile suddenly lighting up our afternoon, "are the drawings I did last week." These are the ones we do at the end of a series of groups, after kids or adults have learned and used the techniques I'll be teaching you—the various kinds of meditation and movement; Guided Imagery and Biofeedback; mindful eating; body awareness and written Dialogues; Laughter, Gratitude, and Forgiveness; ways to find guidance from the people who populate our family trees.

They do this second set of Drawings after they've grown comfortable with themselves and close to one another in the safety of the group circle that our leaders create, a safety I hope you'll feel as you read this book.

Again, the first Drawing is "Yourself." Azhaar's composition this time is simple, balanced. On one side of the page, instead of a tiny stick, there is a larger, solid girl in a bright skirt. On the page, as now in life, brown curls frame a smiling face. An arrow extends from her chest across the page, past flowers with well-defined petals, pointing toward a tree bursting with bright green leaves. In the middle of the page, the arrow pierces a heart with a message carefully lettered in the English Azhaar is learning in school. "I Love Nature," it says. "After these groups, I like to smile," Azhaar tells me. "I love myself."

The second Drawing shows "Who or how you would like to be." In it, Azhaar is wearing what she explains is a doctor's white coat. There is a stethoscope around her neck, its tubes extending from her ears. The disc-shaped resonator, which picks up sounds, is on the chest of the figure who lies on top of a structure that looks uncannily like the grave in her first set of Drawings.

"This is my patient," Azhaar announces. "He is lying on my examining table. I am," she says proudly, "a heart doctor."

"And who are these?" I ask, pointing to the five figures lined up next to her examining table.

"They're my other patients. They're waiting to see me."

I'm amazed and delighted. Azhaar's Drawings tell me that, after participating in nine two-hour groups over three weeks, she has shed her suicidal despair and embraced a future filled with hope. They will soon bring the same message to the fifteen million people who will watch the *60 Minutes* episode.

Of course, Azhaar still grieves for her father. The purple socks she's wearing today are, she tells me with warmth and tears, gifts he gave her. But her terrible losses have been transmuted. Her own heart was broken, but now it has opened in compassion and offered a new life to her. She will be a heart doctor—a doctor, I feel, with heart as well as a specialist in that organ—and she will care for the others in Gaza whose hearts have also been hurt.

The third Drawing—"How will you get from where you are to where you want to be?"—is matter of fact, practical. The girl who delights in Nature is now indoors. A book is open in front of her, a pile of them nearby. "I will study hard so that I can go to medical school," she explains. But here, too, there is a surprise. As I look closely, I see that the grave that became an examining table in the second Drawing of this second set has been enlisted as a desk. What was, nine groups ago, an end point for a despairing child, now supports a student's progress toward a life-affirming future.

IN THE PAGES of *The Transformation*, I'll share with you the practical tools and techniques of self-care that Azhaar learned, the ones that my CMBM colleagues and I teach. I'll explain how and why they reverse the biological as well as the psychological damage that trauma has done. I'll show you, step by step, how to bring them together in a comprehensive program designed to meet your individual needs and preferences. As we work together, you, like Azhaar, will have the opportunity to discover in yourself the hopeful attitude, the inner strength and ability, and the adventurous spirit that will bring you the best, most satisfying, and enduring results.

In the next chapter, I'll describe the biological, psychological, and social damage that trauma inflicts. This understanding will help you realize and deal with what has happened to you and how it may be affecting you now. It will provide a baseline from which you can measure the positive changes that *The Transformation*'s healing prescription can bring.

In the chapters that follow, I'll share with you the many specific tools and techniques of self-care that I've used over the last fifty years. I'll show you how each of these tools reverses the biological and psychological damage trauma has done and give you the scientific evidence that demonstrates its effectiveness.

Each chapter will encourage you to look at yourself and your troubled mind in a kinder, more generous, more hopeful way. As you practice using the tools I teach, you'll know that you, like Azhaar, have the power to use them to reverse trauma's negative biological, psychological, and spiritual effects, and to help yourself heal. You'll know as well that you deserve to be healthy and whole.

You'll also learn to understand and use trauma as a door that opens a world of wisdom to you, as the catalyst that encourages you, as it did Viktor Frankl and Diana and Azhaar, to embrace Hope and Love, to grow and fulfill yourself.

Azhaar's story makes the point powerfully: a brokenhearted girl finds the meaning and purpose of her life in opening her heart to others and helping them heal their hurt hearts.

I've seen this kind of Transformation again and again in thousands of people I've worked with, and in myself. I'll teach you how to embrace, encourage, and nourish this natural process.

Jane, a sixty-year-old American wife and mother whom you'll soon come to know, had never read Viktor Frankl, but she sounded like him when she spoke: "I would not wish to have had cancer. And it has been the most important experience of my life." Over the years, so many others have said something similar.

This is, as I've shared with you, the insight of indigenous people. It animates shamanic rituals of healing and initiation in Asia, Africa, and South America, as well as the Vision Quests and Sun Dances of the North American Plains Indians. It also informed the tragedies performed at festivals in ancient Greece.

THE STORIES OF the world's religious leaders make clear the connection between early trauma and later enlightenment, between childhood danger and abandonment and world-changing adult missions of compassion, meaning making, and community building. The mother of Siddhartha Gautama, who later became the Buddha, died days after he was born. Abraham, the Hebrew patriarch, had to leave his homeland, and Moses was abandoned by his mother. Jesus's family fled to preserve him from slaughter. The Prophet Muhammad was orphaned.

This same understanding comes alive in the stories of modern women and men who have transformed their suffering into lives of heroism and compassion: Harriet Tubman, the whipped and degraded slave, escaped the South only to return, again and again, to bring hundreds more to freedom and lead a movement for racial and gender equality; an overprivileged Franklin Roosevelt met the challenges of paralyzing polio with unexpected courage and grace, and became a president of uncommon purpose and vision; a committed and angry

Nelson Mandela, growing in humility and wisdom through twenty-seven years of harsh imprisonment, was a world-inspiring exemplar of truth and reconciliation; Scarlett Lewis, whose son Jesse was gunned down at the Sandy Hook school, has become an advocate for mental health services for children who are, like her son's murderer, troubled and violent.

When we talk about trauma, we are, as my sixteen-year-old son Gabriel might say, "talking about a lot of reality." But we're not talking about psychopathology, about mental illness, or about an aberration. Trauma is an integral part, an inescapable part of all our lives.

In the pages of this book, I'll show you that you, too—that all of us—can experience and embrace the path of self-discovery and self-care that trauma opens to us. You'll see that however ordinary and expectable, or overwhelming and exceptional, your trauma has been, it can become the wake-up call for your journey of self-realization.

THIS BOOK, LIKE Azhaar's story, begins in pain and recognition. It unfolds in experiences of self-awareness, empowerment, and Love, in healing and Hope.

I'm talking not about the false Hope of wishful thinking but the earned Hope of lived experience—of knowing that the techniques you're learning, the experiments in exploring and expressing yourself, are making a real, felt, measurable difference in your life.

Reading the stories of people like you who have used this approach to meet challenges that resemble yours or may seem far greater than yours will, I believe, inspire you. High-functioning but troubled and confused professionals, police and firefighters, business people, farmers, clerks, and homemakers have all benefited from this approach. So have college and high school kids, elders with Alzheimer's, and three-year-olds in nursery schools.

You'll see that those who've survived the death and destruction of war—American troops and civilians like Azhaar—have used the approach you'll be learning to rebuild their lives and recover their souls; that threats of fatal illness have brought new life to Jane and many others; that those who have lost treasured jobs and loved ones have found new and often deeper satisfaction and intimacy. Children and adults whose brains and bodies were damaged by rape and other terrible forms of abuse have used this program to recover and live lives filled with Meaning, Purpose, joy, and intimacy. Again and again, you'll also meet people very much like you who followed this book's trauma-healing approach to resolve the common crises of youth, midlife, and old age.

THE TRANSFORMATION MAY require a step-by-step unwinding of layers of forgotten past events and buried feelings. It is a program for accepting and feeling at ease with all the stages of your history. It offers you ways of putting what has happened to you in perspective, of claiming your hurt and anger without being owned and dominated by them. Sometimes, as with Azhaar, the process is astonishingly fast. Sometimes, particularly when trauma is early, steeped in betrayal, and repeated, as it was with Diana, it's a long-distance run, not a sprint. We need to learn to be patient with ourselves and to appreciate all stages of the journey—each layer we uncover and the freedom that comes with it.

Like so many people I've worked with, like me, you'll likely learn to find satisfaction in each step you take: overcoming morning inertia to do an energizing, expressive meditation or mindfully making and eating a tasty meal. I'm amazed, again and again, at the broad grins that appear on the faces of people who are walking this path of Transformation, by their sudden, unaccustomed urge to dance or give a hug.

Your hope for change will be reinforced by your understanding that the techniques you're learning—from slow, deep breathing to active, expressive meditations and mental imagery, from connecting with landscapes and animals to embracing Gratitude and Forgiveness to participating in a healing circle—have been used for millennia by indigenous people and in the great spiritual traditions.

The growing body of modern science I'll share with you will be reassuring and encouraging. It will demonstrate that you can use these tools to reliably produce both the psychological benefits you're looking for and the biological changes that make them possible—and that those changes have been and can be measured.

Most of all, your Hope will come from your experience of this program, from seeing in your Drawings, as Azhaar did, and from knowing in your bones as well as your brain that what you're learning and doing to help yourself is making a difference. Over time, as you'll see, healing and Transformation get easier, less painful, more swift and sure. You'll feel more capable and curious, more open to new understanding, and more likely to feel satisfied and be kind.

THE PROMISE THAT trauma invites us to fulfill is ultimately a spiritual as well as a therapeutic one. It enables us (even if we are agnostics or atheists) to live in harmony with who we are, to discover that we are connected to, graced by, someone or something greater than ourselves: God, Nature, other people, a life's Meaning and Purpose.

I believe you'll see that every technique I teach, every tool you use, and every experiment you do will offer you the opportunity to discover or reaffirm this spiritual dimension. It may come anytime: in blissful, thought-free moments of slow, deep breathing; in an image that reveals a Meaning and Purpose that had always eluded you; in the joyful, childlike freedom that may follow practice of "Shaking and Dancing"; in sharing old, deep pain with a new friend; when Forgiveness unexpectedly lets the chains of resentment fall away; or when you're bringing meditative awareness to each moment of a life that will soon end.

As we learn to accept and embrace rather than flee from or numb ourselves to trauma's challenges, we can discover, as Azhaar, Viktor Frankl, and Diana did, as I and the others you'll meet in these pages have, that our greatest pain can teach us the most important truths about ourselves: who we are and how deeply and inextricably connected we are to one another; what gives our lives Meaning and Purpose; and how we can live with greater wisdom and compassion, joy, and Love.

2
The Biology of Trauma

O UR INITIAL RESPONSES to physical threats, abuse, and loss are healthy and designed to preserve us.

First, we seek out connection and comfort, as we did as infants and small children; we call and look for help. This response, described by the contemporary neurobiologist Stephen Porges, is facilitated by the most evolutionarily advanced part of the vagus nerve, the central element in the parasympathetic half of our autonomic nervous system, the one that's also responsible for helping us to "rest and digest," to relax. This call for connection is aided and abetted by other nerves that control facial expression and speech.

When safety and reassurance are unavailable or inadequate and the threat requires an immediate reaction, we experience the fight-or-flight response. Fight or flight, which the Harvard physiologist Walter Cannon named one hundred years ago, is mediated by the hypothalamus, one of the brain's central switching stations. It's grounded in the sympathetic branch of our autonomic nervous system, and in the amygdala, an almond-shaped structure in our limbic or emotional brain. Fight or flight, which exists in all vertebrates, increases the secretion of the energizing neurotransmitter epinephrine from the medulla, or inner part of the adrenal glands, the small cap-like structures that sit on top of our kidneys.

Fight or flight enabled our ancestors to struggle against or escape from a predator or natural disaster. We feel it when we're threatened emotionally as well as physically, when we're insulted, or when we remember—or anticipate—painful events. When fight or flight's in play, it overwhelms the rest-and-digest functions of the parasympathetic nervous system. Every one of us has—at many points—been in fight or flight.

Fight or flight increases our heart and respiratory rates, raises our blood pressure, and sends more blood to our large muscles, enabling us to successfully challenge a predator or run away. Meanwhile, blood is directed away from our hands, which may become cold and clammy, and from our digestive tract; when our life is in danger, it's not wise to stop for a snack.

Signals from the hypothalamus also reach the nearby pituitary gland, which controls all the organs in our endocrine system: our thyroid, testes, ovaries, etc. This pituitary-governed stress response, which the physician Hans Selye identified in the 1930s, prepares us to meet the challenges life brings. It releases adrenocorticotropic hormone (ACTH) from the pituitary, and ACTH in turn tells the outer part, or cortex, of our adrenal glands to secrete cortisol and other stress hormones. Cortisol helps us retain water, raises our blood pressure, and mobilizes sugar from our cells, activating and nourishing us and stimulating our mental functioning.

When fight or flight and the stress response can't deal with an overwhelming and inescapable threat (think of a woman being raped at gunpoint, or a soldier trapped in a burning Humvee, or a mouse caught in the jaws of your pet cat), a last-ditch survival mechanism, the "freeze" response, takes over. Freezing is mediated by the oldest part of the vagus nerve, deep in our brainstem. It produces physiological collapse and a release of pain-numbing endorphins. When humans freeze, we may experience a self-protective detachment from our helpless, ravaged body, called dissociation. When someone "leaves her body" when she is being raped or beaten, she's in a dissociated state. Diana and others you'll meet in the pages of *The Transformation* have been frozen and have experienced dissociation.

The fight-or-flight and freeze responses are vital and necessary, but they're designed to meet acute emergencies—to be quickly turned on and just as quickly turned off. Picture a nature film: A gazelle is drinking at a water hole on Africa's Serengeti Plain. A lion comes; the gazelle runs. Two outcomes are possible. Either the lion catches the gazelle and the story is over. Or the gazelle, successfully fleeing, appears in the film a few minutes later, happily grazing. Fight or flight has come, done its job, and gone. The same is true of freezing. Most of the time your cat will happily chew the mouse to death. On occasion, however, kitty may lose interest and put the inert mouse down. The mouse shakes her frozen body, revives, and scampers away.

In humans, the fight-or-flight and freeze responses, and all the biological changes that stress brings, can last a very long time: for the duration of a war, while growing up in an abusive household, or enduring a demoralizing marriage, or coping with an ominous medical diagnosis and its painful treatment.

And these responses can persist even when the actual trauma is long over. The gazelle grazing on the plain and the mouse retreating to her mouse hole forget what has happened. We humans can carry the lion or the house cat—the cruelty of an abuser, the loss of a loved one, the threat of a potentially fatal illness, rape and its horror—with us. Our large, complex brain may replay an endless loop of traumatic memories—of loss or abuse, of damage or helplessness, and of the pain and shame that go with them. These memories can affect us just as profoundly as the original trauma, and can significantly prolong and compound its physical and emotional damage. That's how it is for those of us who continue to be preoccupied with memories of past trauma.

High levels of cortisol that persist may destroy cells in the hippocampus, a part of our emotional brain crucial to memory and the regulation of stress. They can also diminish and disturb our immune response, making us more vulnerable to infections and to autoimmune disorders like rheumatoid arthritis. Over time, the adrenal gland of chronically traumatized people may seem "exhausted," unable to mobilize the appropriate response to new stress.

The level of the energizing, feel-good neurotransmitter dopamine, which rose in response to the initial traumatic event, declines, as does the level of serotonin, a calming neurotransmitter that is sometimes deficient when we're depressed. Many people who've been traumatized feel chronically tired.

Trauma diminishes functioning in a number of areas in the frontal lobe of our cerebral cortex and, with it, our capacity for judgment, self-awareness, and compassion. Vital brain connections may be damaged. Sometimes communication between the two hemispheres of the brain—the more linear and rational left brain, and the more emotional, spatial, and creative right brain—can be disrupted, causing us to feel fragmented, unable to put thoughts and feelings together. The visual images of trauma, which are formed in our optical cortex at the back of our brain, may be partially or completely cut off from the area of verbal expression (named Broca's area, after its discoverer) in the temporal lobe of the left hemisphere. Many people are tortured by terrifying images but are unable to put them into words.

Prolonged over time, fight or flight agitates us and makes us feel powerless. We grow angry with little or no provocation and can't seem to reason it away. We cannot concentrate or relax into a sleep that may be filled with nightmares of what we've suffered or might again undergo. Painful images of past loss and future harm recur, invading quiet moments. When trauma causes prolonged freezing, our emotional numbness may make us pull away from those to whom we've been close. We're unable to find relief by sharing our pain with them.

Even when these symptoms do not reach the disabling level of post-traumatic stress disorder, trauma can challenge our ideas about who we are and why we're here on earth. Often enough, it compounds our pain and confusion with feelings that we've been responsible for what happened to us. Feeling guilty for causing harm to ourselves or others, our mind is filled with recriminations.

Traumatized, we find ourselves chained to a past that we feel doomed to forever repeat, like the souls in Dante's *Inferno*. Sometimes, as it did for Azhaar, death feels like the only option. Suicide may seem, in desperate moments, to ratify our despair or demonstrate our loyalty to those we've lost. Twenty US veterans kill themselves every day.

AZHAAR'S TRAUMA WAS overwhelming, but it was not repeated on a daily basis. She suffered greatly and felt, when she first came to our group, that death was her only option, but she had not been betrayed by the father she lost. Very large numbers of American children like Diana are regularly abused and neglected by the very people to whom they look for love and support. The damage to their brains and biochemistry is likely to be far greater, its psychological consequences graver and longer lasting. As adults, 66 percent of the women with high numbers of adverse childhood events and 35 percent of the men suffer from chronic depression; they are fifty times as likely to try to kill themselves as those who experienced no adverse events.

As children we are most vulnerable. Because our brains are still developing, the biological damage may be more deeply embedded, more pervasive, and more difficult to reverse. And because we can't, as very young children, make sense of what's happening and do not have the words to speak of it, we may well, like Diana, grow up with fears and vulnerabilities, fractured and frightening images and feelings that we cannot understand or explain. Without knowing why, we may fear intimacy and be exquisitely sensitive to loss or the threat of it.

Social attitudes can make things worse. In the United States, we've created a society of rugged individualists who find vulnerability uncomfortable, even shameful. In other places where I've worked—Israel, Gaza, Kosovo, Bosnia, Serbia, Macedonia, and Haiti among them—an emphasis on being strong has similar consequences. We push life's inevitable suffering and death—its traumas—to the periphery of our minds and the edges of our social world.

Survivors of rape, adults who were abused and neglected as children, those of us facing the loss of loved ones or life-threatening illness, people dealing with demeaning discrimination, even soldiers whose suffering is obvious and honored minimize and deny their wounds. Concealed, they fester. Unshared, they compound our loneliness and multiply our suffering, deepening and prolonging the biological as well as the psychological devastation. This, in turn, makes us more vulnerable to future trauma, as well as to the vast array of conditions and illnesses—including heart disease, diabetes, immune disorders, cancer, and alcoholism—to which chronic stress contributes.

And the cycle continues, damaging and debilitating us, and perhaps also our children. Trauma can cause epigenetic (*epi* is Greek for "above") changes—alterations in the structure of our chromosomes, which affect the way our genes function and may make us less resilient, more vulnerable. These epigenetic changes can be transmitted to our children and grandchildren and make them, as well as us, less able to deal with stress and prevent illness.

Trauma can also accelerate the shortening of telomeres, structures at the ends of our chromosomes that diminish in size with age; by shortening our telomeres, trauma and the stress it produces may well shorten our lives.

THE COMPREHENSIVE PROGRAM in *The Transformation* directly addresses trauma-induced biological damage. The techniques are the antidotes to the fight-or-flight, stress, and freeze responses. They revive functions that have been compromised: memory, focus, self-awareness, judgment, emotional intelligence, and compassion. Many of these techniques, as you'll learn, stimulate the growth of new tissue, including new brain cells in the frontal cortex and hippocampus.

Combined in *The Transformation*'s comprehensive program, these techniques reestablish broken brain connections and promote the healthy integration of thoughts and feelings; they connect the torturous images of trauma to words that can give you relief from them; they free you from rumination—the loop of hopeless, self-defeating thoughts that bind you to your trauma.

This program can have significant long-term, life-enhancing benefits. It may help prevent the chronic illnesses to which trauma makes you vulnerable. It can reconnect you to the intuitive wisdom that can guide you in solving problems that seemed intractable. It will likely make it far easier for you to be close to others and to feel love from and for them. It may also be a powerful force for extending your life and ensuring that you do not pass along epigenetic vulnerabilities to your children.

Your Gut Under Siege

When experts discuss the biological damage that trauma inflicts, they almost always focus exclusively on brain biochemistry, physiology, and structure. Neglecting trauma's effect on our gastrointestinal tract is incomplete and shortsighted. Trauma disrupts our digestion as predictably and dangerously as it does our thinking and feeling. And what's going wrong in our gut causes further damage to our brain, and this additional damage will, over time, cause more problems for our gut as well as our mind.

The remainder of this chapter maps the biology of this vicious, trauma-magnifying cycle. I'll do it in some detail because the information is so important—and much of it so new—and because you're unlikely to find it in any other book on trauma. Later, in "The Trauma-Healing Diet," I'll show you how to use food and supplements to break the cycle, reverse the damage to your gut and your brain, and enhance your biological as well as your psychological resiliency.

THE DAMAGE TO our digestion begins at the top, in what researchers call the cephalic (the word is Greek and means "head") or mental phase of digestion: how we think about food, the food choices we make, and the way we eat what's in front of us.

Sometimes, especially when trauma feels overwhelming and out of control, we totally lose our appetite. No food appeals. When we do eat, it's like we're chewing chalk. This is common when the freeze response predominates, but it can also come with the anxiety and agitation of prolonged fight or flight.

More often, after trauma, we tend to eat compulsively and fast. When we eat quickly, the enzymes in our mouth don't have time to do their digestive job. The rest of our GI tract suffers and has to work harder. We swallow air, which bloats our stomach.

Hungry for the emotional as well as physical satisfaction that food brings, we often choose "comfort foods," which, as I'll soon explain, briefly reduce our stress, only to later increase it exponentially.

Stress can also make our stomach underperform and even rebel against the food that's entering. Hydrochloric acid rises up from the stomach into the esophagus, causing heartburn. Heartburn doesn't mean we have too much acid. In fact, hydrochloric acid is vital for digestion and the absorption of critical, brain-nourishing nutrients like vitamin B_{12}. When we're stressed, many of us actually have deficiencies in hydrochloric acid. If we take proton pump inhibitors (PPIs) like Prilosec to reduce the symptoms of heartburn, we further compromise our digestion and may make ourselves more vulnerable to trauma's effects.

On occasion and over time, stress can produce ulcers, holes in the lining of the stomach and the duodenum, the first part of our small intestine. These can lead to serious bleeding.

Hydrochloric acid helps our muscular stomach break down food into a lumpy liquid, which then enters the small intestine, a twenty-foot-long tube where more digestion and the absorption of nutrients takes place.

Stress affects the small intestine in many ways. It can damage the villi—the tiny, fingerlike projections from the endothelial cells that line the small intestine—and interfere with the absorption of vital, stress-reducing vitamins and minerals.

Stress can also loosen the tight junctions that connect endothelial cells. As these junctions widen, molecules of food substances that a healthy gut does not absorb pass through our now "leaky" gut and enter our bloodstream. These molecules, among them the gluten protein from wheat and other grains, can in turn cause destructive inflammatory reactions everywhere in our body, including our brain. These in turn may contribute to the anxiety and depression that often follow trauma.

Stress may also interfere with the production of digestive enzymes that the liver and pancreas secrete into the small intestine. And stress can disturb the detoxification processes by which our liver protects us from harmful food by-products and environmental poisons.

Stress and trauma also have a powerful effect on the microbiome, the tens of trillions of bacteria that live in our small intestine. Trauma can turn this dynamic powerhouse from a beneficial, protective friend to a dangerous enemy.

When the microbiome is in balance, its "good," "probiotic," bacteria, like the ones from the *lactobacillus* and *bifidus* families, play important roles in digestion and overall health. The microbiome helps maintain the structural integrity of the gut. It plays a major role in immune functioning, and its bacteria are important in synthesizing B vitamins and vitamin K. Its good bacteria are also crucial to producing the short-chain fatty acids that are the primary energy source for the cells lining the large intestine.

The microbiome appears to have a particularly important role in maintaining brain functioning and helping us deal successfully with stress and trauma. A healthy microbiome stimulates the vagus nerve (90 percent of whose fibers are carrying messages back to the brain) to its optimal, stress-reducing performance. It likely helps ensure that the messages the vagus nerve brings back to our brain promote nerve cell maintenance and the healing of damaged neurons.

The microbiome may regulate our response to trauma and stress in other ways. It's in direct contact with the hundred million neurons (more than in our spinal cord) that live in the lining of our small intestine. These neurons, sometimes described as our "second brain," produce neurotransmitters, including serotonin, dopamine, norepinephrine, and the endorphins, which are vital for coping with stress and stabilizing mood.

Under stress, the population of good bacteria decreases, and the numbers of pathogenic, infection-causing "bad" bacteria increase.

Trauma also challenges the functioning of the final stage of our digestive tract, our colon or large intestine. The colon is responsible for removing digestive waste products and ensuring that adequate water is reabsorbed. It's here that undigested fiber is fermented by bacteria into the short-chain fatty acids (like butyric acid) that protect the colon's lining.

When we're stressed, we may lose the slow, regular colonic contractions that guarantee good bowel movements, and get crampy with constipation or diarrhea. Under stress, bacteria that belong in the colon may migrate to the small intestine, where they cause small intestinal bacterial overgrowth (SIBO), a condition that has been linked to depression and may be responsible for exacerbating psychological stress.

Craving Comfort Foods

The trauma-food interaction is powerful and is built into our evolutionary biology. My colleague Dr. Claire Wheeler uses a cartoon to illustrate it. It's a picture of a smiling woman in a 1950s dress. She's holding a cake, amply endowed with frosting, which people of a certain age may associate with the popular food promoter Betty Crocker. The word STRESSED is written in large block letters. It is, the picture slyly tells us, DESSERTS spelled backward.

This makes evolutionary sense. If we need to run from or fight a predator, we need quick energy—foods easily broken down into the simple sugar glucose, which feeds our hardworking heart and lungs and our activated muscles. And we need to make sure there's enough extra, so that the energy-mobilizing glucose molecules that make up sugar can be stored in our liver as glycogen, for use in an ongoing emergency.

The same thing happens to us moderns when we've suffered a loss or are confronted with stress that feels overwhelming. As I've explained, our cortisol rises and lets us know that our heart, lungs, and muscles need the energy that comes from sugar, that our brain has to be adequately nourished. That's when we reach for foods that are easily broken down into sugar—sweet, fatty, salty concoctions.

These energy-dense, nutrient-poor foods—think of a mac and cheese or a Big Mac, a late-night pint of ice cream or a quart of soda pop—provide jolts of sugar, reduce high levels of cortisol, and stimulate the production of the feel-good hormone dopamine, which stress has lowered. And when we eat sugar or foods that are quickly broken down into it, the amino acid tryptophan enters our brain more easily and increases the level of calming, mood-enhancing serotonin.

These sugary, fatty foods may also directly, if briefly, reduce some of trauma's other psychological consequences. Dishes high in fats and carbohydrates have been shown to impair both short- and long-term memory, including painful memories of traumatic events. And sweet-tasting foods increase our levels of endogenous opioids, our body's version of pain-relieving drugs like morphine. This process of mood enhancement and tranquilization may be multiplied by the good memories and associations that comfort foods bring with them: our mom, or some other loving adult, comforting us with the same or similar dishes.

Unfortunately, the appealing short-term solution can become a serious long-term liability. Studies on humans, as well as animals, show that high-sugar, high-fat diets can easily become addictive. And over time, comfort-food consumption reverses the feel-good effects that it initially stimulated. Cortisol levels may rise and brain serotonin levels fall; dopamine and endorphins are depleted. Brain-derived neurotrophic factor (BDNF), a vital ingredient in healthy brain functioning and the repair and regeneration of neurons, is lowered after trauma; comfort foods deplete it even further. This is particularly damaging in the hippocampus.

Meanwhile, the comfort foods we eat, combined with the stress from which we're seeking relief, produce high levels of inflammation throughout our body. Over time, inflammation may contribute significantly to depression and anxiety, as well as heart disease, diabetes, arthritis, and cancer.

Continued eating of comfort foods, combined with ongoing high levels of stress, can also be a major factor in weight gain. The dangerous combination of comfort food and stress deposits significant amounts of visceral fat—fat inside the belly and around the abdominal organs (liver, pancreas, and intestines)—as well as the fat beneath the skin of our abdomen.

Both kinds of fat add excess weight, which is difficult to lose.

Visceral fat, which may accumulate even in people who appear skinny, is particularly dangerous. In time it may increase levels of blood insulin and triglycerides, which contribute to type II diabetes, heart disease, and other chronic illnesses. Accumulated visceral fat also exaggerates the stress response, producing high levels of cortisol, which in turn increase the amount of visceral fat.

The more we eat comfort foods, the more firmly we become hooked on them. When we make an effort to reduce our consumption of them, we feel worse and may even develop actual withdrawal symptoms, including fearful, agitated unhappiness and a sense of powerlessness and victimization—symptoms that mimic and intensify the trauma-induced feelings that made us reach for comfort foods in the first place.

This is a health-threatening vicious cycle. And you need to know that you can reverse it.

THE TRAUMA-HEALING DIET that I'll give you in chapter 10 is the antidote to the gut-destroying effects of trauma and the damage it does to your brain. It eases withdrawal from comfort food, regenerates the stress-damaged digestive tract and brain, replaces lost nutrients, repopulates the good bacteria in the microbiome, promotes the rebuilding of trauma-damaged brain tissue, reverses visceral fat accumulation, and promotes weight loss. It will help you recover more quickly and easily from trauma. It may also enable you to become more resilient and healthier than you've ever been.

In the next chapter you'll learn a simple, powerful technique that will begin the process of reversing the biological damage trauma has done to your brain, maximize the effectiveness of the Trauma-Healing Diet, and also make it far easier for you to use and benefit from all the other tools and techniques I'll teach you.

3
Soft Belly: Quieting Mind, Body, and Spirit

M EDITATION IS THE antidote to trauma.

Trauma, as you now know, creates storms of fear and aggression in the amygdala and the sympathetic nervous system. It suppresses the executive functions located in the frontal parts of the cerebral cortex, functions that help make us distinctly human, like judgment, self-observation, and compassion. Trauma binds us to the painful past and makes us continually apprehensive about the future. And trauma may override our intrinsic urge to connect with others, forcing us to fear and avoid those whose care and concern could help and heal us.

Meditation frees us from those chains. It brings us into the present moment.

Meditation is not fancy or esoteric. You don't have to change your clothes or your religion, or be a paragon of virtue or patience, or go to the mountains to do it. It is, above all, practical, easy to learn and do, and firmly grounded in science. People of any faith can do it and receive its benefits. And so can agnostics and atheists. No belief is necessary.

When we meditate, we are reversing the biological damage that trauma does. Meditation calms the storm. It quiets the amygdala's frenzy and balances the sympathetic nervous system's fight-or-flight response with the rest and digest of the parasympathetic nervous system's vagus nerve.

Scientists have shown that if you meditate regularly, the tone of your vagus nerve—its level of functioning—increases. And with better vagal functioning, you get better self-regulation, enhanced memory, clearer thinking, greater ability to deal with life's stresses, and quicker recovery from anger and distress. The improved vagal tone that comes with meditation also activates the nerves associated with facial expression and speech, which make it easier for us to recognize and welcome the support that others may want to give.

Meditation enhances functioning in the hippocampus, a crucial structure for quieting agitation and consolidating memory. As you meditate, you also repair the brain connections that trauma has ruptured and rebuild brain tissue that has been damaged and destroyed. In recent years, researchers such as Harvard's Sarah Lazar and Britta Holzel have repeatedly shown that meditation actually promotes the growth of new brain tissue in areas of the frontal cortex that trauma often damages, areas responsible for self-awareness, thoughtful judgment, and compassion.

More than forty years of research on meditation has also demonstrated its capacity to prevent physical illness. Meditation reliably reduces high blood pressure and decreases the inflammation that contributes to so many chronic conditions.

Meditation may help us to live longer as well as calmer, happier, and healthier lives. Researchers at the University of California, San Francisco (UCSF), including Elissa Epel and Nobel laureate Elizabeth Blackburn, have shown that meditation helps preserve the length of the telomeres, the structures at the end of our chromosomes that shorten with age and shorten more rapidly under the influence of stress. When we regularly meditate, we lower our level of stress and maintain or enhance the length of our telomeres—and perhaps lengthen our lives.

We may also be able to pass on the benefits of meditation to our unborn children. Meditation, as researchers at Harvard and UCSF have shown, can help reverse the epigenetic damage from trauma and enhance beneficial and inheritable changes in our resistance to stress and our resilience.

And it's not just Tibetan monks or long-term meditators who can reap the benefits of meditation. In one of Lazar's studies, beginning meditators, just like most of you, created significant changes in brain structure after an intensive eight-week course. And in another study by Fennell, beginning meditators were able to slow their breathing and heart rate, lower their blood pressure, and calm angry reactions just as well as more experienced practitioners—after only one twenty-minute session.

Much of the research on meditation has been done with people who meditate for forty minutes a day or more. However, this recent research, as well as my own experience, strongly suggests that you may be able to reap similar benefits from meditating for briefer periods.

The bottom line: MEDITATION IS MIRACULOUS.

Meditation should be a "treatment of choice" for all of us—for healing trauma, building resilience, preventing illness, enhancing happiness, and prolonging life.

It's safe to say that if meditation were a patentable, profitable drug, every doctor on the planet would be prescribing it for every patient who walked through the door. But don't wait for your doctor to prescribe it. Meditation is easy to teach and learn. ANYONE CAN MEDITATE. I'll teach you how, here in this chapter.

THE POWER OF meditation to help and heal is revealed in the history of the word. *Meditation* and *medicine* come from the Sanskrit and Greek root *medi*. *Medi* means "to take the measure of" and "to care for"—good summary descriptions of the science and art of medicine. In fact, meditation is a central element in all the world's great healing traditions, including our own Greek, Hippocratic medicine.

There are many kinds of meditation. They were created at different times, by different societies, for different purposes. One ancient Indian tantric text (*tantra* is a Sanskrit word that means "method"), the *Vijñāna Bhairava Tantra*, describes 112 different kinds: meditations on the in-breath and out-breath, and on the space between breaths—indeed, meditation on just about every human thought and activity, including sex. One of my personal favorites is "While sitting in an oxcart and swaying, go within the swaying."

Though there are many forms of meditation, all can be divided into three general categories: concentrative, mindfulness, and expressive.

Hindu mantra or sound meditations are concentrative. So, too, are meditations that advise us to focus on a visual image—a picture of a saint, a mountain, a flower—or a sound. Every religion and just about every spiritual tradition includes one or more concentrative meditations. Repetitive prayers—Our Father, Shema Yisrael, Il Allahu, Illallah, and Hare Krishna, Hare Krishna—are also concentrative meditations. When you say them, you're concentrating on the name of God.

Mindfulness meditation is South Asian and owes its origin to Siddhartha Gautama, the Buddha, who called it Vipassana, a Sanskrit word that means "awareness." Twenty-five hundred years ago, Buddha urged his disciples to become aware of their thoughts, feelings, and sensations as they arose, to let them come and let them go. In later chapters, I'll show you how to bring mindfulness into all the activities of your daily life: sitting, walking, eating, dishwashing, and, yes, making love, too.

Expressive meditations, the kind that Shyam taught me, are the oldest ones on our planet. They're central to the lives of many aboriginal and tribal people and continue to be a significant part of modern religions. The Lakota Indians chant and dance. Bushmen in southern Africa and Indonesians shake. Tibetans breathe fast, and Sufi dervishes whirl. Hassidic Jews daven—bow down rapidly, over and over—and dance ecstatically. Saint Ignatius Loyola, the founder of the Jesuit order, prescribed intense physical exercises. The postures and breathing of Indian yoga and Chinese tai chi and qi gong are slow but powerful expressive meditations. In the chapters that follow, we'll practice a number of expressive meditations and discover their capacity to thaw and energize trauma-frozen bodies, to open fear-closed minds.

RIGHT NOW I want to teach you a concentrative meditation that is fundamental to all our work together. It's called Soft Belly, because you breathe slowly and deeply in through your nose and out through your mouth, with your belly soft and relaxed. It is, like its name, unpretentious and nondenominational. But it's also powerful: body relaxing, brain reviving, mind quieting, connection enhancing, Hope promoting. And it's fundamental. It is, in fact, the way babies breathe, their bellies rising and falling with each breath.

I learned Soft Belly forty years ago from the inspiring psychologist and spiritual teacher Stephen Levine. I've done it ever since. It's usually the first technique I teach in my office and in the workshops, trainings, and small groups my colleagues and I have led for hundreds of thousands of stressed-out and traumatized people.

You can feel the benefits of Soft Belly the first time you do it. Seventy to eighty percent of those who do it—even those who have lost family members, or are mourning a lost relationship or struggling with cancer, or have survived a natural disaster or recent rape—report positive changes. After only ten or twelve minutes, tight shoulders relax, heart rates slow, and the torrent of disturbing thoughts abates. Afterward, people say they feel calmer, happier, more stable, more present, and more hopeful. If they repeat it before bed, many people sleep better than they have for years.

Here, for example, is what happened in Haiti a year after the 2010 earthquake. My team and I were leading a July training in Jacmel, a city of artists and craftspeople on Haiti's southern coast. On the morning of day two, while we were baking in the 105-degree heat of a grade school assembly hall, a serious, solid man walked to the microphone at the front of the room. He was, like the rest of us, sweating. And he swayed a bit, as if he were on the deck of a ship.

"My name is Batichon," he began in Kreyol, the language of the Haitian people and of our training. "I am a farmer nearby and a leader in my community.

"I have to tell you about Soft Belly. I was very skeptical yesterday. I am a practical man and a Christian, and I didn't know how this would fit. Still, I liked very much what I felt when I did it. My neck, which was so tight with anger, got loose; and my mind, which was constantly filled with worry about my brother's destroyed house and food for my family, and the survival of the beautiful trees, began to be quiet.

"When I got back to my village, I called everyone together and taught them Soft Belly. 'Try it,' I told them, just like you told us. 'Then, you make up your own mind about it.'

"This morning I gathered my village together again, before they went off to the fields and I came here. And I heard the testimony. Many people said they had the first good night's sleep since the earthquake. Children weren't crying so much and their beds were dry. Now I know Soft Belly works. Thank you."

OKAY. ENOUGH TALK about meditation and Soft Belly. Let's do it.

As I take you through the steps, I'll remind you how Soft Belly is changing your physiology—relaxing your body, quieting your mind, and making it easier for you to connect with others who can help you heal. Repeating the biological facts will inform and encourage you, and help deepen your experience of Soft Belly.

Here we go.

Find a comfortable chair you'll enjoy sitting in. You might want to have some things around that make you feel peaceful and even more comfortable: a work of art, a photo of a loved one, some flowers, a religious symbol. It's better if the lights are dim.

The instructions I give you this first time will lead you in a ten- or twelve-minute meditation. When you do it again, you can go to the CMBM website and listen to me talking you through it. Or you may want to say what I've written here to yourself. You can also record my words slowly and clearly, in a tone of voice that encourages and comforts you. After a few times, you'll know the physiology well and may not need my descriptions of it. You can use a kitchen timer to let you know when the session is over.

Become aware now of yourself sitting in your chair, breathing slowly and deeply, in through your nose and out through your mouth. Allow your belly to be soft. Let it expand on the in-breath, relax even more on the out-breath. You can say to yourself "Soft" as you breathe in and "Belly" as you breathe out. This will help you focus your mind and remind you that you want your belly to be soft and relaxed.

This is a concentrative meditation because you're concentrating on the breath, on the words "Soft" and "Belly," and on the feeling of your belly rising and falling, softening a little more with each exhalation.

Close your eyes if it's comfortable for you. This eliminates a great deal of external stimulation and will probably help you relax even more.

If thoughts come, let them come and let them go. Gently bring your mind back to the phrase "Soft . . . Belly," "Soft . . . Belly."

As you breathe in through your nose and out through your mouth with your belly soft and relaxed, more air goes to the bottom of your lungs, and more oxygen enters your bloodstream—and this oxygen will feed and nourish all the cells in your body.

Breathing in and out like this, with your belly soft and relaxed, activates the vagus nerve. *Vagus* means "wandering" in Latin. The vagus is the tenth cranial nerve. It's long and wide and has many branches. It runs up from your abdomen through your chest, back to your central nervous system, to your brain. It is, you'll remember, the antidote to the fight-or-flight response of the sympathetic nervous system and to the stress response.

Breathing slowly and deeply in through your nose and out through your mouth, activating the vagus nerve, you're relaxing the large muscles in your body, slowing your heart rate, decreasing your blood pressure, and improving your digestion.

The vagus nerve is also quieting activity in the amygdala, the part of the emotional brain that is concerned with fear and aggression. It helps promote activity in the frontal cortex, in areas of the brain concerned with judgment, self-awareness, and compassion. And one branch of the vagus nerve stimulates activity in the nerves responsible for facial expression and speech, nerves that help us record and respond to others' words and facial expressions.

As you continue Soft Belly breathing, you're relaxing your body, quieting your mind, decreasing your fear and anger, and enhancing your judgment. You're becoming more compassionate to yourself and to others, allowing yourself to connect more easily and closely to them.

Breathing slowly and deeply, in through your nose and out through your mouth, with your belly soft and relaxed, sets the stage for relaxation in all your muscles. I'm going to help you relax those muscles now.

Each time I guide your attention to a muscle group or a part of your body, breathe twice, slowly and deeply, and become aware of the relaxation in those muscles.

Breathe slowly and deeply and, as you exhale, feel the relaxation in your pelvis and your buttocks.

Now breathe slowly twice more, and feel your thighs and knees relax; now your lower legs and feet.

Breathe twice more and, as you exhale, feel the relaxation in your back.

Breathing twice more, feel your chest and shoulders relax as you exhale. Continue breathing slowly and deeply. Relax.

As you continue to breathe, feel the relaxation in your upper arms; your forearms; your hands. With each exhalation, you'll feel more relaxed.

Breathe twice more and as you exhale, feel the relaxation in the muscles of your neck, face, and head.

Continue breathing slowly and deeply for another few minutes, feeling your whole body relax with each exhalation.

To encourage and deepen this process, continue to say to yourself "Soft" as you breathe in, and "Belly," as you breathe out.

If thoughts come, let them come and let them go. Gently bring your mind back to "Soft . . . Belly."

After about ten or twelve minutes, slowly, gently open your eyes and let your attention come back into the room.

I RECOMMEND YOU begin by doing Soft Belly once or twice a day for about ten minutes each time. As you get familiar with Soft Belly, you can vary the amount of time, practicing for more or less time and doing it once or several times a day, depending on your need and the time available.

It's great to have a special place where you can do Soft Belly, where you can close the door and be by yourself. And it's good to have at least one regular time. A regular place and time make it easier to practice. And knowing that you're going to be doing Soft Belly gives you something to look forward to, a reliable relief from stress. It also helps give some reassuring structure to days that may be disturbed and disordered by trauma.

I love using the words *Soft Belly* because they remind me so specifically of the part of the body I need to relax and of the feeling I want to create. But if for some reason, and after some practice, these words are really difficult for you, you can use others that will help you do the same slow, deep breathing. The other day a teacher on the Pine Ridge Reservation in South Dakota said her third-grade students loved to say "smelling roses" as they breathed in and "blowing out candles" as they breathed out.

You can do Soft Belly anytime: when you're anxious or agitated, growing impatient in the supermarket line, or stalled in traffic (closing your eyes is not an option here). Soft Belly will help free your mind from painful repetitive thoughts and memories and relieve preoccupation with what's happened to you, or how "bad" you've been, or how hopeless your situation seems. And it is, as Batichon the Haitian farmer discovered, great for helping you sleep—and getting back to sleep if you've awakened in the middle of the night.

If you feel agitated when you sit to do Soft Belly, get up and move around. Do some chores, go for a walk. Or maybe do the Shaking and Dancing that I'll describe in a later chapter. Then sit down again to do Soft Belly, perhaps on a bench in a park after you've walked for a while, or in a coffee shop or library or church or back home. Movement will decrease the tension, and relaxation will be easier.

Breathing this way, with your belly soft and relaxed, is grounding. As all your muscles relax, you connect to a place of calm and stability in your body. You feel the support of the earth.

When you're doing Soft Belly, don't try to resist unpleasant thoughts or force them away. That will only give your painful thoughts more power than they deserve. It will perpetuate the struggle against them and actually reinforce the memory of the trauma you've experienced.

Meditation is not about having a totally empty mind, though occasionally those moments of grace will come. It's about allowing the thoughts, including the disturbing ones of trauma remembered and reexperienced, to be there. The idea is to let all thoughts come, and let them go, to relax with them, to accept them.

RESEARCH BY THE University of Wisconsin's Richard Davidson, and the experience of many people, clearly show the trauma-dissolving power of meditative practices like Soft Belly: disturbing thoughts gradually lose their hold on you, becoming what Davidson describes as "less sticky." Your mind clears. It functions better. Your mood lifts. You realize you can help yourself. Your comfort with and appreciation for others may grow.

Many people I've worked with have begun by thinking Soft Belly is weird or unlikely to be of help or not worth the time. But when they experience Soft Belly, their minds change.

Medical students, who are anxious about devoting even ten minutes of their crowded day to meditation, discover that Soft Belly enhances their capacity to function. They concentrate better and assimilate information more easily, and they study and sleep better. When they do Soft Belly, they feel less anxious and get better grades. They're more hopeful about becoming doctors. A small investment of time pays off handsomely.

Many of the people you'll meet in later chapters, who've been traumatized in childhood and youth, do it daily; and then they do it again when harsh words or rejection triggers past pain. Azhaar taught Soft Belly to her family and does it with them.

If you practice Soft Belly regularly, you'll likely decrease your levels of stress hormones and improve your mood, along with your concentration and sleep. Soft Belly will help you to respond rather than react to scary situations that might previously have triggered your trauma. Regular practice of Soft Belly may give you your first experience of freedom from traumatic memories and obsessive and painful thoughts, from the guilt that so often clings to them, and from the crippling worry that the future will repeat the traumatic past.

In addition to its direct benefits, Soft Belly breathing brings you an additional blessing: it tells you, every time you do it, that you're not helpless or hopeless. You can, with just a few minutes of focused effort, make a difference in how you feel and think and look at the world around you, and relate to other people. And Soft Belly creates the calm mind and hopeful attitude, which form the rich soil that will nourish all the other trauma-healing techniques that you'll learn.

EVERY DAY OR TWO, someone at least as surprised and pleased as Batichon tells me about Soft Belly's benefits.

Not long ago, Shirley, a fifty-one-year-old widow and government worker, came to see me. When I'd met her a month before during a brief workshop on grief and mourning, her face was blotchy, her body shapeless and slumped; her crossed leg was jumping up and down with anxiety, and her eyes were focused on the floor. She had confided, "My blood pressure is off the charts. I'm headed toward diabetes. I can't sleep, and I think I'm going to die of chest pain—and sometimes I'm miserable enough to want to speed up the process."

Now she was sitting in my office, her back straight, neat, alert, looking right at me. I hardly recognized her. She was still grieving for her husband, who had died a few years ago, and was uneasy about her son, who had just left home to live on his own. She was lonely in her empty nest. And her boss, overbearing and unappreciative, was still an irritant.

Now, though, she was moving through, not drowning in, troubled waters.

"When I did the Soft Belly breathing in the workshop," she told me, "I felt quiet. As you talked us through it, I realized, 'I'm in fight or flight all the time.' Sitting there, even that first time, my mind started to slow down, my boss seemed to shrink in size. And then the thought popped into my head: 'You can be healthy.' That got me started. I decided to do the breathing every day, sometimes once, sometimes two or three or five times.

"It was like cleaning out my mind so new ideas could come in. Then I started walking and breathing slowly and deeply, holding my head up so I could see the 'real world' around me. I'd forgotten the beautiful trees and the grass, and even the people. My blood pressure came down, and I got off the meds, and I started sleeping at night. It felt so good. 'This is me,' I thought. 'I have feelings, even some good ones.' That made me laugh. And then I called you."

And as I was editing this chapter, I received an email from Terri, a forty-year-old accountant: "Although learning to breathe with a Soft Belly initially seemed ludicrous," my correspondent began, "it has been THE most helpful thing I learned. . . . I have practiced every day since returning home.

"Since my husband's death by suicide this past June, I have found running, an activity I have loved all my life, difficult—especially, it seems, when my heart rate would hit a certain point and all the memories of that day come back in a flash and cause me to hyper-ventilate.

"Practicing the Soft Belly breath has been so helpful. I have been able to do it even while I run. . . . I have run more than a half dozen times now without a single hyperventilating panic attack. I know this is just the very beginning of the healing process for me, but it is a huge step forward. . . . I will be forever grateful."

THERE ARE TWO questions that people frequently ask about Soft Belly and other meditations.

The first is whether they can be harmful. Not, I say, if they are done properly. Still, there are important cautionary notes. The relaxed awareness that meditation, or indeed any mind-body practice, might bring can sometimes open us up to long suppressed disturbing thoughts and feelings. Most often, you'll be able to relax with them, letting them come and go. If, however, you're feeling overwhelmed, you should open your eyes; usually the anxiety will dissipate. You can do the practice again on another day, perhaps for a shorter period of time. If you discover after several attempts that a particular technique is still disturbing, you might want to contact a therapist who can help you deal with the feelings or memories that are emerging (I'll give you some guidance on selecting a therapist in the Appendix "Finding Other Help"). Or you might want to stop the technique and use one of the many other tools that you'll be learning in *The Transformation*.

On the other hand, some people find that mind-body practices work so well that a dose of a medication they've been taking that was adequate might now be excessive. Because your body is in a more balanced and relaxed physiological state, an anti-anxiety drug that was mildly calming is now putting you to sleep. So, if you're taking medication for anxiety, depression, insomnia, pain, hypertension, or diabetes, you should check in periodically with your physician to make sure the dose is appropriately regulated.

The second question is whether Soft Belly is the same as or somehow different from mindfulness. It's a good question, and here's my answer: all forms of meditation, including the active expressive techniques that I'll teach you later, like Shaking and Dancing, ultimately encourage relaxed moment-to-moment awareness—mindfulness. And all the other techniques I'll teach—the Drawings and the Imagery; the walks in Nature; choosing, preparing, and savoring healthy foods; exploring the tense and troubled places in our bodies; cultivating Gratitude and Forgiveness—are also facilitated by, and grounded in, mindfulness. Doing these activities mindfully is what changes them from unwelcome chores to interesting, satisfying challenges and effective tools for self-care and healing.

Soft Belly—quieting your mind and enhancing your perception, judgment, and compassion—makes mindfulness so much easier. It's foundational.

AND SOFT BELLY, with its gifts of balance and ease, makes it much easier for us to embrace Hope, the great healing force that we'll explore and activate in the next chapter. And Hope, as you'll see, can inspire and sustain every step on your life's journey.

4
Embracing Hope

TRAUMA'S MOST EXQUISITE torture is the hopelessness it brings, the fear that its pain will never end, that we will always be assailed and limited by its terrors. As Soft Belly breathing quiets our mind, it gives us a reprieve. We may realize, like Shirley and Terri, that we can, at least for a few moments, stem trauma's assault, tame its terrors. We know that relief is not someone else's theory or a nice idea. It's our experience.

The glimpse of Hope that Soft Belly gives us is a revelation and a promise. It can be the beginning of the end of our worst suffering. Now our mind understands that if one change is possible, so, too, are others. Now we're ready to make Hope our sustaining reality.

Hope includes our expectation and desire that something will happen. It is also, more deeply, our trust that what happens will somehow serve and benefit us.

Hope is powerful medicine. Over the last sixty years, scientific studies have shown that placebos (the Latin word means "I shall please"), the biologically inactive sugar pills that we invest in for hope of healing, are 30–70 percent as potent as the active drugs to which they're compared. The faith-enriched Hope of sugar pills can improve the breathing of asthmatics and reduce the excruciating pain of heart attacks. Placebos can calm the anxiety, raise the depressed mood, and reduce the fear that are the hallmarks of post-traumatic stress.

Recent research on the biology of placebos is beginning to help us understand why. Placebos affect many parts of our brain that mediate pain, anxiety, mood, and expectations, including the frontal cortex, the cingulate gyrus, and the hippocampus. And the placebo response releases powerful, calming, pain-relieving, and mood-enhancing neurotransmitters—dopamine, the endorphins, and serotonin among them. Studies have shown that the placebo response may account for 82 percent of the effect of antidepressant drugs.

And of course, it's not just the sugar pills. The definition of placebo includes all the nonspecific factors in healing—our belief in the doctors who prescribe the pills and advise us, and in the institutions where we seek help and healing. William Osler, perhaps the most distinguished physician of the early twentieth century, once observed that more people were cured by Saint Johns Hopkins—by their belief in that august institution—than by any of its therapeutic procedures.

Hope significantly improves performance in life, as well as recovery from illness. Children and young people who are hopeful are far more likely to focus on success rather than being preoccupied with failure; they do better academically and athletically. Students who are more hopeful are less likely to see poor grades as a sign of personal inadequacy, more likely to focus on trying harder or developing alternative study strategies. In one study, "high hope" accounted for 56 percent of the difference between the performances of groups of student athletes.

And the power of Hope endures as we age. Hopeful adults are more flexible, committed, and imaginative; they function better at work. Hopeful older adults are far less reactive to stressful events. Hope decreases suffering from chronic pain and extends our survival from life-threatening illnesses like cancer. People who are more hopeful live longer.

The positive experience we create for ourselves may, as I've suggested, be an even more reliable and sustainable source of Hope than our belief in pills and the doctors who prescribe them. As we feel the change created by Soft Belly breathing, we mobilize Hope. Doing it regularly significantly reinforces our Hope. Successfully using all the other self-care techniques multiplies the effect.

OTHER PEOPLE'S EXAMPLES can also reinforce our Hope. In the midst of personal darkness, they can be illuminating, even life changing. More than fifty years ago, my friend Jenny did this for me.

As a student at Harvard Medical School in the 1960s, I marveled at pediatric surgeons who treated the hearts, brains, and bones of tiny children with tenderness as great as their skill. I had lecturers and lab instructors who had won, or soon would win, Nobel Prizes. When I was desperate, Bob Coles threw me a psychotherapeutic lifeline, and Erik Erikson—Sigmund and Anna Freud's student and Bob Coles's mentor—was a guiding presence. Still, when I look back, I believe my greatest teacher may have been twenty-three-year-old Jenny, whom none of you is likely to have heard of.

Jenny was the girlfriend of my med school buddy, Mike, an elementary school teacher he had known back in Kentucky who now lived with him in Boston. I knew her casually, but I loved her unaffected, down-home lightness, the energized twang of the banjo in her voice, the kind attentiveness she brought into Mike's life and mine. I remember one gray winter afternoon chasing seagulls with her across the frozen Fenway. Our mouths were steaming with cold, Jenny's blond hair barely tucked under a wool cap.

And then one night a truck crushed Mike's VW bug. He was okay, but Jenny—the runner and dancer, the girl who drew on the board and led the class in crafts projects and hugged her little students—was paralyzed from the neck down. It was so horrible, so inconceivable for someone so young and alive and good. I wept then and weep now, all these years later, remembering it.

Once Jenny was stabilized, which simply meant in no imminent danger of dying, I began to visit her. Jenny's hospital, like many rehab facilities, was buried in the back of beyond. Sometimes I hitchhiked, sometimes I took the trolleys that crisscrossed Boston to see her, long rides with time to think about Jenny and what her catastrophic injury meant—about life and to her. Time to wonder how she could survive in this condition and why she would want to. Time, also, to wonder what my life was about. Why I was enduring tedious lectures and labs that seemed hopelessly removed from helping people who were hurting. Why I was no longer able to value or sustain my relationship with my girlfriend.

As soon as I sat down by Jenny's bed, her smile swept away my accumulating gloom and self-pity. She was down, especially about not being able to scratch constant, infernal itches, even despairing sometimes. But through more than a dozen surgeries—most were high degree of difficulty tendon transplants—and endless, exhausting, only minimally successful rehab, she was never out. I sat by Jenny's bed, reaching through IV lines and braces to hold her cold, immobile hands and trace the bony ridges that muscle loss had made mountainous. And we talked.

Jenny, immobilized and challenged in every moment, was, to my wonder, deeply sympathetic to the loves and losses of the doctors, therapists, and nurses who gathered around her bed like chilled travelers at a bright fire. After she had shared their news with me and asked me about my own love life, she would speak of her Hope that her surgeries would someday, somehow—I wanted to but could hardly imagine it—make her functional enough to teach again. She sipped juice through a straw and, unable to move her hands, used her mouth to point that brave instrument, like Franklin Roosevelt's cigarette holder, toward Drawings her students had done for her.

I was amazed at how tragedy had transformed Jenny. She had been my playmate. Now she was my teacher. Under the most extreme pressure, her spunkiness had crystalized into stunning courage. Her good heart was now opening in unself-conscious, unaffected, apparently universal compassion. This, I thought, is what's possible for a human being. What a privilege—how amazing it is to sit with her, to witness who she is.

And what a gift. Being with Jenny, being of some small help to her—scratching one of her itches, listening, being her friend, someone she could rely on—was right, worthwhile. Being with her was also giving me hints about the doctor I might become. I was beginning to feel, along with wonder at Jenny, a sense that Hope could survive almost anything, that change might be possible for all of us, and that I could help it happen.

THE HOPE I encourage in you is not theoretical or abstract or Pollyannaish. I know the fruitless protests that follow terrible injuries and disappointments, the frustration and fury of dealing with the unavoidable limitations of loss and death. I know the relentless guilt and shame of actions taken or not taken, and love not expressed, which can obliterate present joy and cast an impenetrable shadow over the future. I know all of them from working with people in pain during fifty years of psychiatric practice. And like so many of you, I know them in my own life—from the death of people I loved, from my own irrevocable mistakes, and especially, from my unwilling, enforced separation from a child who is as dear to me as my own life.

Many of the people in this book were in despair when I first met them, before they began this program of Transformation. Two weeks before she came to my office, sixty-year-old Jane had been diagnosed with inoperable stage IV cancer and had discovered that her husband of thirty years had long been cheating on her. Months after her fiancé was killed in a car accident, thirty-year-old Patricia was "in shock . . . moving through life like a zombie . . . unable to do anything or to feel anything" for friends or family, sure that she would never be close to another man. Jason, a retired army officer, was haunted by death and destruction, convinced he had "left [his] soul in Iraq." In grade school, long before she became a self-destructive adolescent and a fearful, often despairing adult, Maya was repeatedly raped by a succession of "uncles" while her prostitute mother turned tricks. Howard, who had taken an overdose, was convinced that he would always be a medicated, numbed-out "psych case," a failure.

Many times I have been stunned by these and other terrible stories, by the stooped shoulders, pale, shocked faces, and haunted, burdened words of hopeless people, by their fixed, grim conviction that nothing will or can ever change. But hours of sitting with them—inviting them to share their pain, helping them discover their own enduring strength and wisdom and humor, watching them come back to life—have taught me not to be intimidated or discouraged. Great and unpredictable change, I discovered, could come to all of these people and many, many more, just as it did to Jenny and Diana and Azhaar and to me.

Pictures of Hope and Healing

I'm asking you now to consider that your Hope can grow, that it can, like a thirsty plant, find water in the most parched, devastated ground. I'm going to invite you to use Drawings to discover this truth for yourself, to see that your imagination may be able to help you make Hope's promise a reality.

These Drawings will build on the relaxed awareness, the hopeful foundation that Soft Belly brings. They will help you move beyond doubts you may have about your capacity to be and feel different. They'll show you that it may be possible—even now, when you may feel empty of ideas or in despair—to imagine change.

These Drawings will also serve as a baseline against which you, like Azhaar, can measure your progress as you move through and beyond trauma.

Drawings are one of the simplest, most reliable ways to bypass the fears that arise from our amygdala and the hope-limiting doubts of our "rational" left hemisphere. They give us immediate access to the great storehouse of the right brain's intuitive wisdom.

Drawings are easy for all of us to do and are a safe, playful way to express and share what's going on inside us. I often do Drawings in my first individual or group session with adults as well as children and always at the beginning of our CMBM trainings. I recommend them when anyone is confronting an apparently insoluble problem. And I use them myself. Often.

You may, even as I raise the possibility of Drawings, feel self-conscious, remembering belittling remarks about your early artistic efforts from your third-grade teacher, Ms. Grundy, or your big brother. But, hey, everyone has a Ms. G. We can all laugh about it, and everyone can draw—something. It may be, if you are artistic, that your Drawings will be representational. If you're unskilled, as I and so many others are, you're likely to produce stick figures or abstractions, lines and blobs. All of them are fine. Ms. Grundy has taken a leave of absence. These Drawings are for you.

We'll do three Drawings. All you need is three sheets of blank paper—8½" by 11" is fine—and crayons or magic markers (which I like better because they're so bright and bold). Do the Drawings quickly. "First thought, best thought," as the Zen Buddhists say. That way the Drawings are likely to be uncensored, authentic, surprising, revealing. Drawings are calling your shy imagination, your intuition, off the bench, to play a creative guiding role in your life.

You'll take about five minutes for each Drawing.

OKAY, LET'S GET STARTED.

Begin by doing two or three minutes of slow, deep Soft Belly breathing, with your eyes closed. Relax, repeating "Soft" as you breathe in and "Belly" as you breathe out, noticing your thoughts, feelings, and sensations come and go, then gently bringing your mind back to Soft Belly.

Now open your eyes and do the first Drawing. It's of "Yourself." Don't think about what this means. Just get started. Let your hand take the lead. This first Drawing will get you wrestling with, maybe even laughing at, your self-consciousness. And it will get you out there and down on paper. This is not about skill. No grades. No judgment. Just do it.

Once you've done Drawing #1, you'll likely say, "Oh yeah, that's me—more or less." Now put this first paper aside.

The second Drawing is "You with your biggest problem." Though this may be quite painful, it's always useful. It's good to identify a problem, even if it's only one among many, to make it real and concrete. Putting it out there on the page, you've removed it from the confused, troubled mass that has filled your mind and maybe overwhelmed you. You can, quite literally, see what you're dealing with.

Again, take a few deep breaths. Now do it.

In her second Drawing, Frieda, a middle-aged woman, sketches her daughter, dead of a drug overdose, in a grave. Frieda represents herself as a tiny stick figure kneeling alone nearby. Everything is gray or black. "I am lost," she says. "Alone. Weak. Helpless." Hervé, a Haitian security guard, shows us a garden. The flowers have lost their petals, and the stems of all the plants are drooping. "My wife died in the earthquake," he explains. "Our house was destroyed and our garden, too. There's no life in me."

In Drawing #2, harried law firm associates, young executives, single mothers, and medical students are often sitting under the grim face of a clock or behind prison bars.

Shelly, a middle-aged woman with ovarian cancer, draws a red blob in the belly of her stick figure. "No, it's not the cancer," she says, when I ask. It is, to my and her surprise, her rage at her unfaithful husband.

Will, a Lakota elder whose daughter was killed in a car accident, draws himself, a stick figure with a braid, walking and crying. Above him is "Mother Earth, dying because of all the hate and aggression."

The third Drawing is "You with your problem solved." "Impossible," you may protest. "I've just lost my job and have no prospects" or "My husband died, and my children don't love me." Don't worry. This is not about listing logical possibilities. It's about letting your imagination come up with *its* answer. Once again, just do it. Allow your intuition to guide you to the colors, to move your hand.

Sometimes the third Drawing seems dark—a defeat, not an illumination. Frieda, whose daughter was in the grave, draws herself in bed. Putting it on paper is painful. It certainly doesn't make everything better, but it is definitely a message from her intuition. It lets her know, as she tells me, "that I need to retreat for a while to take care of myself."

More often, the third Drawing is enlivening as well as revelatory. The first hints of Hope clearly appear. A lonely single mother is on a park bench happily sharing childcare duties with a friend; a med student, his back turned on a stack of books, is headed to the gym, no clock or prison bars in sight; a teenage girl has enlisted family and friends to dispel clouds of shame and anxiety that have darkened her days since a sexual assault.

In her third Drawing, Shelly, the woman with ovarian cancer, is sitting opposite her husband, confronting him with the red flames of her hurt and anger. Her eyes are bright. "I look energized," she observes, "and I feel it, too. I guess I was afraid before. Now I know what I have to do. This is the only way forward, the only way to work things out with my husband. I have to let him know what's going on."

In Hervé's third Drawing there are flowers growing and vegetables sprouting from the earth. "For the first time," he says, "I realize that my garden can grow again. My life can go on."

Will, the Lakota elder, is raising his arms toward Mother Earth. Now our planet is in the shape of a heart, shining, not crying, promising a legacy of love and caring to "all our children."

AFTER YOU'VE FINISHED your own Drawings, take some time to look at them.

What do you see on the page? Notice the forms, the colors, the relative size and position of the figures. What's the mood of each Drawing?

Are you surprised at the first picture, the way you drew yourself? So small or big? Without feet or missing a head? Smiling or sad? Alone or with others? What does this Drawing have to tell you about the way you see yourself? What's missing in your picture of yourself? Have you neglected to include aspects of your character, perhaps admirable qualities?

What about the problem that emerged in the second Drawing? Is it an exquisitely painful portrait of life-dominating loss? A predictable acknowledgment of limitations and constraint, like a clock, prison bars, or stacks of unread assignments? An astonishing gift from the unconscious, like Shelly's fiery blob of anger? Were you aware of it before? Does seeing it on the page help you understand and deal with it?

And what do you think about the third Drawing, the solution?

Is there intelligence, even wisdom, in it? Does it point you in a new direction?

It may be a practical solution: reaching out to a friend to overcome loneliness, going to the gym to relieve stress and feel better about your body, sharing shame and feeling it loosen its grip. It may involve, as it did for Shelly, confronting what you've been avoiding. Your solution may take you deep inside, like Frieda, to regroup emotionally. It may point you to a new commitment to life and caring, as it did Hervé and Will. Take some time to consider the solution you drew.

Are there action steps you want to take? Frieda did take time for herself. Shelly spoke honestly to her husband and insisted he go to a therapist with her. Hervé actually planted his garden. Will is devoting himself to teaching traditional Lakota reverence for Mother Earth to the young children of his tribe.

Countless stressed-out people of all ages have followed the guidance of their Drawings to open spaces, energizing physical or creative activity, the welcome company of forgotten friends and family, to a new commitment to helping themselves and others. They have been able to embrace what they've drawn—both the pain and constraint of their problem and the expansive satisfying third picture of what their lives might be.

Sometimes they do it right away. Sometimes it's a gradual process.

YOU MAY WANT to put your Drawings on your wall or refrigerator, or next to your computer, where they can welcome you with possibility and encourage your progress. In any case, hold on to them. Put them somewhere safe. We'll return to them toward the end of *The Transformation*.

You can do this set of Drawings often—whenever you're dealing with difficulty, overwhelmed by fear, uncertain of how to act, unable to do what needs to be done, or simply in need of an image of Hope.

5
Shaking and Dancing

O N   A   C O L D, damp morning in March 1999, while US
bombers roar overhead and UN trucks groan through
the endless rows of tents in Macedonia's Stancovic refugee camp, I
lead a workshop for two hundred Kosovo Albanians who have fled
Serbian ethnic cleansing.

I begin, as I usually do, with Soft Belly breathing. Afterward, I
ask for a show of hands: "How many of you," my interpreter queries,
translating my English into Albanian, "notice any change?" Here, as
elsewhere after war is over or even in the middle of fighting, about 70
or 80 percent of the hands go up. "What happened?" I say, and answers
are shouted out. "Calmer," "Relaxed," "My body's less tense," "Fewer
bad thoughts," "A little less cold"—there are laughs at this.

I explain the fight-or-flight response, asking my audience to tell me
if they've experienced it and what it's like. There's no problem getting
the answers. Their hearts have been racing. Just about everybody
is having trouble sleeping. Older peoples' blood pressure is off the

charts. The close quarters of cold, small tents are filled with irritation. Ordinarily patient mothers are smacking unruly children.

"Does anyone," I go on, "have any questions about fight or flight or this Soft Belly meditation, or any concerns you'd like to share?"

Far away, toward the back of the huge tent, a man with a pale, round face stands and raises his hand. "Doctor," he says, "thank you so much for coming to help us. Three months ago, I saw twenty-one members of our family massacred by Serbian paramilitaries. I cannot get the picture out of my mind. It is always there when I'm awake, the children falling and bleeding, my wife trying to cover the bodies. And it is there in my dreams. It was still there while we were doing the breathing. What can I do to make it leave my mind?"

My own mind stops. My beating heart seems to overwhelm my voice. Finally, I tell him that I'm so sad and moved by what he has told me, and honored that he would share his pain with me. "I do not know what I can do to help," I say, "but I do hope that you will stay with us in this workshop."

"Thank you, doctor," he says and sits.

I speak, haltingly at first, my eyes filled with the face of this questioner whom I think of as the Man of Sorrow, with his unimaginable suffering.

I pause and breathe slowly and deeply, this time to quiet my own shock, and my sadness at not being able to help.

When I'm calm enough to speak, I begin again. "I know there are many of you whose minds are filled with terrible memories that won't go away, whose hearts are heavy with grief. I know that some of you feel weak and stiff in your body, unable to act or even feel. These are all effects of trauma.

"We're going to do something now that will shake loose the tension of your fight or flight and help melt your frozen body. It may help you get rid of some of your anger, raise your energy a little, maybe even lift off some of the troubles that weigh down your minds.

"What we're going to do," I continue, "is technically called an 'expressive meditation.' Expressive meditations are the oldest ones on our planet. All our ancestors did them. They shouted and danced and whirled and jumped up and down. When something terrible had happened or was about to happen, they moved their bodies and let go of their tensions and expressed their feelings. Are you willing to do this?" I'm shouting now.

Hands go up everywhere. I hope it's enthusiasm. Perhaps it's only that right now I'm a diversion in this tedious, troubled tent town of seventy thousand refugees.

"In the first part, we'll shake for about six to eight minutes to fast music. Then we'll stop and stand still for a couple of minutes, relaxing, paying attention to, being aware, 'mindful' of, our body and our breath.

"Then there will be new music. Just let your body move to it. I don't say 'dance' because then you'll have an idea in your head—waltz or salsa or electric slide." Some laughs. "Or you'll start worrying: 'I'm such a poor dancer.' Or you'll start thinking how you're going to show off some new steps." Many laughs here. "It isn't about those dances or any particular dance, and it's not about skill. It's about doing *your* dance.

"Each of us is different. We all look a little different. We have different genes, different fingerprints, different faces, different minds, different preferences. So, if there are two hundred of us here, there will be two hundred different dances.

"Now I'm going to show you how to shake." I say, climbing up on a truck bed so they can see me from the back of the tent. "Put your feet shoulder-width apart. Bend your knees a little bit and relax your shoulders. And now begin shaking from your feet up through your knees and your hips till your whole body is shaking."

I do it and see incredulous looks on weathered faces: a grown man, a doctor, doing *this*? Meanwhile, the team of doctors and therapists I've brought from the US spreads out and shakes with me.

Soon, pretty much everyone is moving up and down, shaking, laughing. "Great!" I shout. "You're very good! This is just practice. We'll start again soon. Relax for a minute.

"Now, this is an experiment," I go on, "and you may remember from science class that every experiment has 'conditions,' things you have to organize so the experiment works the way it should. There is only one condition for this experiment: close your eyes. That's so you don't peek at your neighbor and say to yourself"—and I exaggerate here for comic effect—"'Oh, I really need to teach that woman how to shake.' Or 'I could never be as good as him.' Forget those other people for a while. Leave judgment and comparison outside our tent. This is just for you.

"Breathe deeply and slowly for a minute or two," I say. A few guys at the edge of the crowd shuffle around, puzzled and uncomfortable, but everyone else gets ready. "Thank Nature for this experience, as my teacher, Shyam, used to tell me. Now begin."

The music—fast, driving, rhythmic, electronic—fills the air underneath the huge tent. "Shake up from your feet through your knees, hips, and shoulders to your chest. Let the shaking take over. Let your shoulders go. Most of us have so much tension there." I'm crooning, coaching, coaxing. More and more people join in, masses of men moving like jackhammers, women in hijabs gathering together, bobbing up and down, kids shaking arms and legs as if to bring down rain.

"Let your head go as you shake. Let your jaw hang open. Lots of us have tightness there. If sounds come out of your mouth, let them come." And now there are shouts, howls, a few high-pitched screams. "If you feel silly or bored or tired—KEEP GOING. Let the shaking take over your whole body. Good. Good. Keep going." I'm shaking as hard as I can now, my head whipping side to side, laughing, enjoying and encouraging my new partners.

After about four minutes, just when everyone is ready to call it a day, I shout the remaining time: "Three minutes left." Scattered groans. "If you feel tired or bored—pick up the pace. KEEP GOING, KEEP GOING. FASTER. GOOD. GOOD. Two minutes." I'm counting down now. "KEEP GOING. GREAT. One minute. 100 percent effort. Thirty seconds. STOP." The music stops and so do the shakers.

"Now be quiet. Pay attention to your breathing. Relax. Be aware of your body, of breathing." Our breath rises in steam toward the roof of the great tent.

After two or three minutes of silence, I speak again, announcing: "WHEN THE MUSIC BEGINS, LET IT MOVE YOU."

A couple of dramatic chords surprise us, and then there's the voice of Jimmy Cliff, at once insistent and angry, upbeat and hopeful, urging us on. It's the reggae anthem, "You Can Get It If You Really Want."

Older people are shuffling in place. Younger ones kick their legs and flail their arms. Some can't resist opening their eyes and grabbing partners—mostly men with men and women in circles of women; children are whirling.

After a few minutes the song is over, but some people continue to move, by themselves and in the lines they've formed for traditional Albanian dances. There's lots of loud talk. Women laugh, and men slap each other on the back. It looks like sleepers have come awake. Eyes are bright.

The air is filled with appreciation and questions. "Finally I am relaxed." "I can feel my body again." "What time of day is best to do this?" "Can I teach it to my grandmother?"

"Morning," I answer, "or any time you are tense." "And yes, it's fine for your grandmother."

Afterward, some people hang around, wanting to tell each other or me more about what has happened. I listen, answer questions.

As the crowd melts away, I see the Man of Sorrow, sitting quietly, apart. He signals to my interpreter, says he wants to take a picture with me.

I sit next to him, our arms around each other's shoulders. I ask him why he wants the photo. "For a few minutes," he says, "after the shaking, during the dancing, those terrible images and thoughts were gone from my mind. It's the first time in three months. It gives me hope that I can live again."

I DO NOT know what happened to the Man of Sorrow. I have, as we say in medicine, no follow-up. Sometimes, though, as I work in other places where tragedy has overwhelmed so many, I look at the picture we took—our arms around each other's shoulders, a little smile turning up one side of his face—and think of him. And often, in these new places, I have had follow-ups that confirm the enduring power, as well as the sudden blessing, of Shaking and Dancing.

It's highly likely that Shaking and Dancing and the other expressive meditations, when done regularly, have the same or similar trauma-healing benefits as physical exercise like brisk walking, jogging, and yoga, which we'll explore in later chapters. These include such biological boosts as increases in feel-good neurotransmitters like serotonin, dopamine, and the endorphins; the creation of new neurons in the hippocampus; and decreased anxiety, greater resilience, better mood, relief from and protection against depression, improved sleep and memory, and greater capacity to focus.

But these outcomes are only part of expressive meditation's happy therapeutic story. Exercise is controlled, goal directed. Though controlled at first, expressive meditation becomes spontaneous, liberating.

While the science is still in its speculative stage, our collective human experience of these approaches is vast—tens of thousands of years of natural experiments with them, by hundreds of millions of us in cultures around the planet. These are the oldest ways of changing and enlarging consciousness, of freeing us from our fears and self-doubt, from the structures of belief and thought and feeling that can limit and cripple us, as well as the societies in which we live.

These were the tools of the shamans of Siberia and of ancient healers and healing traditions around the world. Fast, deep breathing was practiced by the wandering orange-robed sadhus ("spiritual seekers") of India and the Buddhist monks of Tibet. Whirling was used by the Sufis of medieval Persia and Turkey. And physical movement and emotional catharsis are central to the modern expressive forms of Western psychotherapy such as Gestalt and bioenergetics, and their descendants, the various body-oriented psychotherapies. "Archaic techniques of ecstasy" is what the historian of religion Mircea Eliade called these approaches.

Shaking and Dancing is perhaps the simplest and most consistently effective expressive meditation. It's almost always the first one I use. Indigenous people in Asia, Africa, and the Americas use Shaking with Dancing to free tribal members from fear and depression, to promote emotional expression and increase the life energy—"N/om," the Kalahari Bushmen call it—and to bring about spiritual as well as physical and emotional healing.

Shaking breaks up self-protective, leaden despair, melts physical rigidity, and energizes depleted bodies. It is likely that shaking taps directly into a reparative biological mechanism that is part of our evolutionary heritage. When animals emerge from threatening situations, they shake themselves before they resume their ordinary activity. This appears to be true for those who have been in a fight or have successfully escaped from a predator, as well as those who have been immobilized by fear. Think of your dog after an angry confrontation, or the mouse that was limp and frozen in the jaws of your cat; released, she shakes herself and scampers away.

Peter Levine, a researcher who has long used body-oriented

therapies, suggests that shaking facilitates passage up the evolutionary ladder from the immobilization of "fear paralysis" through the fight-or-flight response to a more balanced state in which awareness, imagination, and social engagement are possible.

The second phase, of standing still and experiencing and observing your breath and your body, provides a few precious moments, often a first experience, of relaxed mindfulness.

And the third stage of dancing allows you to express the buried feelings that shaking may have brought to the surface, to delight in newfound freedom as you move in ways that satisfy your body's need to express itself.

Nobel Prize winner Ilya Prigogine's work on dissipative systems in chemical reactions provides a useful perspective on energy-mobilizing, tension-breaking expressive meditations like Shaking and Dancing. At certain "far from equilibrium" points, Prigogine observed, the "perturbation," the disturbance of physical and chemical systems, can bring about a profound and creative change. Out of this chaos, a new, more highly integrated order can emerge. This is a natural process, a result of the unfettered evolution of a system (chemical or physical) and of the free exchange between that system and the world around it.

The analogy seems pretty clear to me. When we've been traumatized, the natural processes of biological and psychological growth and evolution are inhibited. Our muscles are tense and tight, our breathing shallow, our thoughts and feelings limited and constricted. Expressive meditations like Shaking and Dancing create the far-from-equilibrium states that disrupt fixed physical, mental, and emotional patterns. Chaos arrives, and with it the possibility of creating a new, more open and flexible order.

My CMBM colleagues and I have taught Shaking and Dancing to hundreds of thousands of children and adults. We've taught it to soldiers at Walter Reed Army Medical Center and to civilians who are hoping to de-stress; in hotels and churches, synagogues and mosques; to tense health professionals in med school amphitheaters; to firefighters and police officers who regularly face danger and death; to amputees in wheelchairs and bedridden hospital patients; in shelters in the middle of wars; and in the living rooms of suburbanites whose children were murdered in school shootings.

Once they get over their fear of feeling foolish, resistant teenagers, self-conscious medical students, solemn soldiers, harried working moms, tense Washington lawyers, and even politicians all learn to look forward to Shaking and Dancing. Children love it and are likely to teach it to their parents. And parents often teach it to their stressed-out kids. Every day you do Shaking and Dancing, you'll make new discoveries about yourself and reclaim your rightful emotional and physical territory from trauma's tyranny. You'll feel a new sense of freedom.

OVER THE YEARS, Shaking and Dancing has been a turning point for many people, giving them, as it did the Man of Sorrow, a glimpse of possibility and Hope, even in the midst of despair.

Darcy, who joined my weekend workshop on Trauma and Transformation, is thirty-one years old, smart and attractive, squared away in tailored khakis and a crisp blouse but unhappy, embarrassed. She nods with understanding, painfully serious, as I explain the biology of stress. She's as earnest and armored as a knight. Actually, Darcy is a kind of knight, a firefighter—the first woman in the department of her southern city.

"My body," she says in a thin, strained voice, "works fine when I have to run into a burning building. But I can't really feel it." She has been "dissociated" for two years, since her longtime boyfriend broke up with her. It's gotten worse since she joined the department. "A woman in a man's world. Guys are grabbing my ass, brushing up against my breasts. One guy in particular. He's older, he's big, and he's my supervisor. He just smiles innocently, with hurt in his face, looking surprised that I'm angry that he's touched me. In my profession, you don't talk about depression or PTSD, and you definitely don't rat out a superior officer. I can't feel my body and I've lost my voice."

Darcy stands still for the first thirty seconds of the shaking. Grudgingly, she begins to move, at first only her upper body, until I remind her that shaking needs to go from her feet up through her knees and hips. Dutifully, she shifts into another gear. She's moving faster now, arms windmilling, thrusting her pelvis. When she dances after the pause for mindful breathing, there's a lightness to her step, color in her face. Afterward, her voice is deeper, resonant. "I've been holding on so tight, trying to control everything. This is the first time in two years I've felt my body, really heard my voice, I feel present and clear, I feel me again." And Darcy's not the only one.

A sixty-five-year-old Jesuit priest, a dean at Georgetown with a reputation for solemn disapproval, surprises me by joining a group of anxious medical students during an orientation week workshop. I watch him warily as he Shakes and Dances in his black clothes and clerical collar, wondering whether this will be the end of my participation in welcoming medical students. Afterward, though, he announces with childlike wonder: "I haven't danced like that in fifty years."

As they shake, one hundred Haitian nursing students cry for the first time since ninety of their classmates—sisters and friends—died in the 2010 earthquake. Then they dance and sing, laughing as well as crying, to Bob Marley's "Everything's Gonna Be Alright."

A gangbanger imprisoned in San Quentin finds himself crying as he shakes with sixty other inmates, and smiling sweetly after he's finished.

And not long ago, after Shaking and Dancing in a workshop on South Dakota's Pine Ridge Reservation, a Vietnam vet stands slowly and speaks deliberately of watching Ken Burns's series on the Vietnam

War. "I went through all the emotions—angry, sad, afraid, mostly just pissed off. I realized as we shook that because of the anger I've had since Vietnam, I've lost my connection to myself, to Mother Earth. I've been an empty shell of a man who just continues to exist. Then when Bob Marley came on, for the first time in all these years, I really relaxed. I feel a little more connected to myself and to Mother Earth. I know now I can heal myself."

FOR MANY THOUSANDS, Shaking and Dancing has become a daily practice, prying people loose from the terrible memories that have oppressed them, enlivening their bodies, bringing them, day after day, more and more of the relaxed awareness, the meditative mind that dispels trauma and allows them to savor each moment.

Before a near-fatal car accident, Moira had been a successful, strong executive, fearless in dealing with bureaucratic obstacles, effectively challenging men who tried to derail her career. Since the accident that fractured her skull, she's become uncertain and fearful of cars, conflict, and even social contact.

The first time Moira shook and danced, she was skeptical, inhibited, and anxious, terrified of reinjuring herself. Afterward, she felt "a little more energy, a little looser," and decided to do it regularly. Within a week she discovered that "my daily dose was the only pick-me-up that worked." Whenever she shook and danced in the morning, she moved through her days with confidence. When, on occasion, she didn't, she could feel the fear creeping back in, reminding her to "get my butt up and start shaking."

A high-ranking US government official says that regular Shaking and Dancing allows him to be sensitive to, but not overwhelmed by, decisions that may save or cost hundreds or thousands of lives. Howard, who's done expressive meditations for twenty-five years, likes Shaking and Dancing because it dissolves his stubborn self-doubt

and "helps me take myself less seriously." An older woman has transformed the Parkinson's disease shaking that shamed her into an energizing morning celebration.

Stressed-out medical students who practice regularly tell me that
just before an exam, when they're taut with tension, they sometimes
go to the bathroom, lock themselves in a stall, and shake for a few
minutes. Why? "Better concentration." "Easier exams." "You feel a
little lighter." "You don't worry as much." "Better grades."

After my own losses, morning Shaking and Dancing has let me
cry and then move more easily into my day's activities.

This chapter's message: You can make Shaking and Dancing a
revelatory and celebratory part of your life. Anyone can do it.

I'm hoping that now you'll join me and everyone else who's done
Shaking and Dancing—all the people I've just introduced you to and
those you can see in the videos on our CMBM website, perhaps resistant and self-conscious at first, a little goofy later on, energized and
smiling afterward.

HERE AGAIN ARE the instructions.

If you're making your own playlist, leave a couple of minutes
of silence at the beginning so you can relax into the experience. For
Shaking, you can use the first segment of the "Kundalini" CD listed
in the Notes, or you can substitute similar driving, wordless rhythmic
music. Begin with five or six minutes of this. Then silence for two or
three minutes. Then add three to five minutes of music that makes
you move.

Sometimes I use African music for this third part—by Youssou
N'Dour or Oliver N'Goma—sung in a language I don't understand.
The melody energizes, delights, and moves me. As you've read, I often
use reggae songs, such as Bob Marley's "Three Little Birds (Everything's Gonna Be Alright)" or Jimmy Cliff's "You Can Get It If You

Really Want." The message for me is upbeat, inspiring. The music feels like it comes from and connects me to the earth.

Of course, musical taste is individual. Choose any song whose words and melody are helpful to you. Several years ago, three women who were patients in my private practice independently chose to use the same tune for the third stage: Carly Simon's "You're So Vain." Not surprisingly, all of them were dealing with hurt and betrayal in relationships. The song helped them feel buried, righteous anger, express it with their bodies, and release it.

After a while, or if you're feeling particularly frustrated or stuck, you may want to move for longer periods—ten to fifteen minutes each of Shaking and Dancing.

OKAY, LET'S BEGIN.

Start by planting your feet shoulder-width apart, bending your knees slightly, and relaxing your shoulders. Even if you're alone, close your eyes so you're not distracted. If you have trouble with balance, you can keep them open and look at a wall or out a window. Breathe deeply and slowly for a minute or two. Thank Nature, as Shyam long ago advised me, for this opportunity to move, and to move through and beyond where you may be frozen or stuck.

As the first rhythmic music goes on, begin to shake your whole body. Shake up from your feet, through your knees, hips, and shoulders, through your chest. Shake to your capacity—vigorously, strongly. Let your shoulders relax and bob up and down with the shaking. Let your head go as you shake. Let your jaw, which can carry so much tension, hang open. If sounds come out of your mouth, let them come.

If you feel silly or bored or tired, that's okay. Many of us do. Just keep going. Remember to shake from the feet on up. Do it faster, wholeheartedly. Let the shaking take over your whole body. Keep going.

Now stop. Pay attention to your breathing and your physical sensations. Breathe deeply. Relax. Be aware of your body, of your breath. Stay this way for two or three minutes, breathing, relaxing.

Now comes the music for moving. Let it move you. Don't follow a particular pattern or dance step; just let your body move as it will, freely and spontaneously. If you feel awkward or silly, notice that . . . and keep moving. You're doing this just for you. No one is watching or judging you.

When the music stops, relax for a few moments, standing, sitting, or lying down.

Afterward, you may want to write down what you've experienced.

IT'S GREAT TO do Shaking and Dancing first thing in the morning, or when your energy is low, or any time you feel particularly tense or discouraged. It's also a wonderful way, late in the afternoon or early evening, to shake off the burdens of the day. But don't do it right before you go to bed. It may be too energizing—unless of course you want to loosen your body and clear your mind before you make love.

And be sure to give yourself some time afterward to recall the memories and images, the thoughts, and especially, the emotions you felt and expressed. In the next chapter, you'll start using new tools to explore these emotions and new methods for learning the lessons they teach.

6

All Emotions Are Innocent

NOT LONG AGO, I led a workshop on the West Coast for fifty successful, good-looking people, mostly in their thirties and forties. Almost all women. They dressed with the casual elegance of the cool kids in high school now grown up. We talked about stress and trauma. We did slow, deep Soft Belly breathing, which helped quiet their anxiety and clear their minds. Some were brought to tears they couldn't explain. Then we shook our bodies and danced out self-consciousness and tension. Smiles blossomed on many faces. Toward the end of our time together, we watched the *60 Minutes* segment featuring Azhaar.

A dozen women who spoke afterward told similar stories of suppressed trauma now demanding attention. Enough recalled childhood sexual abuse to make me wonder if even the shocking reports that it happened to 25 percent of American girls were underestimates. Many remembered neglect by parents so preoccupied with their careers or marital combat or a troubled son that they seemed to look past their daughters. These women had made strenuous efforts in school, earning high grades, tennis tournament trophies, soccer scholarships, and outstanding performance awards. They did well later, in college and in graduate school, in law, business, and engineering, and on the ground floor of surging start-ups. Many married. Many had kids. Some divorced.

Just about all of the women said they became aware during the workshop, or earlier, before they had signed up for it, that they'd been traumatized. "I've realized it's not working," said Patricia, a software engineer. "Losing my last job was my wake-up call. Nine a.m. to 7 p.m. six days a week. Stellar evaluations. More money in five years than my parents made in a lifetime. I knew it wasn't my fault. Just another start-up imploding. Still, it was a blow. How could this happen to me?"

She felt now that she was in a hole much deeper than unemployment had dug. "After all, I have a dozen job offers." Some pain of long ago, now reawakened rejection seemed to be filling her whole body, seeping out in the tears she had rarely allowed herself. She had a feeling that she'd done something wrong, or everything wrong, or hadn't done anything right. "I didn't care enough for my parents, so they rejected me; maybe I somehow led on the guy who raped me when I was thirteen. It feels like I've been in denial all these years. You know, 'I'm fine. No problem.' Let me take my parents on vacation, forget about the rapist, make allowances for the boyfriend who says he's just about to leave his wife, and then tough it out when he decides to stay with her. I'm realizing it's me. I was hurt, and now I've become a victim. I don't trust myself to make good choices, and I'm scared to be close to any man."

When the others spoke of buried trauma, they, like Patricia, said that "denial"—they almost all used that word to describe the way they had defended themselves from pain—had kept it from surfacing. And then there were the other symptoms of trauma that suddenly seemed so clear. One woman told me about the hypervigilance that made her fearful of walking a few blocks to work. Others questioned the laser focus and coiled energy they brought back home, as well as to their jobs. They weren't able, they realized, to let down their guard, even with husbands or lovers.

It seemed to me, as I listened to them, that agitated, urgent achievement and self-protective numbing had combined to override, obscure, and bury their emotions—sadness especially, but also anger, fear, and joy. In the safety of our workshop, it was occurring to them, as it was to me, that if they were ever to be truly happy—to become who they were meant to be—they had to first recover those long-buried and denied feelings.

Believing emotions are life shattering, relentless, and unending, as well as shameful, we fear and suppress them. "If I start crying," several of these women and hundreds of other women and men have told me, "I'm afraid I'll never stop." "My anger is so great," I have heard many people say. "I don't know what I'll do. And I certainly can't talk about it. How could anyone else possibly deal with it?"

The lesson I shared with these traumatized achievers—the one that's important for all of us—is that our emotions are not our enemies. They can, in fact, be friends and allies on our healing journey.

MANY OF US, like many people in my workshops, have learned or decided that emotions are dangerous, and likely self-indulgent as well. Our parents have suppressed or denied their own feelings in the name of toughness or proper behavior, or looking good or being strong for others. They—and later, teachers and bosses—may have dismissed our feelings as distractions from academic achievement, impediments to superior work performance, flaws rather than valued facets of our character.

Sometimes we have learned to ignore our own feelings to accommodate those of another family member. Not infrequently, an alcoholic parent expresses feelings loudly and emphatically, and his children grow stoic and supportive, tuned in to nuances of parental emotions but suppressing or denying their own.

Trauma compounds our difficulty in dealing with our emotions. Prolonged fight or flight turns up fear and anger to hard-to-control levels, while disabling the parts of our emotional brain and frontal cortex that could put them in perspective. The defenses we use to deal with overwhelming loss and grief may distance us from and numb our feelings. They prevent us from accepting, experiencing, and ultimately, finding relief from painful feelings; these defenses also keep us, as they did Diana and Patricia, from being joyful and loving.

This can be lethal as well as limiting. A number of parents, including Marlene, a fifty-something rural school bus driver, have told me that children who killed themselves had "kept everything inside" until the suppressed emotions exploded in self-annihilating action. And loved ones, traumatized by suicide, also find themselves avoiding feelings that now seem dangerous.

Marlene confided that before her son, Clay, a soldier back from Afghanistan, shot himself, she was "a free spirit—up for any adventure. Not afraid of jumping out of planes or rock climbing or falling for some guy and getting my heart broken; ready to cry or laugh with friends or at movies." Since he died, "I've become a control freak. Nobody's going to get to me—I'm like that Paul Simon song, 'I Am a Rock.' I can't stand not knowing the ending of a TV series, like *Sons of Anarchy*, which I loved. It makes me too anxious. I've got to read all those 'spoiler alerts.'"

But emotions are not really the problem. They are an utterly natural part of human life. The problem is the way we have learned to deal with them, to protect ourselves from them.

For example, anger need not be lethal or even dangerous. If we simply acknowledge, experience, and express our anger, we'll find that it's like wind. It will shake us, but also blow through us and leave us refreshed, lighter, more aware. On the other hand, if anger is suppressed, compounded with guilt and shame, it can curdle into body-destroying, soul-souring resentment.

The sadness that comes with loss may be overwhelming, but fully admitted, experienced, and shared, it may leave us tender and vulnerable without stagnating to depression; it may even make us kinder to ourselves and more compassionate to others who also deal with loss and death.

Only when we are stuck in our emotions, when we replay them endlessly, like a needle jumping in the scratched groove of a vinyl record, are they likely to warp our minds, damage our bodies, and distort our relationships.

THE EVIDENCE FOR this is becoming increasingly convincing. In the early 1970s, cardiologists Ray Rosenman and Meyer Friedman described the angry, time-obsessed type A personality. Anger, they hypothesized, was a primary cause of the high incidence of heart disease, depression, and death they saw in type As. More recently, Redford Williams and his Duke University colleagues have refined these earlier observations. Blazes of anger that flare and subside are not the primary culprits. It's chronic, powerless frustration and smoldering, life-spoiling resentment that do the greatest damage.

Trauma often provokes anger. This makes sense. Anger is the emotion that accompanies the fight half of fight or flight. It's far more likely to be dominant if the trauma has been caused by violence or injustice. However, problems arise when those fires burn unabated, always ready to flare. Gina, a high school student whose brother was murdered in the 2016 Pulse nightclub shootings, told me that she now "takes everything to heart" and is poised to pounce at the slightest hint of a friend's misunderstanding. When I asked a dozen family members of others killed in the shooting if they felt similarly, most nodded their heads.

Sadness and fear are similar. Sadness, even profound, heartbreaking, life-shattering grief at a death or the loss of a loved one, is normal. So are its disturbing and sometimes dramatic biological and psychological manifestations: parasympathetic "freezing" and emotional numbing, weeping, hopelessness, lethargy, indifference to what once gave us pleasure. The far greater destruction comes when this state persists, when, as Freud observed a century ago, acute and natural mourning stagnates to chronic melancholia—what we would now call major depression.

This condition, which often follows trauma and affects close to twenty million Americans, is characterized by persistent hopelessness and ongoing lack of interest or pleasure in oneself or the world, a sense that nothing will ever change; shame; self-blame; difficulties with sleep, digestion, and sexual activity; agitation and fatigue; and a preoccupation with death and dying. It's depression, not sadness, that makes us so much more vulnerable to heart disease, immune disorders, infections, diabetes, drug abuse, and early death.

Fear, and the fight-or-flight response that it provokes, are natural and necessary. Fear is an important evolutionary development, making us alert to the potentially lethal dangers of predators and high places. Fear continues to ensure that we will take care when we confront situations that may do us harm.

But when the fear that drives fight or flight long outlasts its cause— when we carry the attacking lion with us out of the jungle and onto the grazing land of safe, everyday life—then it becomes self-limiting and self-destructive.

After the car accident that fractured her skull, Moira, the accomplished executive, became terrified to drive or to ride in the front seat of someone else's car—or, indeed, to enter situations whose newness or strangeness somehow evoked the feelings of powerlessness that she had felt in the moments of her accident. Chronic unresolved fear dragged a confident, assertive, sociable woman into tentative, doubt-ridden isolation.

Fear continues to provoke and stoke rage in many veterans who return from combat. Unable to distinguish a passerby's innocent glance from an enemy's surveillance, or an inadvertent bump from a life-threatening attack, they brace for combat or launch a blow.

Making Friends with Your Emotions

Many of you—like Diana, Patricia, Moira, and Darcy the firefighter and Clay the warrior and Marlene his mother—have been trying to eliminate or subdue fear and anger and sadness and have become stuck in them. Perhaps you've made some short-term gains in productivity or conflict-free coexistence. But, like them, you may be paying dearly for it—ever vigilant and overcontrolling, distant and guarded, and fearful even in close relationships.

There are, however, life-giving, trauma-relieving alternatives that can help you safely express, deal with, and learn from your emotions: natural resiliency-building processes that sustain and support your psychological and biological integrity. What follows is a process for befriending your emotions, for making them your partners in healing trauma. I, along with my CMBM team and those we've trained, have taught it to hundreds of thousands of children and adults. At first this process of emotional friending can be challenging. But it's straightforward and over time becomes easy to use.

There are three parts to this process: *Relaxation* with our emotions; *Awareness* of them; and *Emotional Expression*. At different times, one of the three may be more accessible to you, a better starting point. Each facilitates the next, in a virtuous cycle that can become an ongoing, sustaining part of your life.

Here's what it looks like.

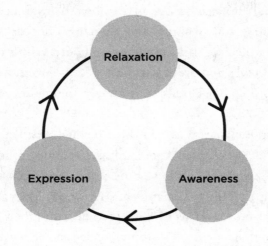

The techniques we've already learned—Soft Belly, Drawings, Shaking and Dancing—will go a long way to making each of these strategies and the healing they bring a reality. And of course, as we discuss more techniques, you'll likely want to include them.

Relaxation. Meditation is fundamental here. Soft Belly quiets the stress response, making it easier for us to accept and put our emotions in perspective. It enhances activity in the hippocampus and frontal cortex, which allow us to gain perspective on our emotions, to integrate them more easily with our memories and our ongoing experience.

When our brain function is restored by Soft Belly, we are able, little by little, to quiet the flood of painful memories and fearful anticipation. Now our feelings inform but don't overwhelm our thoughts. We react less and respond more.

Shaking and Dancing uses intense, disruptive effort and free movement to help us shed stress and tension and bring up and release emotion. This expressive meditation uses activity to bring us to a place of relaxation, balance, and acceptance that is similar to the one we find when we do Soft Belly. Both meditations show us that emotions need only be temporarily overwhelming. They really do come and go.

Awareness. Relaxation opens the door to Awareness. Both Soft Belly breathing and Shaking and Dancing offer us safe vantage points from which we can experience and observe our emotions. As we breathe slowly and deeply, we can watch our emotions rise like bubbles or pass by like clouds. As we shake them loose, we feel them storm up and out.

When emotions arise as I do these meditations, I'm reminded of the episode in *The Odyssey* where Odysseus is able to listen safely to the beautiful but death-dealing Sirens' song. Ordinarily, their melody lures listening sailors to a watery death. However, Athena, the goddess of wisdom, wants Odysseus to be their student, not their sacrifice. She counsels him to have his crew stop up their ears. However, Odysseus, beloved by and in love with life-illuminating wisdom, is told to safely listen. "Have your crew," Athena instructs, "tie you to the ship's mast so, your hearing unimpaired, you can listen."

Concentrative and expressive meditations and the mindfulness they promote are our mast and the ropes that tie us to it. They make it possible for us to safely hear, accept, and learn from the Sirens' song of threatening emotions.

Imaginative exercises can also help us become aware of long-buried emotions without being overwhelmed by them. In the second Drawing you did in the chapter on Hope, you may have discovered previously unspoken, maybe even unacknowledged, fear, grief, or anger. Perhaps you felt satisfaction as you encountered what you had previously avoided, or a small growth in understanding and maturity as you claimed an abandoned and feared part of yourself. Later we'll use a variety of other techniques to mobilize our imagination to help us accept our emotions. For now, remember that you can use Drawings to reveal emotions and find ways to move through and beyond them.

Expression. Freud famously wrote about the importance of bringing painful emotions and the experiences that provoked them into our consciousness and, through words, up and out into the world. He said this process was cathartic (the word is Greek and means "cleansing") and that it's crucial to healing the damage that dammed-up—consciously suppressed and unconsciously repressed—emotions had caused: phobic avoidance, depression, sexual dysfunction, and psychologically caused physical disabilities, like pain and paralysis.

Freud's insight struck a revolutionary note in modern Western psychiatry. This insight is also a legacy of our aboriginal heritage and of Rituals everywhere on the planet. It informed healing ceremonies in Greek temples and the collective experience of ancient Athenian theatergoers.

And now, in the twenty-first century, we can appreciate the modern science that explains the healing power of emotional expression, as well as the ancient wisdom that urges us to it.

As we express what's been inside, we're quieting the agitated amygdala and bringing online parts of our brain that have been damaged by trauma: the dorsolateral prefrontal cortex, which gives meaning and context to our experience; the hippocampus, which holds and shapes memory; and the medial prefrontal cortex, which facilitates self-awareness, thoughtful judgment, and compassion. Putting into words what we've seen and felt and held inside helps reanimate Broca's area, the part of the left temporal lobe responsible for verbal expression; it nourishes healing linkages between Broca's area and the visual cortex, the source of confused, terrifying, and previously inexpressible images.

When we welcome and express our emotions, we are, like ancient Greeks in the amphitheater, inviting these painful feelings to possess us for a while and then leave us. As we do, we free up the compassion and love, the joy and creativity that have been buried with our painful emotions.

The Gnostic Gospel of Thomas, a two-thousand-year-old scroll found seventy years ago by a peasant in a cave in upper Egypt, describes this healing process in an urgent, compelling way: "Jesus said 'if you bring forth what is within you, what you bring forth will save you. If you do not bring forth what is within you, what you do not bring forth will destroy you.'"

Here again is the circle—a simple visual reminder.

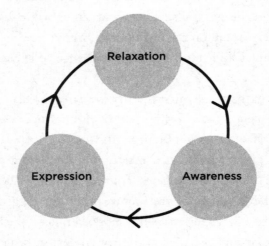

Remember the circle. Perhaps draw it, and put it on your refrigerator or next to your computer. Welcome your emotions. Adopt this healing process as a reliable practice. Experiment with it. Enjoy it.

Putting Feelings into Words

Words, Drawings, and movement are all effective ways to bring out and learn from our emotions, heal from their pain, and make them our friends. In the next chapter, we'll focus on sharing our story with others. Later on, we'll work once again with Drawings and with ways to express our emotions physically. We'll also use Guided Imagery to inform and instruct us. Right now, I want to teach you two techniques for using the written word to express, relax with, and become aware of your emotions.

Keeping a Journal. Simply recording what you're feeling is a safe and private way to begin. And it's remarkably effective.

The instructions and the practice are simple: Buy a Journal—an elegant, leather-bound volume or a simple spiral notebook, according to your taste and budget. Put your name on it. Begin each entry by noting the date. Write down what you feel. Don't censor. Do it every day, even if it's only a shout of protest: "I can't stand this !@#$%^ journal."

As you write, you'll discover painful and pleasurable experiences and the emotions that go with them. Some will tumble freshly on the page. Others, forgotten, repressed, or previously regarded as weird, shameful, or self-pitying, may emerge only with effort. As you write them down, you'll have a sense of relief and release. What was jammed up inside you is now out there on the page.

University of Texas psychologist James Pennebaker and his colleagues have done many studies on the psychological and physical benefits of writing about emotionally charged experiences. Just three or four days of twenty-minute writing sessions, or even three twenty-minute sessions in one day, have repeatedly and reliably lowered stress hormones in people who've been traumatized and enhanced mood in those who are depressed. And expressing emotions in writing has produced other measurable benefits: improved breathing in asthmatics and decreased pain and greater mobility for people with arthritis.

When we've been traumatized, many of us are terrified of being overwhelmed by the feelings that trauma has aroused. Often we're ashamed to share them and the events that caused them with others. Writing down events and feelings gives us a sense of safety with and control over our feelings, even as we experience the healing benefits of emotional self-expression. Just about everyone I work with keeps a Journal and, perhaps after initial resistance, finds it enormously helpful.

Keeping a Journal will give form and meaning to your feelings. It will allow you to create something out of the void that may threaten you when you've been traumatized. And writing gives you proof that you can actually *do* something. Many traumatized people begin their writing exhausted and desperate, and ten minutes or a half hour later feel energized.

I've found, even when I've been most desolate, that my Journal is a faithful, reliable companion. It focuses my attention, cuts short rumination, and produces surprising insights and answers. Its physical presence is comforting, even defining: This is my Journal. I'm carrying it. I'm the one writing in it. I write, therefore I am. It's also, as I mentioned earlier, the place where I record the steps I'm taking to help myself.

Dialogue with an emotion. You can also have an active verbal engagement with your emotions, wrangle as well as express them. Chase each one down, as if you were a cowboy or cowgirl and it was an unruly calf. Lasso it. Jump off your horse. Tie it up. Look at it closely. And ask, insistently, what its message is. If you do, you'll discover that emotions, like skittish calves, can be overtaken. When confronted, they have much to teach you.

We're going to use a written Dialogue to do the job. It's an all-purpose method of inquiring that you can bring to any symptom, problem, or issue (SPI) you'd like to learn more about. It could be a physical symptom (pain, limitation of motion, an upset stomach) or a problem, such as a craving for food or alcohol or obsessive thoughts. Or it could be an issue in your life—difficulty in a relationship, memories of past abuse, inability to get started on a project. Or it could be what we'll focus on here: emotions, like fear, anger, loneliness, or frustration.

All you need to do is write down a letter to denote the SPI, in this case your emotion, and one that stands for you. Then, once you've identified your emotion, imagine it's sitting across from you in a chair and you're about to have a Dialogue with it.

If I'm having a Dialogue with my sadness, I'm "J" and my sadness is "S." I close my eyes and take a few deep breaths. When I open my eyes, I begin writing and let the dialogue unfold. I start by asking a question of my emotion. I let it respond. Then I ask again. I keep going, writing down the questions I ask and the answers I receive.

As you do this Dialogue, trust your intuition and imagination. Write as fast as you can. Don't censor yourself. Again, let the Zen motto "First thought, best thought" guide you. If the answer isn't satisfying, push for clarification. Insist. You have a right to know why you're feeling what you are and what you can do about it.

Welcome whatever your Dialogue reveals, even if it seems harsh. Perhaps because I'm from New York, my emotions are often confrontational. The voice responding may be insistent, sarcastic, reminding me of waiters from Lower East Side delicatessens insisting I should order dishes I'd never considered. This is my unconscious using muscles and guile to get through to me.

I've learned not to be offended, to enjoy the perspectives that this bracing humor gives and the liberation that comes with laughter.

Continue your Dialogue for about ten minutes or until you come to a natural stopping place.

Here's an example. Jake, a successful, handsome, happily married, but fearful thirty-five-year-old magazine art director, had a Dialogue with his feeling of insufficiency, which he explained is "really just my abusive father talking to me." He put down "J" for Jake and "I" for insufficiency. At first, he found himself engaged in a painful Dialogue with his father, the man who originally caused him to feel insufficiency, rather than the feeling itself. Still, the results were satisfying.

J: Why am I insufficient?

I: Because you're a pain in the ass (this is my father speaking) and annoying and not what I want you to be.

And it went on like this. His father kept repeating the angry, demeaning, hateful things he had long ago said to Jake: "You can run in the lake and drown." "You're nothing. You shouldn't have even been born." "You're a terrible person." And Jake, accusing his father of cruelty and neglect, presented the case for his own skill, competence, and kindness.

This Dialogue gave Jake some relief. Standing up to his imagined father and arguing were liberating. "These are all the things that are just sitting in my body. I've never said things like this to him. It felt amazing, like if you have a long day and you go for a run and it's super-hot out, or it's pouring rain. And you come back and just say 'Ahhh.'" But Jake knew there was more and asked for my help.

"This time," I told him, have the Dialogue with your actual feeling, with the insufficiency, not the man who made you feel it.

The results were even more helpful to Jake.

Here again "J" is for Jake and "I" for Insufficiency.

J: Who are you?

I: A part of you.

J: Why are you here?

I: I want you to suffer and fail.

J: That's terrible. What good are you?

I: Without me you would've been dead.

J: What? How could that be?

I: I kept you anxious, eager to please, a good boy. Otherwise your father might have beat you to a pulp.

J: But that was a long time ago. I'm a grown-up now—out of the house.

I: So?

J: So, why do I need insufficiency now?

I: You use me as an excuse to hide out. You can take the easy way, so you won't fail.

J: But I'm tired of that. I'm tired of being afraid.

I: So?

J: So what do I do to get free?

I: Stop worrying about me. You know when you run or meditate I don't bother you.

J: Yeah.

I: So run and meditate more. Just watch me out of the corner of your eye. You're a big guy. I'm really kind of small. Don't take me so seriously.

J: You mean maybe even laugh at myself when I feel insufficient?

I: Now there's an idea.

In fact, Jake is laughing as he tells me this.

TIME AFTER TIME, your Dialogue will tell you, as it did Jake, what you need to know about why an emotion persists so painfully, what it gives you, as well as what it takes away. And if you insist, your problematic emotion will tell you, as it did Jake, what steps to take to deal with it.

As you write about your suppressed emotions, you are quite literally putting your damaged brain back together, putting your trauma in the larger context of your life. You will soon realize an important truth: "This happened to me, it's not happening now. I'm more than this painful emotion, this suffering past. These emotions and the trauma that provoked them are parts of my life from which I can learn. They're not all of it."

Over time, you'll grow more comfortable bringing your emotions up and out and onto the page. You'll likely find, as Jake did, that one insight leads to another. And the more you express yourself on the page, the more likely it is you'll want to tell others what you're feeling and discovering. We'll talk about this in the next chapter—about the extraordinary benefits of sharing yourself with others and the ways to make it easier for you.

7
Only Connect

THERE ARE TIMES when just about all of us need to reach out, to connect with other people. It's an essential part of what makes us human. It's built into our biology.

As infants we would not have survived without a nurturing, sustaining connection with our mother or other caregivers. In fact, researchers, beginning with René Spitz in the 1930s, have observed that without this kind of warm, human contact, even babies who are adequately fed, clothed, and housed may waste away and die—"hospitalism," Spitz called it. We can still see these dying children in some orphanages or in homes where neglect drains kids of life.

When we're traumatized, the need for connection is reawakened, heightened. Remember that our first biologically programmed response to trauma is to reach out and scan the world around us for support and comfort. When that urge is temporarily overwhelmed by the agitation of fight or flight, or the numbing and withdrawal of freezing, it doesn't go away. It becomes even more compelling.

The medical literature tells us that social support—connections with other people—helps prevent illness; when we are ill, it makes recovery more likely, easier, and faster. Highly sociable children are significantly more able to withstand stressful early lives. Lack of these social connections has been shown to be as great a risk factor for early death as smoking and twice as likely to kill us as obesity.

When we are traumatized, social support is even more critical. Trauma numbs and isolates as well as disables us. Even when we know intellectually that other people have been neglected or abused, or had their careers short-circuited, or lost spouses or children, it feels to us as if we're the only ones. This sense of isolation is a direct consequence of trauma's self-protective biology: when we're fighting for our life, it doesn't serve us to trust; when we're overwhelmed by inescapable threats, we're programmed to withdraw. Even in the aftermath of a war that has killed thousands, I've seen survivors feeling alone with their loss and grief, constrained and thwarted by their biology.

The sense of isolation and powerlessness can be significantly compounded by others who ignore, dismiss, or minimize the reality of our trauma. People who've been raped or sexually abused or harassed often confront disbelief or are accused of causing what they could not prevent; children who've been abused by one parent are too often dismissed or ignored by the other parent, who is unwilling to confront the reality or take action to change it. Soldiers overwhelmed by death and destruction they have caused or witnessed are often advised to "suck it up." Many people have told me that as painful as their trauma was, it was less demeaning, less destructive, far less soul slaying than the reaction of the people and institutions with whom they tried to share it.

WHEN WE ARE finally able to connect with others who do believe and have compassion for us, everything begins to change. As we share ourselves and our stories with them, we find and feel safety. This can happen with a therapist or in an organized group—we'll talk about it in the chapter "The Healing Circle," which describes Mind-Body Skills Groups, and in the Appendix, "Finding Other Help," where I'll provide guidelines for choosing a therapist and snapshots of other therapeutic approaches. Here, however, I want to emphasize the importance of friends and families, clergy and colleagues, as embracing refuges. Many are or have been just as troubled and hurt, as confused and vulnerable, as we are. They know what we're going through, and can often help sustain and support us on our journey.

As we share with others, we assert ourselves as people worthy of being heard—men, women, and children whose sorrows and sufferings can be understood, people to whom attention should be paid. In sharing ourselves and our story, we're also overcoming the fear of judgment, the pride and the shame that have fed the isolation bred by trauma.

These caring, trustworthy people let us know that it is right for us to care for ourselves, that we deserve it. We begin to feel that if these others can appreciate us with all our clumsy contradictions, our unlovely pain and shame, then perhaps we can appreciate ourselves. As we look into the mirror of their eyes, we see ourselves more kindly, more generously. Self-protectiveness falls away. Sharing our burdens, we lighten the load.

I FIRST BEGAN to understand this in my twenties, in the 1960s, when old fears and hurts were making it just as painful to stay with as to leave my girlfriend, when I was still looking for a way to wholeheartedly embrace medical school.

I spoke, hesitantly at first, with new friends about what was happening to me. I felt shy, ashamed that I wasn't as cool as I hoped they believed me to be, that I didn't have it all together. But it seemed important that they understand. Though I couldn't have put it into words at the time, I felt that if they could accept me, I could better accept myself.

My friends were surprised that I'd been feeling so lost, but they treated me with kindness and in turn opened up about themselves. My vulnerability became an invitation for them to be more open, closer to me.

None of them—not Marshall, the political scientist with his world-class mind, nor Judy, the wry, much-published writer, nor Barry the historian, with his graceful body—was unfamiliar with what I was discovering. Neither brilliance nor wit nor beauty had exempted them from times of terror as children. Even now, underneath their impressive exteriors, they could be as uncertain, as haunted by the past, as I was. I felt bad for them, but what a relief! I was realizing that everyone suffers. All of us had been traumatized. Sharing what had happened to us brought us closer, and our closeness felt like good, soothing medicine.

And then there was William Alfred, who had been my college English professor. When I was an undergrad at Harvard, he was my beloved, inspiring tutor and mentor. Now he was my dear friend. Bill was at home for me whenever, in my medical school confusion, I needed him, and then for thirty-five more years, until his death.

Soft voiced, stooped, oldish, and baldish even in his late thirties, Bill was unfailingly kind and hospitable—to Nobel laureates, Cambridge's homeless, and stressed-out students like me who appeared, clamorous and often unannounced, at the warm, dark, wooden front door of his Athens Street home.

Bill welcomed me with stories of old-time Brooklyn priests and politicians, with the latest news about his feckless, funny, bricklayer father, and memories of his saintly Irish mother and all their formidable female forebears. There was always time for me to tell my own sad and happy stories and feel Bill's kind curiosity, his unwavering acceptance. And there were glasses of bourbon, and often lamb chops, which Bill charred with garlic in a cast-iron skillet on an ancient stove. Sometimes we talked till morning, when Bill and I went to the Mass he never missed. And occasionally, when I needed it, there was a bed for a night or three.

I've had other friends as well who, over the years, have helped me through loss and death, men and women to talk to about anything. George and Maha sat with me as my silent, paralyzed mother was dying, and held me close when I cried for her. At her memorial service they told funny stories. Friends like these are lifelong trauma-healing treasures.

THE FIRST TIME I see patients, I ask them what and who helps them feel better. Sometimes the answers are immediate and obvious. Then I encourage them to do what's already working. "The Soft Belly breathing you taught me," said Teresa, a forty-year-old lawyer who was grieving the loss of the man she believed to be her last hope for fathering her children. "It quiets me when I'm freaked out. And yoga. And of course," this with a big smile, "my friend Barbara. I look forward to her calls and her visits. I can look like hell or repeat myself and say self-pitying things. But she's there for me. She loves me and she doesn't take me too seriously. We're friends." Sometimes when no one comes to mind, I suggest a simple experiment with Guided Imagery to facilitate the process. You can do it now if you'd like. Here it is:

Set aside a few minutes for slow, deep Soft Belly breathing. As your thoughts start to slow and your body begins to relax, ask a couple of questions: "Who do I want to visit, or see, or call, or write to? Who will really be there for me?"

At first, Dorothy, who had been gearing up to leave the self-absorbed, womanizing US Senator who was her husband, drew a blank. She was sixtysomething and had colon cancer, and she was terrified of being on her own without the security, status, and power conferred by the senator's position. There was no one in gossip-saturated Washington whom she could trust to understand—and also keep her secrets.

That was Dorothy's anxious, conscious mind speaking. But after a few minutes of breathing, Dorothy relaxed, and her intuition offered her an answer. When she opened her eyes, there were tears in them. Later in the day, she called the old woman who had appeared in her mental image. Aunt Grace listened for a few minutes and let out the closest thing to a war whoop Dorothy had ever heard. "Child," Aunt Grace fairly shouted, "that man's been death on you from the beginning."

Though she'd hardly spoken to her in years, Dorothy discovered that she trusted this woman as she did no one else in her busy, all-too-public life. Too old to be impressed by anybody and too ornery to be intimidated by conventional wisdom, Grace was remarkably clear-sighted about her niece and, it turned out, very gratified to be useful to her. For years afterward, they spoke almost daily.

SOMETIMES THE PEOPLE we need just show up, and our job is to recognize them when they appear. When a man she knew from work invited her to dinner, Moira, the executive who fractured her skull in a car accident, stopped just short of saying no. Since the accident, she'd only left her apartment for work. Feeling damaged and inadequate, fearful, and ashamed of her fear, she'd routinely turned down social engagements. This time, she heard my voice encouraging her and trusted the intuition that Soft Belly breathing and Shaking and Dancing were nurturing. Her evening out—dinner and, afterward, goofing at miniature golf with a group of gay guys—was a first step away from fearful, frozen immobility.

As a general rule, I suggest that you, like Moira, assume that just about everyone who appears in your life may have something to offer you. This perspective, which I feel is valuable under any circumstances, is particularly useful when you've been traumatized or feel depressed, when you're devaluing yourself, your experience, and life itself.

If you're willing, at least as an experiment, to regard those who appear in your life as potential sources of support and instruction, you're automatically reinvesting in and valuing other people and, with them, the world and life itself. Human beings are no longer simply reminders of your inadequacy or alienation or unhappiness, or of terrible things that others have done to you; they are a part of your community and also your teachers. These encounters can yield lessons. Even at your most fearful, discouraged, and gloomy, you're still a student, prepared to learn and maybe grow and change.

It may seem strange at first, even naive. Still, I think you'll find that if you adopt this point of view, many of the people who come into your life will provide support and guidance, helping you move through and beyond trauma.

There's an old story that may encourage you to welcome those who appear. It's told about faith, but it's also very much about recognizing help and being ready to accept whoever may bring it.

A man in the midst of a flood is clinging to the top of his floating house. The man prays to God for help. Shortly afterward, a raft appears. The pilot asks the man if he wants to climb aboard. "No," he says, "God will take care of me." The man's home sinks a little more. Along comes a boat. The captain calls out: "Come aboard." "No, thank you," says the man, "I'm waiting for God to save me." The captain shakes his head and continues on his way. Now the man's whole house is going under, and he is barely clinging to his roof. He prays harder. A helicopter appears. Once again the man refuses the ride.

Drowned and in heaven, the man proudly tells God that he faithfully awaited his rescue. God greets him with a thundering rebuke: "Idiot, who do you think sent the raft, the boat, and the helicopter?"

THE MORE TRAUMATIZED we've been, the more anxious and fearful, numb and withdrawn, the more important it is for someone else to see us, to hear and appreciate what we have to say, to know us as we are, to love us.

This is how it was for my friend Maya, who felt her childhood was lived in a huge and ever-widening "gap"—a barren space empty of caring.

Maya's mother was a prostitute, preoccupied with alcohol and the men who paid her. Maya never knew her father. When she was three, she watched her mother's brother shoot himself.

From then on, Maya knew, with the uncanny instinct that children have, that her very survival depended on finding people to "fill the gap." And often, when she most needed them, people did appear to fill it, people whom Maya thought of as "angels who wore skin."

At five it was her upstairs neighbor. "I was home alone on a Saturday morning on my front step. As usual, kids were teasing me. When I tried to get away, I broke the glass on the apartment door and cut my hand to pieces. I knew my mother would beat the crap out of me.

"And then this neighbor appeared and cleaned up the floor and repaired the window, and bandaged my hand, and took me upstairs for lunch. She lived in our building for only five months, but I still have the little ring she gave me.

"When she moved away, I sobbed in her arms, and she held me and said words that let me keep breathing: 'You're a good girl, and I would take you with me if I could, but I can't. You need to learn how to take care of yourself. Life is everything. And,' she added, 'you can also trust other people.'"

A few years later, Maya's innocent hopefulness called out great kindness in another woman, a clerk in a store.

"I used to watch the TV show *Queen for a Day*. I'd see the women on that show and imagine that they were my mother. One day—I must have had such a need—I sang the coronation song from the show to a store clerk and asked her to come with me to a coronation in the backyard. She did. For the next year, she came almost daily"—like one of those kind queens—to be with Maya, to help her with her homework.

Maya's troubles didn't disappear. She continued to feel shame for her mother, for her own victimization by "uncles" who paid her mother for her little girl's as well as her own sexual services. Maya "punished" herself by cutting her wrists and taking overdoses of pills. But somehow she always managed to find someone to help her across the bridge back to life—to fill the gap. And over the years, practicing the techniques of Transformation that you're learning and continuing to reach out have helped her continue to heal.

Remember Maya's lessons: there are people who comfort and care. They may well be there for you, too.

THERE'S AN ADDED, unexpected bonus to reaching out to others. You'll discover, if you pay attention, a natural wonder, a symmetry between your need for help and their desire to offer it. Your asking for help often turns out to be a gift to those who are giving you help.

Barbara was happy to be Teresa's friend; giving to Dorothy gave meaning to Grace's life; and Bill seemed to enjoy having me around. And it was perhaps as important for the long-ago neighbor to love Maya as it was for the little girl to feel that love. When Maya visited her in the last days of her life, my now grown friend told her how much her kindness had meant. This skin-wearing angel smiled and spoke: "Now that I know that I've helped one person, I can die in peace."

TERESA, DOROTHY, AND MAYA continue to use Guided Imagery to help them decide who to reach out to and how and when to do it, who to trust and who to avoid. So do I. In the next chapter we'll explore some other ways to use this ancient, effective technique to mobilize our body's intuition and understanding as well as our healing responses.

8
Accessing Inner Guidance

IMAGERY IS THE language of our unconscious mind. It can be auditory, kinesthetic (feeling), gustatory (taste), and olfactory (smell), as well as visual. Images are powerful. When we create mental images, the areas of our brain associated with that sense light up with activity, just as if we were actually seeing, feeling, tasting, hearing, or smelling something in the outside world. Imagery also reawakens right-brain activity that trauma has turned down or off.

The brain centers where images are formed are intimately connected with the limbic or emotional brain, which includes the amygdala and hippocampus, and with the hypothalamus, which controls the autonomic nervous system and its fight-or-flight and freeze responses, as well as the endocrine and immune systems. These intimate, biological connections—often only a few synapses need to be crossed—make possible imagery's remarkable power to improve physical and mental functioning, reverse the damage done by trauma, and help us chart a path to ongoing healing and happiness.

Forty years of published research has demonstrated that we can consciously use these connections to create mental images: people of all ages have used imagery to decrease anxiety and pain, enhance digestive functioning and immunity, promote mental concentration, and alleviate depression.

Imagery, we now know, reduces the biological and psychological symptoms of post-traumatic stress. It decreases the intensity of traumatic events and memories and puts them in perspective. As you mobilize your intuition and imagination, the images you create can provide guidance in transforming trauma from disaster to opportunity.

In this chapter you'll learn to harness the trauma-healing power of imagery.

Imagining a Lemon

This first experiment with imagery will give you a direct experience of how images can affect your autonomic nervous system and, through it, your physiological functioning. I like to begin with this one because it gets you comfortable with using imagery and gives you an immediate felt sense of imagery's power.

If you're going to use imagery most effectively and most creatively, you need to be relaxed. So, once again, we'll start with Soft Belly breathing. Here's a brief review of the instructions:

Sit comfortably, breathing in through your nose and out through your mouth, allowing your belly to be soft, relaxing into the chair in which you're sitting. Feel yourself connected to the chair. Feel your back against the back of the chair, and your seat on the seat of the chair, and your feet on the floor. Let your breathing deepen. Let thoughts come and go. Gently bring your mind back from them—to "Soft . . . Belly." Continue for two or three minutes. Keep on breathing, slowly and deeply.

Now imagine that you're in a kitchen. It could be your own kitchen, or someone else's, or one you've just created. Look around. What does it look like? What does it feel like to be there?

Now imagine yourself standing in front of a cutting board. On that cutting board is a nice, big, ripe lemon. Pick up the lemon. Feel what it feels like, the weight, and the texture of the skin. Is it firm or soft? Look at it. Perhaps you'll want to rub it on your own skin. What does it feel like? How does it smell? Inhale the fragrance.

Put the lemon back down on the cutting board. Now take a sharp knife and cut the lemon in half. Let the two halves fall apart. Look at the exposed surfaces. Perhaps there are drops of juice glistening. Notice the flesh of the lemon, the white lining of the skin, the pits. Now, take one half of the lemon and cut it in half. You'll have two wedges now, two quarters of that lemon.

Imagine now that you're picking up one of those wedges. Again, smell it, feel what it feels like in your hand.

Slowly bring it to your mouth. Put it in your mouth. Now bite down on the lemon, feeling your teeth breaking the flesh of the lemon, feeling the juice go into your mouth.

Notice now what's happening in your mouth, what's happening to your face. What are you feeling in your body?

Put the lemon back down. Breathe deeply for a few moments. Open your eyes and write down your experience.

What was the smell like, the color and texture? How did it feel to hold the lemon in your hand? Was it smooth or rough?

What was it like to rub it against your skin? To smell it? And then, when you bit into it, what was that like? Could you taste it? Did you feel your lips, maybe your whole face puckering up? Perhaps you were salivating more, maybe even shivering a little. Write down whatever experiences you had.

Salivation and puckering are functions that are mediated by the autonomic nervous system. By creating this image, you've directly accessed and affected your autonomic nervous system. And you've likely had many of the same responses that you would have if you'd actually bitten into a lemon.

I remember doing this exercise with a group of US military veterans, mostly tough, grizzled older guys. I'd been talking to them about post-traumatic stress and how mind-body approaches and mobilizing the imagination could reduce it. They were leaning back in their chairs, arms folded across their chests, as if to say, "Yeah. Yeah, sure."

Imagining the lemon and biting into it turned everything around. "Goddamn," one of them said, in what I could only consider a vote of great confidence, "this shit really works."

Autogenics and Biofeedback Therapy

Many years ago, Mary Lee Esty taught me a simple way to become aware of the biological consequences of stress and trauma, and to use imagery to reverse them. It's called Autogenics and Biofeedback Therapy (ABT).

The autogenic (the word means "self-generating") phrases you use create images that are designed to give gentle but firm instructions to your autonomic nervous system. They "tell" your vagus nerve to do its job of quieting and calming. Biofeedback is the way you measure the changes you've produced. By recording the temperature in your finger—it rises as you balance out the fight-or-flight response—you get feedback about whether the phrases you're saying are producing the relaxation for which you're hoping.

I was skeptical at first. It seemed an awkward, modern version of meditation. But I did it, and did it again, and marveled at how easy it was to repeat these six Autogenic phrases and change my physiology— increasing vagal tone and quieting sympathetic overactivity, raising the temperature of my finger, and relaxing.

Ever since, ABT has been an integral part of our trainings and groups and my own practice. Initially some people, like me, find the process a bit mechanical. Many others, including hard-headed types like engineers, doctors, lawyers, and military, take to it right away. You can see the results, and it's simple. Kids love it, too.

I'm going to tell you a little bit about Autogenics and Biofeedback. Then I'm going to lead you in a session.

Autogenic training was developed in the 1920s by a German neurologist and psychiatrist, Johannes Schultz. Apparently, Schultz came up with the idea after reading about the ability of Indian yogis to control their physiology, dramatically slowing heart rate, lowering blood pressure, and raising their body temperature. Schultz, who must also have been tuned in to Cannon's work on the fight-or-flight response, reasoned that these changes were the result of increased vagal tone. He came to believe that in a relaxed state, anyone could instruct her nervous system to produce the required relaxation.

Together with Wolfgang Luthe, a psychologist who popularized Autogenics, he developed and refined a series of phrases that evoked the changes that came with parasympathetic stimulation—for example, saying "my arms are warm and heavy" to relax blood vessels.

Schultz originally used six phrases, which I've modified slightly, but subsequently developed many more, to encourage biological change and promote therapeutic effects. In the more than eighty years since, thousands of papers have been published, most in European journals, on the usefulness of Autogenics in lowering blood pressure, decreasing pain, enhancing immune function, decreasing anxiety, improving mood, and most dramatically, treating migraine headaches and the cold hands and feet that result from the vascular constriction of Raynaud's disease.

Biofeedback—the use of signals registered by our senses to affect physiological functions that were believed to be beyond our conscious control—was developed in the 1950s and 1960s by several different groups in the United States. In his laboratory at Yale, Dr. Neal Miller and his colleagues did experiments with animals which showed that with feedback of information about their biological functioning, dogs and rats could "learn" to control heart rate, blood pressure, and salivation, and reverse urinary incontinence. Later, he showed that humans could do the same.

At about the same time, Elmer Green, a physicist, and his wife, Alyce, a psychologist, traveled to India to visit with yogis and observe firsthand their capacity to control physiological functioning. The Greens were deeply impressed by the changes that the yogis made, lowering their heart rate from sixty to fifteen beats a minute and respiration from twelve to three breaths a minute, increasing and decreasing their body temperature at will.

The Greens continued their study of yogis at the Menninger Clinic in Topeka, Kansas, but quickly became interested in whether ordinary people could, with the aid of instrumentation, become aware of their physiological functioning and achieve similar results. The Greens decided to use feedback about temperature—Thermal Biofeedback—to achieve the goal.

This inventive and intuitive couple decided to combine the Autogenic phrases they'd read about with the Biofeedback procedures they were developing. ABT was born. The elegantly simple idea was to observe the temperature in your hand, do some deep breathing to relax, say the phrases to yourself, open your eyes, and check out the potential change in temperature.

The Greens' daughter, Pat Norris, and her husband, Steve Fahrion, both psychologists, spent many years studying the therapeutic effectiveness of the procedure. Before she taught it to me, Mary Lee had learned it from Pat and Steve. In the years since, I've recognized Elmer and Alyce and Pat and Steve as visionary colleagues and friends on the journey of self-care.

Autogenics and ABT. In order to do ABT, you're going to have to order the temperature-sensitive Biodots (called "Stress Squares") as directed in the note at the end of *The Transformation*.

While you're waiting for your Biodots to arrive, you can begin by practicing the Autogenic phrases I've provided on the next page.

Even without Biofeedback, these phrases are an excellent way to quiet yourself in the middle of a stressful situation. And they can be quite effective in repairing troubled sleep, allowing you to nod off while you're repeating the phrases.

And every time you do Autogenics, you're rediscovering and reexperiencing your power to use images to control your autonomic nervous system and reduce your stress.

Once your Biodots have arrived, you can do the complete ABT practice.

Biodots are like the mood rings some of you may remember from your youth. They change color with temperature. During a challenging precalculus class, when you were in sympathetic overdrive and your hands were cold, your ring might have been yellow, brown, or even black. But when you saw the guy you had a crush on, your hands got warm, and the color changed to green or blue or deep purple. It's the same principle here.

I want you to take one of the Biodots and put it on the muscle between the thumb and forefinger on the back of your nondominant hand. This place is convenient, easily visible, and secure. Now take a look at the color of your Biodot. Remember what it is.

Begin breathing slowly and deeply, with your belly soft and relaxed. After a couple of minutes, you can start to repeat the Autogenic phrases. You'll say each one to yourself, very slowly. You'll repeat each of these six phrases six times. Afterward, take another thirty seconds or so to breathe deeply. Then notice how you feel, open your eyes, and look at the color of the dot.

The idea here is to relax. And of course, you want to change the color of the dot to show yourself that you *have* relaxed. It is, I know, a contradiction—between relaxing and trying to make a change. I suggest that you have the intention to make the change, and then let it go. Bring to this exercise the quiet, unforced attention of meditation—the "effortless effort" described by the Chinese Taoist sages. And remember, this is an experiment. You're hoping that you'll be able to relax—and whatever happens is of interest.

Here are the six phrases.

My arms are warm and heavy (*pause*) . . . . I am at peace
My legs are warm and heavy (*pause*) . . . . I am at peace
My heartbeat is calm and regular (*pause*) . . . . I am at peace
My abdomen radiates warmth (*pause*) . . . . I am at peace
My forehead is cool (*pause*) . . . . I am at peace
My breathing is calm and regular (*pause*) . . . . I am at peace

After you've repeated each phrase six times, notice how you feel. Then open your eyes and look once again at the Biodot.

Many of you will notice that you feel more relaxed and there has been some change in color—from brown or yellow perhaps to green. Others of you may notice much more dramatic changes: moments of deep peace and a purple color that is equally deep. Some of you, especially if you're trying too hard or the worries you brought with you are unwilling to loosen their hold on you, may feel tense, and your temperature may go down. Or you may feel much more relaxed, but your temperature doesn't change or goes down. All these responses are okay.

The idea is to notice what happened and write it down. The entire exercise should take about fifteen or twenty minutes. The more you practice, the more likely you'll be to produce significant relaxation and also color change.

It's interesting, too, to wear your dot for a day and notice what interactions, anticipations, thoughts, and feelings change the color.

This is a wonderful way to get feedback about which aspects of your life are most stressful; to notice when you're being triggered by a traumatic memory; and to give yourself practice breathing through these troubling thoughts and events.

Creating Your Own Safe Place

Next, we're going to do Safe Place imagery. This image can be particularly important in giving you relief when troubling memories are surfacing, or you're facing an experience that evokes previous trauma, or you're just living through a stressful time.

When you create a Safe Place, you draw on happy memories—or the imagined end of distress—to create a place and a feeling of calm and peace. You're using your imagination to take you away from current anxiety, unhappiness, or danger, to take a mental and emotional time-out. When you successfully go to your Safe Place, you learn that even in the midst of traumatic memories and pain and helplessness, you have the power to create your own reassurance, joy, and security.

Almost everyone I've worked with enjoys and benefits from the Safe Place imagery (kids, incidentally, are often able to use this and other images far more easily than adults). Occasionally, however, someone becomes anxious as she allows images to form. If this happens to you, just open your eyes. Don't force it.

Some people, for whom there really is no safety—for example, those who feel unable to leave a violent, abusive intimate relationship or people living in a war zone—prefer, at least at first, the words *comfortable* or *special* rather than *safe*. If that's true for you, feel free to use these alternatives. Many people, even in these situations, discover places to which they return, again and again, for peace and rejuvenation.

Read through the following instructions several times, slowly, until you're familiar with them. Then you can record this exercise yourself or use my version of Safe Place imagery on The Center for Mind-Body Medicine website (cmbm.org). Soft music will likely encourage images to come to you. I like Carlos Nakai's "Shaman's Call." Its gentle Native American flute music evokes a peaceful journey of discovery. But, of course, you should choose whatever music feels right for you.

As the music begins, breathe more deeply and slowly, in through your nose and out through your mouth, letting your belly be soft and relaxed. Breathe this way for a few minutes. Feel yourself connected to the chair on which you're sitting or, if you're lying down (it's fine to do this lying down if you're not too sleepy), to the floor or bed on which you're lying. Breathe deeply, relaxing, trusting that your imagination will do the work it needs to do, that it will take you to a place that's safe, one that's comfortable for you. Breathe deeply and relax. Feel yourself supported by the chair on which you're sitting or the floor or bed.

Now allow the music, and your imagination, to take you to a place that feels safe and comfortable to you. It may be a place in Nature, a spot you particularly love. It may be indoors, in a room that feels just right for you. It may be a place that you know well or one you've never seen before. Allow yourself to go there, to relax into this place.

If you happen to find yourself moving from one place to another, that's fine. Enjoy that as well. After a while, let yourself come to rest in one place.

Look around you. What does it look like? What's the landscape like or the scene indoors? What does it feel and smell like to be there? If there are sounds, what are they?

Make yourself very comfortable wherever you are—sitting against a tree, enjoying a favorite chair, a lovely view. Notice what you're wearing on your body, on your feet. Are you by yourself or is someone else there?

If there's anything you would like to take out of this place—an annoying piece of furniture, a part of the landscape that's blocking your preferred view—please do so. Is there anything or anyone else you'd like to bring in? If there is, please do it. This is your Safe Place, your special place, your comfortable place. You can make it look and feel just the way you want.

Breathe deeply, enjoying this place, the feeling of your body relaxing, the comfort your Safe Place provides. Take some time to enjoy it—several minutes or more—breathing deeply, relaxing. Know that this is a place to which you can return anytime you want, to relax, to be replenished, to be safe.

And now, knowing you can return whenever you like, slowly bring yourself back into the room where you started. Begin by becoming aware of yourself sitting in your chair—or lying down—breathing deeply, connected to where you are. Breathe deeply for a few moments more. Slowly open your eyes and let your attention come back into the room.

Take a few moments now to write in your Journal. Here are some questions to consider: Was there any difficulty getting to your Safe Place? Did you go from one place to another? Where did you go? What was the safe or comfortable or special place like? What did it look like around you? Were there sounds? How did it feel and smell? Was anyone else there? How were you dressed? Were you sitting or lying down or standing? What did you bring in or take out? What was it like for you to simply be there, relaxing in your own Safe Place?

Remember as you write all this down that you can always return, that this place—or another Safe Place that you may find—is there for you, whenever you need it, whenever you want it. And know, too, that even those who have difficulties when they first use this image can usually find a reassuring, calming Safe Place the second or third time they do it.

The Safe Place image can be relaxing and reassuring when you're anxious and depressed or preoccupied with past or anticipated hurt or loss. I've used it often, with good results, with victims of abuse, refugees, and even with terrified children in the midst of wars, as well as with people who are depressed or unhappy. It will show you that peacefulness and control are possible, even in overwhelming situations.

Meeting Your Wise Guide

Having had some practice with Guided Imagery, you're ready to meet your Wise Guide. Your Safe Place, as you'll soon see, is an excellent place for this meeting.

Traditional healers—the shamans of Siberia, the *curanderos* of Latin America, the medicine men and women of North America, the healers of Africa, as well as the physicians of ancient Greece—have used this kind of imagery for millennia. Carl Jung brought the practice into modern psychiatry and psychology. I first learned Wise Guide imagery forty years ago from the late Ruth Carter Stapleton, a Protestant minister who was President Jimmy Carter's sister. I've been meeting my own Wise Guides ever since and have been introducing traumatized people to their Guides for almost as long.

For aboriginal healers, the Guide's words are a communication from the Spirit World. Some people are sure, when they meet their Guides, that they are contacting a Higher Power. For Jung, the Wise Guide was an aspect of the collective unconscious, the great reservoir of planetary thought and experience that Jung believed all of us could access. Most scientific researchers believe the Wise Guide is an Inner Guide, a manifestation of our own unconscious wisdom, the creative right hemisphere of our brain, our intuition. I agree. However, because my Wise Guide is so often so spot-on, I sometimes suspect that it could also be bringing me a communication from some source far more intelligent and knowledgeable than I am.

Any of these and many other explanations may be helpful and true. But you don't have to believe any of them to reap the benefits of Wise Guide imagery. All you need to do is approach this experience experimentally, with an open mind.

As with the Safe Place image, read through the words below until you feel familiar and comfortable with them, and then record them with the appropriate music—or feel free to use the version I've recorded on our website (cmbm.org). It's best if you record the Safe Place imagery and then continue with the Wise Guide image so you can move easily from one to the other. After a while, you'll find that doing them without interruption will deepen your experience of both.

Set aside twenty or thirty minutes for your meeting with your Wise Guide and time to write down what you experienced. Make sure the light is soft. Close the door so you won't be interrupted. Put a sign up if you need to. Sit in a comfortable, relaxing chair or lie down.

Begin as you did with the Safe Place image, following the same instructions I gave you in that exercise, exploring and experiencing your Safe Place in the same way you did in the previous image. It may be the same Safe Place or a different one.

After you've found and explored, perhaps rearranged, and fully experienced your Safe Place, take some more slow, deep breaths, and prepare yourself to meet your Wise Guide.

Here are the new instructions you'll want to record:

The Wise or Inner Guide who appears in your Safe Place may be a wise old man, or woman, or a child; someone you know or someone you've read about; or someone who emerges now for the first time from your imagination. The Guide may be human—a friend or mentor or immediate family member or dimly remembered ancestor—or a figure from a religious text, or a fairy tale, or a pagan god or goddess. It may be an animal or a spirit, a natural phenomenon like a waterfall or rainbow, or a creature you've never seen before. Whoever or whatever appears is a Guide who can teach you.

Breathe slowly and deeply for a minute or two with your belly soft, and invite your Wise Guide to appear. Accept whoever or whatever comes, even if he or she or it seems surprising or peculiar. Your Guide is here to teach and support the part of you that may be lost or frightened or just curious. You may want to consider this Guide a representative of the part of your mind that knows what you need to know, that is here to help the part that doesn't yet know. Let your Guide appear in your imagination. Perhaps it will be a bird flying by, a figure who appears at your side, a voice speaking softly to you.

Introduce yourself to your Wise Guide and ask the Guide to introduce him- or her- or itself to you. Wait for your Wise Guide to communicate in words, or gestures, or through feelings that you're having.

Now ask your Wise Guide a question, perhaps one that has been vexing you for some time—about difficulties in your present life or some painful, depressing memories, feelings, or thoughts. Or a question may just pop into your mind. Whatever question you ask is fine.

Wait for the answer. It may be clear and powerful. It may be quirky, or even, at least for now, incomprehensible. Accept whatever answer comes and whatever form it comes in—words, images, sounds, feelings, impressions. This is just the beginning of your communication with the inner wisdom that will slowly grow into a sure and reliable guide.

If you want clarification, ask for it. If you need more information, tell your Guide. Don't be shy. This is your Guide and you deserve answers.

Let the dialogue continue, asking questions, paying attention to the answers, asking more questions.

When you've heard what you need to, or the dialogue seems over— this may take five or ten minutes or more—thank your Wise Guide and say good-bye for now. Know that you can return to this place, and that this Wise Guide, or another, is there for you whenever you want, whenever you need help on your journey through and beyond trauma.

Now become aware of yourself, sitting in your chair or lying down, breathing deeply in through your nose and out through your mouth. Keep on breathing, deeply, slowly. Let your belly be soft. Feel your back against the back of the chair, your seat on the seat of the chair, your feet on the floor—or feel yourself lying down, supported by the floor or your couch or your bed. Breathe deeply with your belly soft and relaxed. Slowly, as you're ready, allow your eyes to open and become aware of yourself back in the here and now.

TAKE SOME TIME to record your experience with your Wise Guide in your Journal.

Here are some questions to consider as you write: Did a Guide come? Did you see, hear, or feel your Guide? Who was it? What was your response when you first encountered him or her or it? Was it surprise, gratitude, discomfort, or something else?

The first Wise Guide who emerges from within our unconscious mind is almost always the one most appropriate to this moment. But you may have had trouble fixing on one. That's okay, too. If more than one appeared, which one did you reject, which one did you accept, and why? What is the Wise Guide's name?

Write down the questions you asked your Wise Guide and the responses you got and how they made you feel. Do it as close to word for word as you can. Wise Guides are often quite precise in the way they speak. Responses that are hard to understand immediately may become clear later.

Write down what the discussion with your Wise Guide brought up for you—feelings, thoughts, new ideas, etc. For example, "The wise old woman said I should 'make a change in my job.' At first I thought she meant to change one aspect of what I'm doing in the job, and then when I asked, she said I may need to consider changing from my present job to another."

If you experience difficulty . . . Sometimes, in the beginning, no Wise Guide appears. Notice what you do see and feel. The image of a bright winter's day may bring as much understanding—perhaps of the need for quiet reflection—as a wise old man. A feeling of sadness may give you access to an emotion you've neglected and need to honor.

The second or third time you do the experiment, a Guide with whom you can speak will likely appear.

The Guide who appears but remains silent, refuses to answer, or walks away is actually responding. His, her, or its nonresponse may mean that you already know the answer, or that you need to do some more work on your own before an answer will be given, or that you simply have to sit with your question for a little longer.

Sometimes we reject the Wise Guide who comes. One of my patients, who prided herself on her strength, independence, and nonconformity, was shocked and offended when a gentle deer appeared to her. "I wanted a lioness or a wise old witch," she complained, "not Bambi!" She pushed Bambi out of her imagery. No one else came. She was "pissed off." I suggested that perhaps Bambi—gentle, loving, vulnerable—was the one, who at this moment, she needed to see and hear and learn from. Try trusting your inner wisdom, I advised her; let go of your preconceptions. See what Bambi has to say.

YOU CAN DO this experiment—combining the Safe Place and Wise Guide images—whenever you feel confused or down or stuck. In the beginning it's good to set aside half an hour. With practice, communication and useful guidance will come more easily—and perhaps faster. You may, after a while, want to do the experiment without a recording. Remember to write down the guidance you get. And notice how, over time, it may change and evolve.

It can also be helpful to share your images with a trusted friend. You may gain a new understanding of their meaning just by saying out loud what you've seen and felt. And sharing will likely deepen your connection with this person. Just ask her to listen. You don't want or need interpretation or analysis. These generally well-meant assists will likely interfere with what you can learn; they'll make you feel self-conscious and may create an unhealthy imbalance in your relationship with your friend. Your friend's not there to "treat" you, but simply to be a compassionate witness to who you are and what you're discovering.

Often a Guide will appear the first time you do this experiment, and the information he or she brings is revelatory. The tough old bird—it looks like a turkey—who comes to guide Jane, who is terrified by her diagnosis of metastatic cancer, reminds her that in leaving her faithless husband she is living more fully, less fearfully, more freely than she ever has. "Live your bravery," the bird tells her. "It's time to move farther out of your comfort zone, to help others."

Jason, the Iraq vet who's devastated by grief and haunted by guilt, sees his dead buddy's skull, with snakes slithering in and out of it. His initial fear dissolves as he questions his Guide. "Why did you die?" Jason asks his buddy plaintively. The answer comes back immediately. "So you could live and help the rest of us." A ten-year-old boy who lost his brothers and father in the war in Kosovo recognizes that a big dog is his Guide: "You can hold me tight at bedtime so you can sleep," his Guide tells him. "I'll be with you during those scary school exams."

Sometimes the Wise Guide imagery evokes whole scenes. Tara, a midwestern high school senior who'd been sexually abused, felt belittled by her mother's blame. She finds her Safe Place on the porch of her grandmother's house. There's the familiar smell of pies baking. Her grandmother, her Guide, is in a chair, rocking; her hair, as it always was, is in a gray bun. "Your mom doesn't know better. I'm proud of you. Now you be proud of yourself. I love you," she says as they embrace. Tara, telling it, cries.

WHAT YOU'LL LEARN from your Wise Guide is almost always helpful and comforting. It sometimes draws on reservoirs of wisdom that are miraculous. Over the years, I've worked with a number of terribly traumatized people who've received guidance and comfort that turned them away from the suicide to which their loss and shame and guilt were urging them. Meeting their Guide for the first time, they discovered ways and means to live again.

This was the experience of fourteen-year-old Ahmed, a Palestinian boy living in Gaza. Ahmed was big for his age, awkward in the way that boys are when they're overweight, and shy. He told me about his experience with imagery and other mind-body skills with a mixture of embarrassment and wonder.

A teacher at his school in Jabalia, a neighborhood north of Gaza City and close to the Israeli border, had suggested that Ahmed join a Mind-Body Skills Group. The teacher was concerned because Ahmed seemed, in recent months, to be distracted, unable to answer the kinds of questions that had never before stumped him. Sometimes he fell asleep in class. Perhaps, the teacher thought, the group would help him to relax and focus.

Ahmed was skeptical and uneasy about learning mind-body skills. He believed his problems went way beyond anything that the teacher, or the counselor who led the group, could address. And he knew he wasn't going to talk about his biggest problem—with anyone. Still, he was an obedient boy and didn't want to attract attention.

Ahmed was surprised to find himself enjoying the Soft Belly breathing he learned in his first group. It seemed to help him sleep a little better and longer, and to stop fidgeting in class. He thought, too, that it would help him feel confident while he fulfilled the "mission" to which he believed he was called. Autogenic Training and Biofeedback also pleased him. ABT showed him that he could use his mind to control his body.

Practicing Soft Belly breathing and ABT for a couple of weeks made it possible for Ahmed to relax and be confident enough to do the Wise Guide imagery. However, nothing prepared him for the Guides who appeared or the answers they gave.

"The first Guide who came," Ahmed told me, "was my grandfather, whom I loved very much. He said to me, 'Ahmed, you're a good boy.' It was good to hear that, but I wanted something more.

"Then, the Koran came, and I heard passages about finding peace, passages that I didn't think I'd ever read. Then the Koran disappeared.

"And then there was a third Guide, my best friend. I was so surprised to see him and so glad, because he was dead. Three months ago he and I were at the border, throwing stones at Israeli tanks, when one of the soldiers shot him. And I held him as he died. His head was in my lap, and there was blood everywhere, and his face was all white.

"And ever since then—and this is the first time I am telling anyone—I've been going out once or twice every week and throwing stones at the Israeli tanks, hoping the soldiers would kill me, so that I could die a martyr's death and be with my friend.

"And now here was my friend, and it was like he was alive again. And I asked him what I should do, just as I had asked my grandfather and the Koran. And he looked at me and he said, 'Ahmed, do not throw stones at the Israeli tanks. That's not the way to honor me. That's not your mission. I want you to grow up and be a good man and a strong man and marry and have children. And then, when you are old, you will die. And then we will be together in Paradise.'

"And since that day two weeks ago, I have not thrown stones at Israeli tanks."

REMEMBER, YOUR IMAGINATION can create places of safety and comfort, even in the midst of distress, disorder, and danger. If you relax and pay attention, it can put the world of your habitual thoughts and behaviors in a larger context; comfort you with long-forgotten, now revived possibilities for fulfillment; and give you glimpses of new truths that shine like welcoming stars.

9
Befriending Your Body

Trauma turns our bodies against us. Long after the threats are over, trauma may constrain us in a continual loop of fight or flight, flooding us with the stress hormones that damage cells in our hippocampus and prefrontal cortex, brain areas that are crucial for memory, judgment, and compassion; diminishing our immune response and making us more vulnerable to infections, and perhaps also to cancer; disturbing our sleep; and contributing to debilitating pain syndromes.

Trauma may have forced us to distance ourselves from a body that is being violated. After a skull fracture, Moira, like soldiers with traumatic brain injury, felt her thoughts were scrambled, her emotions out of control, and her body numb. Many people who've been raped recall that in a kind of involuntary, last-ditch effort at self-protection, they left their bodies, dissociated. Afterward, they often continue to feel numb, detached from their bodies. And sometimes those of us who have numbed ourselves also "forget," repressing the memory of the traumatic assault we were protecting ourselves against.

The chronic stress that is trauma's most consistent consequence can also expose previously hidden biological vulnerabilities. It can push our blood pressure and heart rate into dangerous zones and open gaps in our small intestine that release proinflammatory proteins to the rest of our body. Chronic stress can contribute to insulin resistance and type 2 diabetes, and fell us with migraine headaches.

Sometimes the symptoms and illnesses we develop point to a clear causal relationship between past trauma and present problems: recurrent urinary infections and pelvic pain are common in women—like Maya and Sally, whom you'll meet in chapter 13, "Make Love, Not War"— who were sexually abused long ago. Asa, who as an infant had a cancer removed from his neck, becomes "choked up," or hoarse, when asked to speak publicly.

Many times, the connection seems more symbolic than literal but is still very real. Some of us who felt neglected and abandoned when very young become more vulnerable to asthma as children or develop it in response to adult losses. Clutching at breath, wheezing, we sound and feel like we're crying for help. It happened to Emma, a supercompetent corporate executive, loyal wife, and devoted mother, during a divorce she didn't want.

All these effects on our body can be compounded by the damage trauma does to critical parts of our brain, including the medial prefrontal cortex, which helps us tune in to what's happening in our body. As trauma has pushed our bodies to run dangerously out of control, we may have become clueless about what's happening and feel unable to do anything about it.

If we are to heal the physical devastation that trauma may bring, to rebalance our stress-disordered biology and reclaim our physical being, we must first make friends with our body. This is likely to be a gradual, respectful process, particularly if we've been physically or sexually abused or have a painful, chronic illness. We started this work in the chapter "Shaking and Dancing." Now, in "Befriending the Body," we're going to approach this project more comprehensively.

Here are some ways to begin.

Bathing. Water is a time- and tradition-honored way of removing trauma and restoring our appreciation of our body. Indigenous healers often use it to cleanse warriors of the physical and psychological harm of being wounded, killing others, and losing comrades. And bathing can give us comfort as well as cleansing.

Long, hot showers are good, and mindful baths—slow, appreciative twenty- to forty-minute soaks in hot water, perhaps with a pound of magnesium-containing, muscle-relaxing Epsom salts—are even better. Soothing and energizing essential oils, like lavender (twenty to thirty drops in a tub), can enhance the experience.

Baths are a daily lifesaver for eighty-year-old Sharon. They give her a chance to once again appreciate a body that injury and illness have turned into a source of disappointment and pain. As she uses a sponge to rub body parts that have given her trouble, she talks sweetly to them. "Thank you, dear legs. I know I sometimes shout at you for being swollen and painful, but I rely on you to help me walk downstairs and work in the garden.

"It feels a bit goofy," she confesses. "But I've never found self-hate particularly helpful. My legs seem to enjoy it, and it does make me smile."

Detoxification. Toxic substances are, by definition, damaging to us. When we're under stress, we're more vulnerable to their assaults on our brain and the excessive demands they place on detoxifying mechanisms in our liver and on the beneficial bacteria that inhabit our GI tract—our microbiome.

The Trauma-Healing Diet that I'll give you in the next chapter will go a long way to reduce the burden of environmental toxins. It will also greatly enhance your capacity to eliminate any toxins you do take in and improve your biological and psychological resilience. Still, there are a few additional easy steps you can take to avoid and remove toxins.

Aluminum is widely distributed in nature and used in manufacturing processed food, as well as in antacids and deodorants. In large amounts, it can be toxic. The evidence for damage to brain functioning is mixed. Some researchers have been impressed by correlations between aluminum levels and Alzheimer's disease; others point out that there's no definitive cause-and-effect relationship. Still, there's no benefit in using aluminum pots and pans. Switch to cast iron, enamel, or stainless steel.

If you're on the Trauma-Healing Diet, you'll be eliminating the aluminum in processed foods. You'll also be unlikely to need antacids, which are high in aluminum. And you can definitely find substitutes for aluminum-containing deodorants. In fact, as you continue with the Trauma-Healing Diet, you may find you no longer need any deodorant.

Plastic. Stay away from canned foods and don't keep your food in plastic containers. Bisphenol A (BPA), which is present in plastic, including the plastic on the inside of cans, interrupts nerve cell signaling and may damage mental and emotional functioning.

Genetically modified organisms (GMOs). GMOs were invented because they produce high yields and are resistant to powerful, toxic pesticides. The most obvious reason to shun GMOs is the glyphosate used in the pesticides that are lavished on these crops. Glyphosate, which was patented by Monsanto and marketed as Roundup, causes oxidative stress, is harmful to our microbiome, and is, moreover, carcinogenic.

There may be other reasons to avoid GMOs—including gene transfer from these manufactured organisms to the gut microbiome and possible sensitivity to the synthesized proteins they contain. The jury is still out on possible dangers. But we certainly know enough about glyphosate to stay away from GMOs—and insist that genetically modified foods be labeled, as they are in Europe.

A Few Other Hints for Detoxifying:

- Remember to breathe deeply. The lungs are important organs of detoxification. And of course, slow, deep breathing lowers our stress level, which in turn leads to more effective digestion and better gastrointestinal detoxification.

- Work up a sweat. Exercise, which we'll be discussing soon, is great for detoxification. Saunas are also good. Our skin is an important organ for detoxification.

- Drink plenty of water. Dividing your body weight in pounds by two gives you the right number of ounces per day (not including juice, tea, and coffee).

- Add a filter to your faucet. That way you'll eliminate high levels of chlorine and any brain-damaging heavy metals, like lead, that may be in drinking water.

A few words about posture. At the risk of sounding like your mother, let me invite you to stand up straighter—not rigid like a soldier on guard, but relaxed, knees a little bent, head up, chin parallel with the ground, shoulders rolled easily back, breathing slowly into your Soft Belly.

This isn't primarily a matter of aesthetics, though you *will* look better. When we're feeling burdened with stress, depressed, or troubled by guilt or shame, we tend to stoop and hunch, and to breathe shallowly in our chest rather than deeply into our belly. If you assume this slumped posture, which I suggest you do now so you'll know what I'm talking about, you'll likely feel a little depressed and depleted.

Standing straight makes you feel more capable, more alert, better about yourself. It lifts your spirits as well as your head. It may take a little effort to go against the grain of the tension and sadness that's making you slump and to break bad postural habits, but it's really worth it. Try it now. And do it sitting as well.

If you need some encouragement, take a look at some recent studies on the effect of posture on attitude and mood, and particularly at one from New Zealand that describes how better posture leads to improved mood and energy in people who are depressed.

Massage and touch. Massage can be a beautiful way to release tension and improve mood, and also to rediscover the kindness of touch. The scientific literature on the benefits of massage for anxiety, depression, and physical pain is robust and includes pioneering studies by University of Miami researcher Tiffany Field. The research will reassure you, if you are fearful of touch.

My own experience working with sexually abused teenage girls and delinquents, adults with chronic illness, and people who've been tortured has shown me the enormous reparative power of receiving massage and other forms of therapeutic touch. My colleagues and I have also taught traumatized children and adults—in US schools and women's groups, as well as in refugee camps—to massage others. We've seen how this kind and generous touch can be healing for the giver as well as the receiver.

Movement and Exercise

All of us can move. Even those confined to wheelchairs and hospital beds have felt new energy from gentle stretching and seated or horizontal Shaking and Dancing. And movement, especially if it's carefully individualized to meet your needs and preferences, will give you a wide range of trauma-healing psychological and physical benefits.

Even if you're bed-hugging tired as well as traumatized, you can, like Dorothy, the cancer-challenged senator's wife, learn to enjoy moving. After some quite eloquent protests, she began with a half-block walk to the corner, then very gradually increased her daily range.

Once she'd overcome the pull backward and bedward, Dorothy began to feel more alert and able. More energy came as she closed the front door behind her. With each satisfying fall of foot on pavement, a sense of accomplishment—and even, she had to admit, power—filled her.

For a while she did ten or fifteen minutes at odd times during the day, then as she grew more fond of it, thirty to forty minutes every morning.

Dorothy enjoyed the crispness of the fall air, the shadows the trees cast on her street, the sound of birds, and the children on their way to school. "You know," Dorothy told me after several months, "it has changed me. My body feels stronger and more energetic, and I have to admit, my mood is better. But I also feel *myself*. I've never taken time like this for myself, for my body, or met a challenge that is just my own."

Aerobic exercise—the kind that requires oxygen and stimulates energy—increases stress-relieving, resiliency-building hormones depleted by trauma, including dopamine, serotonin, and the endorphins. Very good clinical research has shown that a variety of aerobic exercises—including jogging, swimming, and the brisk walking that Dorothy eventually did—increases brain-derived neurotropic factor. And BDNF stimulates the creation of new brain cells and improves functioning in the hippocampus, which modulates the stress produced by trauma.

Clinical trials have also shown that exercise directly addresses the loss of focus and increased fatigue, anxiety, and depression that so often follow trauma. One fascinating study of female military veterans demonstrated significant improvement in PTSD symptoms after twelve weeks of fast walking for only thirty to forty minutes, four days a week.

Recent scientific studies on the postures of hatha yoga and the yogic breathing techniques of pranayama have repeatedly demonstrated improvements in symptoms of post-traumatic stress disorder. The Chinese moving meditations qi gong and tai chi appear to have similar benefits.

And exercise, as we continue to discover, can play a major role in preventing as well as treating the chronic illnesses that may follow in the wake of trauma and chronic stress, including heart disease, cancer, type 2 diabetes, arthritis, and chronic pain.

Exercise, in all its forms, also gives us a sense of increased control over bodies that trauma has agitated and made alien to us, as well as confidence and pleasure in them. For many people like Dorothy—and Sharon, who describes her daily twenty minutes of stretching as "my religion"—exercise becomes a mighty engine of trauma healing.

Exercise can also be a meditation. Mindful walking is a pleasurable, healthy exercise that can bring more awareness and appreciation into your life. Buddhists have been practicing it for centuries.

It's simple, too. Just walk slowly—really, really slowly, at a quarter your normal pace. Notice your thoughts, feelings, and sensations as you walk, and say them to yourself—for example, "Foot falling on the ground . . . interesting bark on the tree . . . feeling the sun on my face . . . thinking of my abusive husband . . . wondering why I'm bringing him with me to spoil the lovely day . . . breathing deeply."

When my first-year Georgetown medical students do mindful walking for twenty minutes, they are often astonished at the results. "I never knew there was a tree in that place," says one. "I never saw that statue before," adds another. And sometimes young men and women who've walked the territory a thousand times will admit, "I never knew that building was there."

Running, jogging, or playing tennis, assuming yoga postures, and relaxing into the movements of tai chi can all be done in meditative ways. Jenna, a court clerk who had been sexually abused as a child and was overwhelmed by her work, discovered that mindful weight lifting—slow lifting accompanied by deep breathing and appreciation of every ounce of effort—relieved tension, released the rage her trauma brought, and gave her new eyes to see her life. After each session, she felt more relaxed, more comfortable in her body, less preoccupied with angry, guilty, ashamed thoughts. Ominous deadlines became manageable. Judges and lawyers who made sexual remarks had threatened her; now they seemed pathetic. Earlier she had retreated in cold silence; now she told them off.

As we befriend our bodies, the watchwords are, once again, *individuality* and *uniqueness*. I could never have predicted that bathing or stretching would be so important to Sharon, that walking would give Dorothy such joy, or that Jenna would discover liberation through mindful weight lifting.

Studies may show that yoga is good for post-traumatic stress—and they do—but if you cringe every time you think of getting on the mat, it's not likely to help. Find a form of movement that suits you and . . . practice, practice, practice.

Start in whatever way feels comfortable, perhaps ten, fifteen, or twenty minutes a day. Or thirty to forty minutes three or four times a week. Gradually increase the time. We humans evolved as hunter-gatherers, people who were continually bending, lifting, and carrying—and of course, walking everywhere. The genes we carry welcome the stimulation that movement brings. Interestingly and importantly, the older we get, the more we benefit from exercise.

Pounding pillows. Words, as you've probably discovered, are effective but not always sufficient to release us from the bonds of unexpressed emotions. When they're suppressed, fear and anger can tie our muscles in knots, even as they lay siege to our thoughts. Sometimes, physical effort is the surest way to loosen the knots and free ourselves.

Pounding pillows, which has long been a part of the repertoire of body-oriented psychotherapies, is simple—and may seem simplistic and weird—but it's effective. If you're feeling tense and tight, put upon, or frustrated, or if you're nursing a grudge or feeling sorry for yourself, you're a good candidate for this experiment. If your shoulder dislocates easily or you've had major injuries to your upper back, head, or neck, this one's not for you. Otherwise, you're good to go.

Here's how to do it:

Find a place in your home where no one will bother you, where you can close a door so any sounds you make don't disrupt your household. Actually, if anyone's home with you, you should let them know that any noises you make are harmless and they needn't worry.

Now kneel in front of a pile of pillows (not the ones you sleep on). Make fists, and raise your arms above your head. Bend back and bring your arms and fists down on the pillows as hard as you can. Do it over and over, putting your whole body, your whole being into it. Shout and scream as you pound. Plan on five minutes and make sure you have time afterward to rest.

You're likely to resist at first. And once you start, you'll have to exert considerable will, as well as effort, to keep going. If emotions are slow to rise, you're likely to feel even more frustrated. That's okay. Keep going, push harder, take it out on the pillows.

At some point, you'll start feeling something. At first it may just be anger at doing this experiment. Your frustration may increase. "Why the hell am I doing this?" Keep going. Once emotion begins to break through, it will keep coming—if you don't force it back down. Keep pounding harder and faster, pushing through whatever comes up— anger, fear, or fatigue. Tears may come. Keep going.

You may feel out of control. That's okay, actually good. You're not hurting anyone else. You're unwrapping your body's bonds, blow by blow, freeing your mind. Your momentary loss of control is opening the door to more of who you are.

Afterward, you're likely to be tired, maybe exhausted, but also relaxed, renewed, perhaps even joyful with newfound freedom. Take some time now, sitting or lying down, breathing deeply, letting feelings and thoughts continue to arise. Write what happened in your Journal.

I suggest you pound pillows every day until you're satisfied that bound-up anger, resentment, and fear have drained away. I've pounded pillows many times over the years; I always begin with great reluctance and end with gratitude.

A Pause for Mindful Eating

Eating is, of course, a fundamental physical function, a necessity of life, a treat for our taste, an opportunity for communion with other diners, and a joy for our spirit. Trauma of all kinds twists and tortures our relationship to food, even as it disrupts every aspect of digestion and the physical, emotional, and mental functions that all depend on what and how we eat.

In the next chapter, I'll give you the plan for the Trauma-Healing Diet: the knowledge about which foods to eat and which ones to cut out, and why, and which spices, herbs, and supplements to add. First, though, I want to give you a taste of the Trauma-Healing Diet's "secret sauce," an ingredient that can restore joy to your spirit and harmony to your home, as well as health to your body. If used liberally, it will transform your healthy eating from a bland duty to a tasty celebration.

The sauce, and it's really not so secret, is, once again, mindfulness: becoming aware of, more sensitive to every activity related to buying, preparing, and eating food. Mindful Eating will make you more aware of the food choices you've been making out of habit, and the emotions and associations, as well as commercial seduction, that urge you to make these choices. Over time, mindfulness will help you choose and prepare foods with more independence and imagination, skill, and joy. You'll discover which foods are truly delicious. And you'll become more sensitive to the effects of all food on your body and mind. Mindfulness will also make the knowledge about trauma-healing foods and nutrients that I'll share with you more real and personal. And the focus and appreciation that accompany mindfulness will actually enhance the healing power of the foods, herbs, and spices you do eat.

You'll need fifteen minutes for this experiment in mindfulness, this tasting.

Begin by putting a grape or a quarter-size piece of banana or apple on a plate. Put a piece of chocolate next to it (dark chocolate, which has more nutrients, would be good).

Now, close your eyes and do Soft Belly breathing. In through your nose and out through your mouth, with your belly soft and relaxed. Do it for two or three minutes. Feel your body and all your muscles relax with each exhalation. Notice your thoughts, feelings, and sensations as they arise. Let them come, and let them go. Bring your attention gently back to your breath. You'll soon feel more relaxed and more alert. You'll be more capable of effectively using all your senses and your imagination.

Now, open your eyes and look at what's on the plate. Notice what thoughts come to you. Do you feel more drawn to the fruit or the chocolate? Do memories come up of times when you had one or the other? Any concern about what you see on the plate—for example, old prejudices against or preferences for "healthy fruit" or "sinful chocolate"?

Now, proceeding slowly, mindfully, pick up whichever piece you're most drawn to. . . . Hold it in your hand. . . . Feel the texture. . . . Bring it close so you can see all the surface details. . . . Smell it. . . . Maybe touch it to your face and lips. . . . Notice how it feels. . . . Any thoughts or memories or emotions?

Now, close your eyes and put the fruit or chocolate in your mouth.

But don't bite down. How does it feel? What's happening in your mouth? What's the taste and the texture? Roll it around with your tongue. Play with it for a minute or two. Slowly.

Begin to chew . . . slowly, slowly—at about a fifth or a tenth of your customary speed. Continue chewing for a few slow, interesting minutes, noticing all the tastes, textures, and sounds, the feelings and thoughts that are coming—about what you're chewing and anything else, past, present, or future.

Slowly swallow, feeling the thoroughly chewed or melted morsels slipping down the back of your mouth into your throat. Chew until all the fruit or chocolate has disappeared from your mouth.

Now open your eyes and write in your Journal everything that happened during this experience. Why did you choose what you chose? What was the smell, feel, texture, and taste? How did the flavors change or stay the same? Describe all the thoughts and memories that came. What was the whole experience like? How was it different from the way you usually eat and experience your food? What did you learn?

The results are often eye opening, sometimes amazing. Time after time people realize how little they taste, or appreciate, or are even aware of the food they're eating, and how fast they ordinarily eat. Many people who've been traumatized become aware of the anxiety that has accelerated their eating and denied them a full portion of pleasure. Others are just astonished by the joy of the experience.

I'll always remember the huge man who stood up at one of our Haiti trainings to share his experience with a small piece of banana. "I grew up," he announced, "on a banana farm. We have twenty-four varieties of bananas on our family farm. I have eaten bananas every day of my life from the time I was a baby until now, when I am sixty years old. I eat bananas for breakfast, lunch, and dinner, and bananas in between, for snacks. But I have never," and here he breaks into a great grin, "eaten a banana before."

To make sure you've got the message of, and greatest benefits from, Mindful Eating, do this experiment again in a day or two. Also, take the time to eat a whole meal mindfully, slowly, in silence, without distraction. If you're eating with others, invite them to do the experiment with you.

You'll start freeing yourself from old habits and food manufacturers' propaganda. You'll read the labels on processed foods with renewed awareness, likely rejecting ones that contain multiple colorings, flavorings, and preservatives. You'll start choosing foods that really look good, are good for you, and taste good.

At Eskenazi Health, Indiana's largest safety-net hospital system, the three hundred employees we've trained in the model of self-care you're learning, and the many they in turn have taught, have begun to speak with wonder about the changes that Mindful Eating has brought them. Every time I return, people—doctors, therapists, security guards—pull out their belts to show me new waistlines. They tell me about the dozens of pounds they've lost, the new foods they've discovered, the medications they've been able to reduce or discontinue, the energy they feel. Their stomachs are now signaling when they've had enough, and they're listening. They have a peaceful feeling at meal's end. And their pleasure in, and success with, Mindful Eating has encouraged them to persist with Soft Belly, Shaking and Dancing, and a comprehensive program of self-care.

Before we brought this program to Eskenazi, health care costs for Eskenazi's 4,500 employees were increasing by 5 percent each year; two years after beginning to include our approach, they are only increasing by 1 percent.

No monetary incentives were necessary at Eskenazi Health, no nagging. All it took was some of the basic information I'll give you in the next chapter and a commitment to awareness, to Mindful Eating.

Like the Eskenazi employees, you'll begin to bring mindfulness into every aspect of your relationship to food. Food preparation is likely to become fun, as you appreciate the cutting and dicing, enjoy the sizzle of sautéing, choose spices you never before used, and create and appreciate new balances of color, taste, and texture.

And if sometimes you find yourself eating fast, losing track of taste, don't beat yourself up. It happens to all of us. Take a few deep breaths. Slow down. Become aware of what moved you out of your mindful groove—worry about work, or annoying dinner-table talk, or a tone of voice that reminded you of past trauma. Take another few breaths and return to your food with friendly pleasure.

SOMETIMES MINDFUL EATING can change your world, as well as what and how you eat, your weight, and your level of stress.

When I talk with kids about their experience with mind-body skills, I ask which one is their favorite. In 2015, not long after Hamas and Israel's war, I asked an eight-year-old Gazan girl who lived in an area devastated by bombs. She looked up at me, checking to make sure I really wanted to hear her answer, then grinned.

"Mindful Eating," she said.

"Why?" I wondered, surprised as well as curious. Kids most often prefer Soft Belly breathing, Shaking and Dancing, or Drawings.

"Because," she continued, powered by her enthusiasm. "When we did it in our group, the date I ate was so delicious. And when I went home, the food my mother cooked tasted so much better. And then I taught my whole family." She draws out the word *whole* and extends her arms to indicate a large number.

"They liked the food better, too. And," she pauses to catch her breath, "best of all, it's so much more peaceful now. After the war, my mother was always scared, and my dad was very nervous and angry. And every dinner, it was like a little war going on. But since the Mindful Eating, everyone eats ver-r-ry slowly and enjoys the food more—and we are all so much nicer to each other. And not just at dinner. So that's why I like Mindful Eating."

10
The Trauma-Healing Diet

BOOKS ON TRAUMA, even the very best of them, have little or nothing to say about the damage that trauma and chronic stress do to our digestive tract, and how that damage compounds the toll trauma takes on our mind, our brain, and the rest of our body. And few therapists who work with traumatized people give guidance about nutrition or make referrals to nutritionists. These are serious, even dangerous omissions.

Chapter 2 told you about the damage that trauma does.

This chapter tells you what you need to know to reverse the damage and heal yourself. It fills the void.

This chapter is easy to read and use, but it's long, by far the longest in *The Transformation*. This is because everything we eat—and I mean everything—can either enhance or hinder trauma healing. I want you to know which foods are best for you but also why they are. That way, as you choose your foods and prepare your meals at home or order them in a restaurant, you'll have a clear sense of what's good for you.

That knowledge will enhance the quality of your choices. And acting on it, mobilizing the placebo response that comes with engaged self-care, will maximize the healing potential of the foods.

Before you read this chapter, you might want to do a quick reread of chapter 2, "The Biology of Trauma." It will remind you of the damage trauma does to digestion, and it will strengthen your understanding of how the Trauma-Healing Diet reverses that damage.

How the Diet Works

This Trauma-Healing Diet is designed to significantly decrease the level of stress that trauma causes and to help reverse the damage it may have done to your brain as well as your gut and the rest of your body. It will improve your digestion and quiet your mind, balance your neurotransmitters, and increase the production of brain-derived neurotrophic factor.

Eating in a trauma-healing way will reverse the inflammation caused by trauma and feed your microbiome. It will ease you away from the comfort-food addictions I described in chapter 2 and help you lose the weight that stressed eating may have put on. It will improve your mood and the way your mind works. It will decrease your vulnerability to memories of past trauma and increase your resilience in the face of present and future stress. And keeping to a Trauma-Healing Diet will go a long way to preventing the chronic illnesses that so often follow in trauma's wake.

If you've been self-medicating with comfort foods, the first few days of healthy eating can be difficult. The withdrawal may make you tired and testy. After five or six days, however, your gut will be calmer and symptoms of constipation or diarrhea will likely be subsiding. You'll be more focused and energetic, less anxious and agitated, better able to sleep. These changes will give you the reinforcement you need to keep eating in a trauma-healing way.

The ground rules of the Trauma-Healing Diet are below. They're simple. Think of them as guidelines or ingredients in a recipe. Read them slowly. Digest. Return to them again and again. Enjoy. Let all of them nourish you.

And if you fall off the trauma-healing wagon and make some poor food choices, don't spend a lot of time blaming yourself. Take some slow, deep Soft Belly breaths. Become aware of why it happened. And when you're ready, get back on.

EAT WHOLE FOODS

When food is processed, it loses vital nutrients and most of the nourishing fiber that goes with them. Meanwhile, it's being contaminated by the toxic chemicals—preservatives, colorings, and flavorings—that seduce our eyes and taste buds, prolong shelf life, amp up profits for manufacturers, and compromise our health.

For example, grinding and bleaching flour breaks down the cell walls of the wheat grain and creates an acellular, stress-inducing, insulin-demanding, fat-depositing, nutritionally depleted, powdery white carbohydrate. (Doesn't sound very good, does it?) Refined flour may also interfere with leptin, a hormone made by our fat cells that tells the brain we're full and it's time to stop eating.

The end result, as we discussed in chapter 2, is the empty calories of comfort food. Comfort foods, like a soda and a mac and cheese, make us feel good for a while, giving us jolts of sugar and feel-good dopamine and serotonin, and lowering our cortisol. They soon become "discomfort" foods, increasing our stress, depleting dopamine and serotonin, increasing cortisol, and interfering with trauma recovery in our brain and the rest of our body.

Study after study has shown that a variety of whole foods diets, all of which are more in harmony with our genetic programming, can reverse this process, reducing stress, preventing and treating chronic illness, and prolonging life.

MAKE NONSTARCHY VEGETABLES A MAJOR PART OF YOUR DIET

There is an amazing, colorful variety of health-promoting vegetables, all with vastly different tastes and textures. Imagine each as I name it, perhaps recalling its image, texture, and taste: green beans, tomatoes, leafy greens, squash, onions, snap peas, cucumbers, asparagus, artichokes, broccoli, cauliflower, mushrooms.

All contain antioxidants, which offset the effects of stress, as well as soluble fiber, which feeds the good bacteria in the microbiome and promotes good bowel movements. They all have a low glycemic index, which means they are slowly broken down into the sugar that feeds our cells, subtracting from, rather than adding to, the burden that stress brings.

Each veggie also has plant or "phyto" nutrients, with specific benefits for trauma recovery. For example, many mushrooms enhance our stress-depleted immune response, and cruciferous vegetables, such as cauliflower and broccoli, improve our liver's challenged detoxification system.

Make nonstarchy veggies—steamed, sautéed, or raw—30 to 50 percent of your daily diet.

INCLUDE STARCHY VEGETABLES

The sweet potato, a starchy vegetable that is rich in antioxidants and phytonutrients, is a wonderful alternative to white potatoes, pasta, and rice. Okinawans, who use purple sweet potatoes as their primary starch, live far longer and are healthier than the rice-reliant inhabitants of other Japanese islands.

Corn and peas—vegetables often disparaged as "just starch"—are in fact nutrient rich and healthy. So, too, are white potatoes—if you don't overcook them, and you eat them with their nutrient- and fiber-rich skins.

The main potato problem is with preparation. Overcooking potatoes (when mashed or baked) depletes them of nutrients and increases the jolt of sugar they give us.

If, however, you cool the potatoes after you cook them you get a more resistant (hard to digest) starch that nourishes your microbiome.

Fried potatoes and chips contain omega-6 oils, which in large quantities contribute to inflammation. Frying also brings out acrylamide, a carcinogen. If you really want a few fries or chips, take a small portion, eat them slowly, mindfully, and enjoy them thoroughly. I learned to do it from one of our recent presidents, and some of my friends have learned it from me.

Crunchy raw potatoes can also be delicious as well as filling. You can grate them, season them with lemon, salt, pepper, culinary herbs, and spices, and put them in a salad.

FRUITS

Fruits are high in sugar, but they are gut- and mind-healthy—if they are eaten in moderate amounts. Fruits contain a wide variety of phytonutrients that help reverse the oxidative stress and inflammation that trauma provokes. I favor berries and, in particular, blueberries, which are a superfood for the friendly bacteria in our microbiome.

Because fruits are sugary, I recommend drinking fruit juices sparingly—an ounce or two in eight or ten ounces of water—and eating only small portions of dried fruit, in which the sugar is highly concentrated; a few apricots, dates, or figs can be a special sweet treat.

You can also use fruit, along with nuts and spices, to vary the taste of salads and in cooking with protein of all kinds.

GRAINS

Grains play a major role in feeding the earth's population. They can, however, be a problem, especially when your gut has been challenged by trauma or long-standing stress.

It makes sense: grains of all kinds are a thirteen-thousand-year-old introduction to our million-year-old human diet, and one to which we're not well adapted. Grains that are high in gluten—the combination of proteins that give bread the stickiness bakers appreciate and the chewy texture diners enjoy—are the most problematic. Wheat, in particular, has been bred to be gluten rich, and wheat is present not only in breads and cakes but as a hidden ingredient in many processed foods.

People with celiac disease—perhaps one in one hundred of us— have a dramatic and damaging immune reaction to gluten. When someone with celiac disease takes even the smallest amount of gluten, she's likely to experience bloating, constipation or diarrhea, and belly pain. If you're having these symptoms, ask your doctor to test you for celiac disease. You can definitively diagnose celiac disease with a blood test and a biopsy of the small intestine.

But it's not just people with celiac who are extremely sensitive to gluten. Perhaps 6 percent of us in the US have non-celiac gluten sensitivity (NCGS), an intestinal immune response without a distinctive biopsy picture. The cytokines, the immune cells stimulated by NCGS, create celiac-like symptoms in the gut. They also damage the intestinal wall. Gluten particles may then enter the bloodstream, provoking inflammatory reactions everywhere in the body, including the brain, where they may produce depression, anxiety, and a decrease in cognitive functioning.

Gluten can also multiply the gut-damaging effects of stress in people who don't have celiac disease or NCGS. When we've been traumatized and eat gluten, it may pass through the intestinal wall, which high levels of stress have made "leaky," and increase inflammation in every part of our body, including our brain.

The bottom line: stay away from gluten while you're working on resolving trauma and reducing stress. At least for several months.

Many traumatized people who stop eating gluten—even those who don't have any digestive symptoms—find they feel more energetic, think more clearly, and are happier. If after a few months, you'd like to resume eating gluten, notice your response. If you feel fine after two slices of bread or a meal of pasta, you can probably safely eat gluten-containing foods—in moderation. If you feel sluggish or anxious, your joints ache, or your ankles or any other part of your body swells, ask your doctor to test you for gluten sensitivity.

If you need to forgo gluten, don't be downhearted. There are many nongluten grains and grain-like foods you can eat, tasty ones that traditional people have long used, like amaranth, buckwheat, wild rice, and quinoa, as well as brown and white rice. A vast array of gluten-free options are now available, including pasta, bread, and pizza crust that are actually quite good. Oats that are certified as gluten-free are also fine for breads, as well as for oatmeal.

EATING ORGANIC

Organic foods are definitively better for you. A number of studies have shown that an organic food diet is less carcinogenic. And many of the pesticides and herbicides that are typically used on plants may have negative effects on our brains, our mood, and our thinking processes.

However, organic fruits, vegetables, and grains can be expensive. You can stretch your food budget, while sparing yourself health risks, if you use the guidelines prepared by the Environmental Working Group (EWG). The EWG strongly recommends putting your organic food money on the "dirty dozen," now expanded to what we can call the "filthy fifteen": the fruits and veggies with the most pesticides. On the other hand, you can safely eat the nonorganic versions of the "clean fifteen," fruits and veggies that are less burdened by toxic chemicals. Below is the EWG's chart for you to consider.

You may want to make a copy of this chart and put it in your purse or wallet.

CLEAN 15	FILTHY 15
Avocados	Apples
Sweet corn	Strawberries
Pineapples	Grapes
Cabbage	Celery
Sweet peas (frozen)	Peaches
Onions	Spinach
Asparagus	Sweet bell peppers
Mangoes	Nectarines (imported)
Kiwi	Cucumbers
Eggplant	Cherry tomatoes
Grapefruit	Snap peas (imported)
Cantaloupe	Potatoes
Cauliflower	Hot peppers
Sweet potatoes	Blueberries (domestic)
Papayas	Lettuce

Reorder Your Protein Priorities

PLANT PROTEIN

Make beans and other legumes (lentils, chickpeas, and soybeans) a foundational part of your diet. That's what many traditional societies do. Legumes have a low glycemic index, are high in vitamins and minerals, and have lots of fiber. Soaked overnight and prepared with salt, cumin, and ginger, they're easier to digest. Adding sautéed onions and garlic while cooking, as Indians routinely do, makes them even tastier and healthier.

Seeds and nuts are excellent sources of protein and are rich in the fats we need for brain health (I'll discuss them later). Walnuts, pecans, Brazil nuts, and almonds, as well as pumpkin, sesame, and sunflower seeds, are particularly nutritious. Each has its own nutritional virtue (high omega-3s in walnuts, selenium in Brazil nuts, zinc in pumpkin seeds, etc.). Combine them freely and use them often. They make healthy, tasty additions to fruit and vegetable as well as animal protein dishes.

FISH: YOUR BEST FRIEND FOR ANIMAL PROTEIN

Fish are rich in the anti-inflammatory omega-3 fatty acids that make the membranes of brain cells more flexible, optimize the transmission of electrical signals from one cell to the next, and promote maximal resilience and enhanced mood. The more fish a population eats, the less likely it is to be depressed. And one dramatic experiment showed that the omega-3s, in which fish are so rich, significantly reduced stress after a traumatic event.

Small fish are far less likely to have mercury and other heavy metals, which are toxic to the brain and can inhibit trauma healing. Anchovies, sardines, and herring are your best bets. Salmon, mackerel, cod, and rainbow trout are also good.

Seafood, including shrimp, mussels, clams, and oysters, is a great source of protein, vitamin B_{12}, and minerals like magnesium and zinc that contribute to brain health. Mussels are underrated for taste and health, and have the added virtue of being inexpensive.

EGGS

Eggs have had a long and undeserved bad rep. It turns out that the cholesterol they contain—and dietary cholesterol in general—is not likely to be a risk factor for heart disease. On the other hand, eggs are an excellent source of nutrients, as well as the amino acids that are the building blocks of protein in our body.

If you can afford the slightly higher cost, make sure you get eggs that have been "pastured"—ones that come from chickens that roam free and haven't been fed the grains, hormones, and antibiotics that are routinely given to caged chickens. "Certified Humane" and "Animal Welfare Approved" are the labels to look for.

You can also raise your own chickens (I did this for ten years). Their eggs are delicious and an altogether different experience from any kind of store-bought. There's real satisfaction in foraging for, finding, and eating the eggs that your chickens hide, and lots of laughs in getting to know the particular and peculiar ways of chickens. And some goofy exercise shooing them back home at night.

MEAT

When they could, our hunter-gatherer ancestors ate meat. It was wild (animals weren't domesticated until ten to fifteen thousand years ago). It was lean (wild animals are always on the move) and, of course, free of the hormones, chemicals, and antibiotics that fatten up and contaminate modern feedlot cows, pigs, sheep, and chickens.

The fat composition of wild animal meat was in harmony with

our genetic programming and good health: approximately 3:1 pro-inflammatory omega-6 fatty acids to anti-inflammatory omega-3s, rather than the dangerous 10:1 omega-6 to omega-3 ratio we find in modern beef. Modern meat also contains saturated fats that violate our genetic programming and feed the bad bacteria in our gut, producing toxins that make our gut leaky and adding significantly to the stress we already have.

If you do eat beef, pork, or lamb, it should be grass fed or organic; chickens should be cage free. This meat will be far less fatty, and the omega-6 to omega-3 ratios will be much closer to what we're genetically programed to handle. It will be free of chemicals, antibiotics, and hormones, which, of course, are toxic to us, as well as the animals. Also, if animals are free to roam and are quickly and humanely killed, their meat won't multiply your stress by the large doses of stress hormones the animals put out before they die.

Instead of making meat a habit, let it be more of a treat. Cutting way down on meat will improve the balance and health of your microbiome, decrease your body's burden of proinflammatory omega-6s, and contribute to your overall well-being. Lower intake of meat has been correlated with a decrease in the incidence of a variety of chronic conditions, including depression, heart disease, cancer, and diabetes.

You'll probably enjoy the meat you eat much more. And if you decide not to eat meat at all, you can get all the protein you need from legumes, seeds, and nuts, as well as eggs and dairy.

FATS

If we choose fats and oils wisely, they can be powerful trauma-healing allies. Olive oil, a healthy monounsaturated fat, is my go-to for cooking and salads. It's a staple of the Mediterranean diet that has been repeatedly shown to help prevent depression and inflammation, as well as heart disease and strokes. Extra virgin olive oil—oil from the first cold pressing of the olives—provides the most health benefits and the best protection. It can also be used as a tangy butter substitute.

Other oils that are healthy include coconut oil (a saturated fat), walnut oil, avocado oil, and sesame oil, which has a very nice toasty quality and can be used in small quantities by itself or with other oils.

Vegetable oils, like corn, soybean, cottonseed, safflower, and canola—which are often used for packaged chips, crackers, and cookies—are marketed as healthy for cooking and salads. They're not. In fact, they're high in the omega-6s, which compound the inflammation produced by trauma. When they're present in baked goods, they're usually hydrogenated—that is, they have a hydrogen atom added—to keep the food from spoiling. Then they become trans fats, which are clearly unhealthy. Scientific studies have shown that trans fats contribute to depression and memory impairment, as well as heart disease, high blood pressure, and diabetes.

MILK AND MILK PRODUCTS

We've been told, primarily by the dairy industry, that milk is a "perfect food." Breast milk for babies certainly is, but animal milk for adults is another matter—particularly for people of Asian or African descent who are often intolerant of lactose (milk sugar) and may have serious difficulty digesting milk and milk products.

In addition, the interaction between lactose and our microbiome creates by-products that can disturb anyone's gut. When we're under stress and our gut is leaking, these by-products may enter our bloodstream and cause inflammatory reactions in our brain, compounding the damage from trauma.

Some people drink milk and eat cheese without adverse effects. Still, if you've been traumatized or are under significant stress, I'd stay away from or cut down on milk and milk products for several months.

Then, as you lower your stress level, you can reintroduce them, starting with yogurt, which is rich in the good bacteria (of the *lactobacillus* and *bifidus* families) that enhance digestion. If all goes well—no GI symptoms, headache, or foggy mental feeling—experiment with your favorite cheese or, if you still love and miss it, have an occasional glass of whole milk, which may well be healthier than low fat milk.

FIBER AND FERMENTED FOOD

Fiber and fermented food, prebiotics and probiotics, are all powerful trauma-healing allies.

Let's start with fiber. There are two kinds: soluble and insoluble. Insoluble fiber includes the bran that coats grains; it's a component of nuts, seeds, beans, and the skins of a variety of fruits and vegetables. Insoluble fiber passes through the gut undigested but absorbs water and provides bulk in stools.

Soluble fiber, which also adds bulk to stools, is present in both nonstarchy and starchy vegetables, as well as fruits, legumes, seeds, and nuts. Foods that contain it are prebiotic—that is, they promote the growth of beneficial bacteria in our microbiome.

When we think about fiber, it's useful once again to compare us to our hunter-gatherer ancestors and our contemporary, indigenous sisters and brothers. Their diet of plants, seeds, and wild game contains as much as seventy to eighty or even one hundred grams of fiber a day—think of a baseball-size portion. The comfort food choices we often make when we're stressed and, indeed, the standard American diet (largely processed food) have only ten to fifteen grams of fiber—a dose no larger than a Ping-Pong ball. Even when our stress level is minimal, this kind of fiber deficiency makes us vulnerable to disease. When we've been traumatized, low fiber intake may present significantly greater hazards, making us less able to deal with our stress and even more susceptible to chronic illness.

Probiotics are the healthy bacteria in our microbiome. We can consume them in food and as supplements. Probiotics work synergistically with fiber, restoring the healthy balance in our microbiome, decreasing the intestinal inflammation caused by stress, and helping repair leaks in our gut. Probiotics send messages back to our brain through the vagus nerve, modulating the stress response, decreasing anxiety, and at least in animal experiments, increasing the levels of BDNF in the hippocampus.

Fermented foods act as probiotics. They include sauerkraut, kimchi, miso, yogurt, and the fermented milk drink kefir; indeed, any vegetables, beans, or fruits that have been fermented can all be probiotics; check the labels to make sure they contain "live" bacteria, which will augment the beneficial bacteria that are naturally present in the microbiome. Probiotics have repeatedly been shown to improve mood in depressed people and reduce anxiety in those under stress.

Prebiotics contain plant fiber that nourishes the good bacteria in our microbiome. Onions, garlic, asparagus, and Jerusalem artichokes are all particularly rich in prebiotics. Because prebiotics significantly increase the population of probiotics in the microbiome, they are likely to have the same beneficial effects as probiotics.

In addition to eating foods rich in fiber, prebiotics, and probiotics, I recommend fiber-rich breakfast smoothies and supplementation with probiotics.

A morning fruit and vegetable smoothie can contain ingredients you vary daily. I like to start with one-third water and two-thirds soy milk, but almond, hemp, cashew, and rice milk are also fine. I use blueberries, strawberries, and raspberries, which are high in antioxidants; cucumbers, celery, carrots, and avocado and, on occasion, other fruits and vegetables; and nuts. I add two to three tablespoons of seeds that are rich in fiber as well as omega-3s; chia seeds are the ones I prefer, but flax and hemp seeds are fine, too. An inexpensive blender will usually do the job. One to two ten-ounce glasses of the smoothie will give a delicious, healthy, gut-mobilizing start to your day and can be quite filling.

During the first months that you're dealing with trauma or long-standing stress, I suggest you take a probiotic capsule twice a day. It should contain billions of *lactobacillus* and *bifidobacteria*. Brands that have been used in research include Garden of Life RAW Probiotics Colon Care, MegaFlora Probiotics, and Renew Life Ultimate Flora Extra Care 30 Billion.

SWEETENERS

Added sugar and the sugar into which processed food is quickly broken down are prime culprits in the damage that comes with comfort foods and the standard American diet. Sugar, as I've explained, briefly increases our energy level before depleting it. And it's addictive, too, stimulating the production of endogenous opioids. Sugar briefly makes us feel good when we're depressed, but it soon leads to an emotional letdown. In some animal studies, sugar has proved more addictive than cocaine.

Sugar directly leads to weight gain and also promotes leptin resistance, which in turn keeps us from realizing we've eaten enough. Sugar increases cholesterol and triglycerides, and stimulates the growth of unhealthy, stress-promoting bacteria in our microbiome.

The excessive quantities of sugar that the average American consumes (nineteen teaspoons per day, sixty pounds per year) continually exacerbate our stress response and contribute to every major chronic illness, including type 2 diabetes, heart disease, stroke, cancer, and depression.

When sugar is contained in fruits and root vegetables, any damaging effects are mitigated by high fiber content and nutrients. When sugar is added at the table, in cooking, or most disturbingly and least obviously, in an almost infinite variety of processed foods, it becomes a dangerous, stress-inducing, health-damaging drug. If you do eat processed food, check the labels carefully. Avoid products with added glucose, dextrose, sucrose, rice malt syrup, or fructose; they're all forms of sugar.

High fructose corn syrup (HFCS), which is widely used in processed foods, including soft drinks, and is noted on the labels, is particularly destructive. When fructose is isolated and concentrated in HFCS, it is metabolized differently than when it's in fruits, where it's combined with glucose. There is no fiber to slow the absorption of HFCS; even more important, HFCS goes directly to the liver, where it's converted to fat.

As you clean up your diet, you'll likely discover that your desire for sweets goes way down. HFCS may well become nauseatingly cloying.

Bottom line: stay away from added sugar, and definitely stay away from soft drinks and other foods that contain HFCS.

Artificial sweeteners, including saccharin (Sweet & Low), aspartame (Equal and NutraSweet), and sucralose (Splenda), are a poor substitute for sugar. Each is toxic in its own way, and all make us crave more sweets. Several studies have shown that people who regularly use artificial sweeteners actually wind up consuming more calories than those who use sugar; they put on more weight and may be damaging their microbiome.

A little natural sugar will go a long way. Unfiltered, unheated honey, maple syrup, and blackstrap molasses retain their nutrients. Use them in small amounts. As you clean up your diet, your taste buds will become more sensitive, and a teaspoon in coffee or tea or on cereal will usually be enough.

Stevia is a sweetening leaf that I'm often asked about. There is no obvious toxicity but also very little research on it. However, its extreme sweetness (up to three hundred times as sweet as sugar) may lead to the same sweet craving as artificial sweeteners.

Supplements for Stress Relief

For many years, I've been recommending high-dose multivitamin and multimineral supplements for traumatized and stressed people. Every year, the evidence for their therapeutic importance gets better. It makes sense. When we're stressed, our body's demand for many nutrients increases. The need for B vitamins like folic acid, B_6, and B_{12} is most dramatic. However, since nutrients work in concert with one another, a slight stress-induced deficiency in one nutrient can inhibit the effectiveness of other nutrients.

Recently, researchers from New Zealand and their colleagues around the world have published important but little known papers confirming that a multivitamin/multimineral combination can successfully address many of trauma's most debilitating symptoms. The combination they used in people severely affected by an earthquake is called EMPowerplus. Its demonstrated benefits included significantly lower levels of stress, fewer painful, intrusive memories, and better sleep. The mood of those taking EMPowerplus was better than those who were taking a placebo control, and they had more energy. There were no negative side effects.

These studies are good enough for me to recommend EMPowerplus or a similar but preferably slightly higher dose multivitamin/multimineral supplement like Pure Encapsulation O.N.E. or Thorne, Basic Nutrients 2/day to anyone who's been traumatized or is under significant stress. Below, for your information and to use in comparison with other supplements you might want to buy, is the EMPowerplus recipe.

EMPowerplus Ingredients

AMOUNT PER SERVING	AMOUNT	PERCENT OF DAILY REQUIREMENT
Vitamin A	768 IU	16
Vitamin C	80 mg	134
Vitamin D	192 IU	48
Vitamin E	2.4 mg	160
Thiamin	2.4 mg	160
Riboflavin	1.8 mg	106
Niacin	12 mg	60
Vitamin B$_6$	4.8 mg	240
Folic acid	192 ug	48
Vitamin B$_{12}$	120 ug	2000
Biotin	144 ug	48
Pantothenic acid	2.8 mg	29
Calcium	176 mg	18
Iron	1.8 mg	10
Phosphorus	112 mg	11
Iodine	27.2 ug	18
Magnesium	80 mg	20
Zinc	6.4 mg	43
Selenium	27.2 ug	38
Copper	.96 mg	48
Manganese	1.28 mg	65
Chromium	83.2 mg	70
Molybdenum	19.2 ug	27
Potassium	32 mg	1

Other research leads me to recommend significantly higher doses of some of the vitamins and minerals that are in EMPowerplus, as well as some additional supplements. What follows is a list of them, with summaries of the research demonstrating their effectiveness and a range of doses. If you're a largish person (160–250 pounds), use the higher number for guidance; if you weigh less, take the lower dose.

In Addition to EMPowerplus

Vitamin D. As many as 50–60 percent of Americans may be deficient in this vitamin (actually a hormone), which is created when sunshine acts on ergosterol (a form of cholesterol) in our bodies. Vitamin D is critically important for the production of neurotransmitters, including serotonin and dopamine, and immune regulation. Its deficiency has repeatedly been correlated with major depressive disorder.

The EMPowerplus amount seems to me far too small to help the vast majority of Americans deal with their trauma. Testing for vitamin D levels is now part of routine laboratory screening. Find out your level. If it's normal—50–75 ng (nanograms) per mL—take 2,000 international units (IU) daily. If it's low, take 5,000 IU each day. Test again after three months, and consult your doctor if you have any concerns. And make sure you spend some time outside.

Zinc, which is so important for many biological reactions, blocks dopamine reuptake, as do some pharmaceutical antidepressants. It also supports BDNF production. Take 50 mg a day in addition to the EMPowerplus dose.

Selenium has been shown to decrease the incidence and severity of PTSD in traumatized people. It also reduces oxidative stress and works in several ways to diminish the accumulation of abdominal fat. Add 100 ug (micrograms) daily to the EMPowerplus dose.

Other Supplements That Can Enhance Trauma Recovery

Omega-3 fatty acids, as I've said, improve the transmission of nerve signals and increase BDNF. They have repeatedly demonstrated significant antidepressant effects and are also anti-inflammatory. I recommend 2–4 grams a day of a combination of docosahexaenoic acid (DHA) and eicosapentaenoic acid (EPA). Some research suggests that higher EPA content may be more effective for depression, so you may want to look at that number on the label.

It's easiest to get supplementary omega-3s in fish oil capsules (make sure they meet European standards, which ensure freedom from heavy metals and toxic chemicals), but you can also take a flaxseed oil supplement.

Turmeric, a yellow spice that is ubiquitous in Indian cooking, contains curcumin and other active ingredients. It has been shown to prevent the consolidation of "fear memory," which plagues us when we've been traumatized. Curcumin is also a powerful anti-inflammatory and antioxidant. Make turmeric a staple of your cooking as Indians do, or take capsules, 1,000–2,000 mg, twice a day. Add some black pepper to improve absorption.

Phosphatidylserine is naturally present in many foods, including white beans, soybeans, and cabbage. But if you've been traumatized, the amount you consume may be inadequate. Phosphatidylserine decreases the hyperactivity of the hypothalamic-pituitary-adrenal axis (which, as you probably remember, governs the fight-or-flight and stress responses). It may also increase memory and improve cognitive abilities in older people. Its tablet form is usually isolated from cabbage. Take 100 mg three times a day.

AND

Research indicates the following supplements can also be of benefit. They may, however, have side effects. I would introduce them only after your basic Trauma-Healing Diet is in place, and one at a time. Pay attention to potential negative side effects, including agitation or daytime sleepiness, as well as positive effects. After a week of taking and noting the effects of one of these supplements, you can decide whether to continue. Then, if you feel the need and it makes sense to you, you can introduce another.

Melatonin can be quite helpful for the disturbed sleep that often accompanies trauma and chronic stress. It is produced in the pineal gland, a portion of the brain located behind the point where our eyebrows approach each other. It regulates our circadian (daily waking and sleeping) cycle. An appropriate dose is 3–5 mg about an hour before bed. If you feel tired and hungover in the morning (a few people do), try 1 mg. If you're still feeling groggy, discontinue melatonin.

Passion flower extract can be extremely helpful for reducing high levels of anxiety and making sleep easier—without the side effects or addictive potential of pharmacological antianxiety drugs, like benzodiazepines, or sleeping pills. Take 15–20 drops in the morning, early evening, and at bedtime.

Rhodiola rosea has long been used by indigenous healers as a tonic for mental strain and physical weakness. Also known as golden root, it grows in the Arctic regions of Europe, Asia, and North America. Recently, researchers have demonstrated its benefits for both depression and stress-related fatigue. If you're feeling low in energy or depressed, consider taking rhodiola. Possible side effects include irritability and headaches. Take 100–300 mg twice a day.

What About?

Here, to complete this chapter, is some guidance about the trauma-healing benefits and trauma-compounding dangers of other substances you may enjoy, crave, or look to for help.

Black and green tea both contain caffeine, which can give you a lift when your energy is low. Black tea, which is fermented, has higher levels of caffeine: 60–90 mg per cup versus 35–70 mg in green tea. Both, and green tea in particular, have other virtues: a compound called epigallocatechin gallate (EGCG), which helps regulate blood sugar; and theanine, an amino acid that has been shown to enhance concentration and creativity and reduce anxiety. Most of us can happily drink several stress-reducing and enlivening cups of tea each day.

Coffee. The story about coffee, our most popular beverage, is still unfolding. For years coffee was demonized as a significant contributor to anxiety, hypertension, heart disease, and cancer. The scientific pendulum is now swinging the other way. For many of us, the benefits of coffee, which contains very high levels of antioxidant polyphenols as well as stimulating and energizing caffeine (some 95 mg per eight-ounce cup), outweigh potential hazards.

In recent years, research on the rate at which we metabolize coffee has helped to clear up some of the confusion. The 50 percent of us who clear coffee from our systems quickly—we're called "fast metabolizers"—are likely to benefit from drinking it. If you're a fast metabolizer, you'll feel coffee's stress-reducing and energy-enhancing effects. Enjoy it. If you're a slow metabolizer, high levels of caffeine linger in your body, and energizing benefits are often outweighed by anxiety and agitation. Experiment with small amounts of coffee or stay away from it.

Alcohol, like comfort foods, is a short-term trauma solution with long-term negative consequences.

As I described earlier, when trauma is overwhelming, our brain produces endorphins, which distance us from and numb our pain. When, over time, our post-trauma endorphin levels bottom out, we experience withdrawal symptoms, like anxiety and agitation, and we may be plagued by memories of being powerless. That's when we're likely to turn to alcohol to elevate our endorphins, inhibit the memories of traumatic events, and keep our emotional pain at bay. When stress is chronic, alcohol may also seem like a viable solution; it can temporarily elevate our mood as well as quiet our anxiety.

The most immediate problem is that, in addition to raising endorphins, alcohol also inhibits areas in the prefrontal cortex that promote judgment and compassion, making it too easy for some of us to act impulsively and aggressively. The soldier back home, drinking to subdue the demons of traumatizing combat, winds up punching out the guy who accidentally brushes up against him; the civilian, overwhelmed with economic struggles and memories of childhood abuse, takes it out on his wife and kids.

Over time, there are other problems. Chronic high consumption of alcohol takes a significant toll on our GI tract. It inhibits liver detoxification, disrupts the balance of our microbiome, makes our gut more leaky, and raises stress levels that the alcohol was meant to lower. And of course, with its empty calories, it can contribute significantly to weight gain.

A beer in the evening or a glass of wine for women, two for men, can be relaxing and okay for most of us. If you start drinking more or are increasingly dependent on drink, you know you're headed in the wrong direction. That's the time to cut down or stop. If even a small amount of alcohol makes you more aggressive, it's clearly contraindicated. And remember, if you've been drinking heavily and have stopped, you may well experience withdrawal symptoms, including a flood of stressful feelings, depression, and terrifying memories of trauma.

If alcohol is becoming a problem and you want to stop, as you should, acupuncture is a safe, side-effect-free way to raise your endorphins and reduce withdrawal symptoms.

Tobacco. I remember during the war in Kosovo, the bars and restaurants were choked with smoke. Everyone was puffing away—all the time. And it doesn't happen just in eastern Europe or during a war. The smoking rates among those who've been traumatized are consistently very high here in the US.

It's not surprising. Nicotine and tobacco can, in the short term, reduce anxiety, enhance energy and mood, and even partially suppress memories of trauma. The problem is long-term use. In addition to all the pulmonary, cardiac, and cancer dangers of smoking, it can, over time, increase cortisol levels and even contribute to the consolidation of traumatic memories. Again, short-term symptom relief is eclipsed by the long-term downside.

If you smoke, you may be able to cut down significantly by bringing mindfulness to your use of tobacco. You'll find if you smoke mindfully that it's really only the first two or three puffs that give you the effect you're looking for. The more you bring mindfulness and Soft Belly breathing into your life, the calmer and more energized you'll be. You'll feel less need to reach for a cigarette, and if you do light up, you'll realize that two or three puffs give you the relief you crave. Soon, a few slow, deep breaths will give you an effect that is just about as satisfying and stress relieving, if not as dramatic, as a few hits of nicotine.

Acupuncture has repeatedly been shown to be effective in stopping smoking and dealing with tobacco withdrawal.

And if you're thinking of starting to smoke—don't.

Marijuana. Marijuana (pot, cannabis, weed, boo, chronic, etc.) is often used and celebrated as a remedy for post-traumatic stress and anxiety. This makes sense. The endocannabinoid system of molecules and receptors, with which the pot we smoke communicates, is widely distributed in our brains and bodies, and it is intimately involved with our stress response. Indeed, many people who smoke pot or hashish (which has high doses of cannabis resin) or eat food containing it feel less anxious, happier, more "mellow." Some, however, find themselves more anxious and fearful.

Careful testing is now beginning to reveal the differences among the various strains of marijuana and some of the differences in individual reactions to these varieties. Strains that are high in the minimally psychoactive ingredient cannabidiol (CBD) lower autonomic nervous system hyperarousal (fight or flight) and are tranquilizing. They have been shown to reduce the impact of trauma-induced memories and to lower levels of fear.

High levels of the highly psychoactive compound delta-9-tetra-hydrocannabinol (THC) are anxiolytic (anxiety ending) for many people. They get "high" and happy, find relief from trauma symptoms, connect more easily with other people, and gain perspective on what's happened to them. Others find high-THC pot anxiogenic (anxiety producing); some become paranoid.

Bottom line: if marijuana relaxes you, moderate use may be beneficial. If high-THC pot makes you anxious, you can get a prescription (in the increasing number of states where it's legal) for strains that contain high levels of anxiety-reducing CBD or use a research-tested mixture of CBD-rich pot and hemp called Charlotte's Web.

It's important to note that teenagers with developing brains shouldn't use high-THC pot. It may reduce their stress, but it brings with it significant risks of damage to their developing cognitive functions.

What to Expect from the Trauma-Healing Diet: A Final Word

Sometimes you'll quickly feel the benefits of the Trauma-Healing Diet. Sometimes the effects will be gradual and subtle. The shift to a largely organic, whole-food, plant-based, high-fiber diet is likely to make you feel more relaxed and energized in a week or two. Eliminating gluten or dairy can lift brain fog and increase energy in days. Significantly decreasing highly processed food and sugar, particularly in somebody who's been a comfort-food junkie, can have similarly rapid results. The benefits of eating more good fats and fewer bad ones will appear in weeks or months. The effects of multivitamins, multiminerals, and other supplements may become apparent quickly or slowly, depending on the degree of your deficiency and your individual biological makeup. All these changes will help you begin to lose unwanted trauma-induced weight—within a few weeks or even days.

Eating wisely and sticking to the diet I've outlined and the supplements I've suggested, decreasing or eliminating alcohol and tobacco, combined with everything else you're learning and using, is a reliable path to sure and steady trauma healing. Even if you don't immediately feel that your new diet is making a difference, you can know that it's providing a firm foundation for your comprehensive trauma-healing program. And it's putting you on the royal road to long-term good physical, emotional, and mental health.

11

The Wisdom of the Body

INDIGENOUS HEALERS—the shamans of Siberia and their counterparts around the world—have long known that we can ask our bodies what is happening in them and that our bodies, eager to respond, will tell us how to mend what's been broken and heal what's been hurt. They (and also the Greeks who created Western medicine) understood and continually experienced the inextricable connection between mind and body. They learned to speak the body's language and to listen carefully to the lessons it teaches, when we are ready to hear and learn.

All of us can do what they've done: call on the wisdom of our bodies to help us heal our trauma. This may seem improbable, flaky, New Age-y, or hopelessly primitive. The thing is, it works.

In this chapter, we're going to do three of these trauma-healing shamanic experiments. The first is a demanding, energizing, expressive meditation. It's called Chaotic Breathing. The second is another application of the written Dialogue we did with our emotions in chapter 6, "All Emotions Are Innocent"; this time you'll be in Dialogue with a physical symptom, problem, or issue. The third is an Inner Journey, a guided tour of your inner world that will invite your body to share with you its secrets and its wisdom.

Chaotic Breathing

Chaotic Breathing is fast and deep, as fast and deep as you can possibly do it, in and out through the nose. It's powered by your arms, elbows bent, fists close to your chest, rising and falling as hard and fast as you can force them, like a bellows or the wings of a bird taking off.

I first did Chaotic Breathing with Shyam forty-five years ago as the first stage of an hour-long, five-stage "Dynamic Meditation" that he had learned from one of his teachers, Bhagwan Shree Rajneesh. When, a year later, I asked with considerable apprehension which meditation I should do and for how long, Shyam responded immediately, as if he had been waiting for the question—which perhaps he had: "Chaotic Breathing. Every day. For forty minutes."

I thought I'd misheard. An exhausting fifteen minutes had been my previous limit. He raised his eyebrows à la Groucho Marx: "You asked."

And so I did it, day after day, surrounded by bales of hay on the floor of the barn on the farm where I lived with Sharon, in the DC apartments of friends I stayed with when I worked long hours with runaway and homeless kids, and in hotel rooms as I traveled the country. Occasionally I did it outside, where farm animals would gather to observe me.

Many mornings I groaned in pained anticipation, put it off with coffee, phone messages, and newspaper headlines. And when I finally did begin, I had to push. I pushed and resisted and learned to push harder, through fatigue and fears of injury and the excuse for stopping provided by pain, and also through laughter at my fear and my excuses. On and on for forty minutes.

I did it every day for six months. Every injury and hurt I had ever experienced cried out. Every worry I had ever imagined, and others that were buried too deep for imagination or years of psychotherapy and psychoanalysis, rose to the surface, pumped out by the bellows force of movement and breath.

Occasionally, usually after effort that had seemed beyond my capacity and pain I thought I couldn't endure, something wonderful happened. The rate and force of movement and breath were increasing, but all effort fell away. I was no longer breathing or moving. I was being moved, and "it"—some force way beyond me—was breathing me. It was, I suppose, a small version of what religious mystics have described as ecstasy, a time beside or outside of oneself. And of course, as soon as I began to think about it, the wondrous experience stopped, and once again I was struggling to do the moving and the breathing.

Afterward, I lay down and turned from side to side with a baby's delighted abandon, as free of thought as I'd ever been. On occasion, I moved spontaneously into yoga postures that I could never consciously enter. When I followed Chaotic Breathing with music, I sometimes found myself whirling, my arms extended, happily watching the barn rafters and bales of hay spin around me.

Over six months, I became less fearful and angry. I felt less pre-occupied with and overwhelmed by past hurt and grievances, more agile, observant, and spontaneous, perhaps a bit more compassionate, more able to laugh at myself and at all the dramas of my life.

After what I came to think of as my six months' apprenticeship, I began to know when Chaotic Breathing might be just right for someone, and I taught it to them. At first, hardheaded people like me seemed like good candidates, a journalist or lawyer, a surgeon, a soldier, another psychiatrist; then, it seemed right for people who had buried emotions deeply and had protected themselves with walls of confidence that were beginning to crack; then, for chronically trau-matized, emotionally shut-down, physically tight men and women.

Soon other people seemed appropriate: fearful, lonely, depleted, and depressed men, women, and children, the hyperactive and the easily distractible. Sometimes, people whom I never expected to like it embraced Chaotic Breathing like a long-lost love.

You'll want to create a playlist for Chaotic Breathing, as you did for Shaking and Dancing. Once again, there are three stages. The first stage is the Chaotic Breathing. Best to begin with five to eight minutes and increase the time if and when it feels right (you might check with your Wise Guide if you're in doubt). The second stage is three or four minutes of relaxed awareness. The third stage is free movement to music.

I like to use the first track of Rajneesh's (he is now called Osho) *Dynamic Meditation* for the fast, deep breathing, but you can use any kind of insistent, rhythmic, repetitive music that will push you to breathe faster and deeper. For the third part, you can use, as with the Shaking and Dancing, any music that is energizing, inspirational, or celebratory for you.

Shaking and Dancing is for everyone. Chaotic Breathing may require some of you to make modifications. If you have "malignant" high blood pressure (say a 180–200 over 100–120), a pacemaker, a history of heart disease, metastatic cancer, significant shoulder, neck, or head injuries, or are pregnant, you should simply breathe deeply in and out through your nose, without any other physical exertion. If you have any doubts, consult your physician before you proceed with this experiment.

HERE IS HOW I taught, and still teach, Chaotic Breathing:

You're going to breathe in and out through your nose as deeply and as fast as you can. Don't breathe through your mouth. If you do, you may well hyperventilate. If you breathe in and out through your nose, you won't.

Create loose fists with your hands and bring them close to your chest, so they're about six to eight inches apart, in front of and to the side of your sternum, your breastbone. To deepen and intensify the breathing, raise your elbows and, with them, your shoulders as you breathe in and then bring your elbows forcefully down to your sides as you breathe out. This creates the bellows-like effect that brings more breath deeper and more forcefully into your lungs. Keep going; when you feel like stopping, as you likely will at some point, pick up the pace.

HOWARD WAS ONE of those people for whom Chaotic Breathing seemed right. He had come to me in distress and confusion, discouraged and ashamed of his inability to be as book smart and successful as his father. The LSD and magic mushrooms he had taken to help him find his way only showed him how lost he was: he had risen to grandiose heights, believing that somehow his good intentions could help bring peace to the Middle East, before he crashed in disappointment and despair. He seriously considered killing himself, took a handful of pills, and was hospitalized. A few weeks later, he was discharged, on step-halting, mind-slowing medication, diagnosed as bipolar, and told to expect, and fear, repeats of the cycle of depression and mania.

I listened for an hour to Howard's disordered attempts to meet his family's expectations for intellectual excellence and responsible social action. Sports had always been his great joy, but his prescriptions had made him inactive. Howard felt alone with his pain. In his isolation and inactivity, his grandiosity and shame had grown wildly. Still, I could feel in him an energy that could be aroused and channeled, a steady current of kindness and concern for others who were suffering.

"You are," I apparently concluded (he recently reminded me of it), "fucked up. But you're okay." By which I meant that he was deeply troubled and confused, had been traumatized by injunctions, expectations, mixed messages, and loss. And, yes, he did appear to qualify for the ominous diagnosis of bipolar disorder. But still . . . I told Howard that I believed his condition could be temporary, that there was in him a basic sanity. He needed to find it, appreciate it, live it.

Chaotic Breathing would, it seemed to me, begin to untangle the knots of his self-limiting, self-destructive beliefs and attitudes, the impossible demands he made of himself, his false hopes and his debilitating shame. I showed him how to do it, we did it together, and I wrote it on a prescription pad: "Chaotic Breathing. Twenty minutes a day."

That was thirty-five years ago. Howard still does his Chaotic Breathing—just about every day. "It keeps me going, moving through whatever comes up. Afterward I feel lighter, less worried about the past or future, ready to deal with my day." He combines it with Soft Belly breathing, which quiets him, and yoga, which dispels rumination and keeps him loose. Occasional Shaking and Dancing helps him move through times of increased tension and take himself less seriously. Periodic consultation with his Wise Guide aborts flights toward grandiosity.

Over the years Howard has made money and helped bring peace to many, if not to the Middle East. Always a fine athlete, he found new calm and focus in his games, an ability to conserve his considerable energy and exploit winning openings in squash, tennis, golf, basketball, and Ping-Pong. In fact, he became national champion in Ping-Pong.

Howard does not take or need medications; he has a loving wife and happy kids. Financial setbacks, occasional crises with his kids, and the deaths of family and friends trigger and challenge him, as they might any of us, but they do not disable him.

And Howard is not the only one. I am continuously delighted, and often surprised, by the people who embrace Chaotic Breathing and the many ways it does its healing job.

As a child, Suzanne had erased her own needs so as to comfort and care for her alcoholic parents. As an adult, she had been fearful, embarrassed to assert herself. She took the nursing shifts nobody else wanted, nodded in agreement when she was harshly and unfairly criticized, and wound up with an alcoholic husband who was even more abusive than her father. She told me daily Chaotic Breathing gave her the energy, confidence, and courage to break the stranglehold of past insecurity, confront condescending supervisors, and leave her husband.

In a tent camp for orphans in Haiti, a grinning eight-year-old boy tells me, "I do the breathing that Father Freddie (the camp director and one of our CMBM trainees) taught me. Every evening." For two years, the boy had dreaded the sleep that brought him nightmares of his mother dying under the rubble of their home. Chaotic Breathing ended that nightly torture. "Sometimes I cry after I breathe, and of course, I still miss my mother. But I sleep now, peacefully, and I don't have nightmares."

Dialogue with a Symptom, Problem, or Issue

Dialogue with a physical symptom, problem, or issue—pain in your head or back, rapid heart rate, high blood sugar, a persistent rash, overeating—is very much like the Dialogue you did with emotions: a rapid, written back-and-forth with questions from you and answers from your Symptom, Problem, Issue. Here again, your SPI will mobilize your intuition to guide you to the answers you need.

Often the advice is practical—steps you've thought of but resisted taking. My injury-jammed, arthritically deformed knees remind me that I keep "forgetting" to do the tai chi that I know will loosen them, or that gluten really does cause them to become inflamed and swollen.

Sometimes a simple physical symptom can offer subtle psychological understanding and spiritual guidance. "You're holding on so tight," my knees tell me, one surprising afternoon in Gaza. "Stop trying to make things happen that are beyond your control."

You can do the experiment now. Choose a physical symptom, problem, or issue. Give it an initial—for example, *P* for the pain in my knee, and go back and forth between you (*J* for me) and your SPI. Asking. Listening. Asking again.

Give yourself ten to fifteen minutes. Write the Dialogue in your journal so that you can refer back to it later. Go back and forth as fast as you can. Repeat this experiment whenever you are troubled by the same or another physical symptom, problem, or issue.

The Inner Journey: The Body Scan and Beyond

Chaotic Breathing dissolves fixed physical and mental patterns, and surfaces buried emotions that may have kept you from awareness, change, and Transformation. Dialogue with your SPI engages your imagination and gives you hints of what you can learn from one troubled part of your body. Now you're ready to use a shaman's version of a Body Scan to go farther and deeper on your Inner Journey— to attend to and take in a larger portion of the wisdom that your body can share.

A version of the Body Scan is included, along with mindful breathing, walking, and the postures of hatha yoga, in programs of mindfulness-based stress reduction (MBSR). Lying on your back, breathing slowly, you allow your mind to move up from toe to foot to ankle and through the rest of your body, becoming aware of sensations of tension and lightness. It's a little like the muscle relaxation I taught you when we first did Soft Belly.

MBSR has repeatedly proven the effectiveness of this Body Scan as part of a program that lowers levels of stress and stress hormones, decreases anxiety and pain, and increases immunity. One study that focused on using the Body Scan showed that it was by itself an important contributor to MBSR's effectiveness. A variation on the Body Scan used by physical therapists that involves motion as well as body awareness has been shown to improve overall health and give patients who practice it a more hopeful perspective on their chronic conditions.

The Inner Journey we're going to take begins with the awareness and relaxation of a Body Scan but moves into deeper, shamanic territory that includes active exploration, inquiry, and dialogue. This Inner Journey may bring you surprising, trauma-healing, life-changing discoveries.

Give yourself twenty to thirty minutes for this experiment, then another ten to twenty minutes to assimilate what you've learned and record it in your Journal.

You may want to prepare for this experiment by spending ten or fifteen minutes glancing at anatomic illustrations to familiarize yourself with or remind yourself of your body parts. I like the elegant Frank Netter illustrations we used in medical school and include about fifteen of them in a slide show before I do the experiment with our CMBM trainees. These are bird's-eye views of the body's major systems—cardiovascular, digestive, musculoskeletal, etc.—and regions. You can find the Netter pictures in his *Atlas of the Human Anatomy* or spend a little time with the easy-to-assimilate images in *The Anatomy Coloring Book*. You can also, with a little searching, find appropriate images free of charge on the websites listed in the Notes. You're not meant to memorize these illustrations or to aim for anatomical correctness in your explorations; just get general impressions of the territory you'll be traveling.

You can sit or lie down for this experiment or, if you want, stand. I recommend music with this scan. It will ease your progress through your body and encourage all its parts and organs to yield their wisdom to you. I use a Lapland chant that combines the haunting voice of Mari Boine with drums and flute that soar and fall as the chant rolls forward. You can find it on our website—and, of course, you can use other, similar journey-encouraging music.

After you've read my description, you can listen to my voice speaking over Mari's song on our website (cmbm.org). Or you can, if you prefer, record the instructions I'm giving in your own voice, over Mari's chant or a similar inspiring, encouraging melody.

We'll begin, once again, with several minutes of slow, deep Soft Belly breathing.

Once you've become aware of your breathing, I'll guide you to follow your breath into your lungs and move with it as it enters your blood and flows with your blood through your body. As blood and breath continue their journey, you'll become aware of the organs they reach and the parts of your body. Then I'll guide you back to your heart. You'll become aware of yourself sitting in your heart. Then I'll ask you to start again. This time I'll encourage you to follow your breath and blood, and my words and the music, to a place in your body to which you're being called—a place of pain perhaps, or of curiosity or wonder. Once you're there, I'll suggest you look around, feel, and listen. Then you'll ask that place in your body, "Why am I being called here?" And then, perhaps, "Why are you giving me trouble?" and "What do I need to learn?" You'll ask questions and wait for the answers.

After several minutes of this dialogue of discovery, I'll call you back to your heart.

Next, I'll invite you to travel to another part of your body that's calling to you, where, once again, you'll pay attention to your surroundings and ask questions to uncover the information and discover the guidance you need.

Afterward, you'll return to your heart and become aware of your breathing. Then you'll open your eyes and bring yourself and your mind back into the room where you're sitting.

It may sound strange. "How can my symptoms give me an answer?" "What on earth does it mean for my stomach to talk to me?" I completely understand your skepticism. I suggest that you think of this imaginative voyage as another experiment. You don't have to have faith or even belief. Just do the experiment. And pay attention to the results. I've seen thousands of people astonished and liberated by what they've learned.

There is no wrong way to do this experiment. No experience that is better or worse. Just follow the instructions. Let my words and the music, as well as your breath and blood, take you where you are called or pulled or pushed. Take your time. Slowly. Slowly. Become aware. Ask what you need to know. And listen, feel, and sense the information, the answers that come. Here are a few examples:

Katie, a superconscientious physician who endlessly, exhaustingly checks herself out for personal shortcomings, finds herself joyously "dancing with my amygdala," dispelling her hypervigilance, laughing at her tendency to excessive self-criticism.

"There was a dark knot in my lung," explains Thomas, who has since childhood had asthma attacks provoked by anxiety. "I looked closely and asked what was happening. I saw something I'd totally forgotten: myself almost drowning when I was four. The strands of the knots loosened, fell aside, and I could breathe."

Rhea was shocked to find herself in the cold, damp cave of her vagina. "Why am I here?" she demanded. "This is your place. It's not your father's," came the answer. "Send him away. He's been here for fourteen years since he forced you to have sex." Rhea relaxes and cries, and the cave gently curls around her. "I am yours," it whispers, and Rhea feels an unfamiliar pleasure that warms her everywhere. "It's my body," she says softly, and with strength and triumph, "my body."

LET'S BEGIN YOUR Inner Journey now, giving each stage, each stop on it, your loving attention. As I guide you on this journey for the first time, I'm going to tell you some stories. You'll likely want to omit them when you return, in the future, to this shamanic practice.

Sit comfortably in your chair or lie on the floor—or, if you like, stand easily, with your knees a little bent. Eyes closed, breathing slowly and deeply.

Breathe in through your nose and out through your mouth, with your belly soft and relaxed. Become aware of the breath with its life-giving oxygen going in through your nose, moving through the back of your throat, down through your trachea, into your lungs. Breathe deeply, imagining, becoming aware of the breath entering your lungs, going through the branches of your bronchi down into the smaller passageways, the branching bronchioles, until finally the breath ends in the alveoli, the little sacks at the end of the smallest bronchioles.

Now let the sound of my voice and the sound of the music bring you, along with your breath and the oxygen it carries, through the walls of the alveoli into your bloodstream. Feel yourself flowing now, with your breath and blood, from your lungs to your heart.

Feel yourself now in your beating heart. Become aware of yourself sitting there in your heart, as you breathe deeply in through your nose and out through your mouth.

Now let the sound of the music and the sound of my voice and the movement of the oxygen in your bloodstream bring you out of your heart, up into the aorta, the great artery that leaves the heart. And move with your blood and the sound of the music and the sound of my voice up into your face and head and then down into your back and buttocks. Become aware of the blood and oxygen in your face and head, back and buttocks. Breathing slowly and deeply.

Once again become aware of yourself, flowing with blood and breath, returning to and sitting comfortably in your heart.

Now, feel yourself moving with your blood as it leaves your heart and moves up into your shoulders and then down into your arms and hands and fingers. . . .

After a minute or two, return slowly, easily to your heart and become aware of yourself there.

Now move with your blood and your breath up through your aorta and then as it curves down through your chest, past your diaphragm, which separates your chest from your abdomen, into your belly. Flowing to all the organs in your belly. Imagining them now— becoming aware of blood flowing to your stomach and spleen on your left. Now to your liver and pancreas and gallbladder on your right. Become aware, now, of the blood flowing farther down, nourishing your small intestine first, then your large intestine. Down to your rectum and anus.

Become aware, once more, of the blood flowing down the middle of your body, this time out to your kidneys—and then down through your pelvis and into your bladder.

If you're a woman, feel the blood and its life-giving oxygen bringing you to your ovaries, your uterus, and your vagina. If you're a man, feel yourself moving with breath and blood into your prostate, penis, and testes.

If organs have been removed or altered in any way, become aware of the structures that are present and of what is missing.

Become aware now of your consciousness extending the journey, moving with your breath and your blood down into your thighs, and your calves, your feet and your toes.

Now let the sound of the music and the sound of my voice bring you flowing back up to your heart. Become aware of yourself once again in your heart. Become aware of your heart beating. Rest there for a few moments.

Now let the sound of the music and the sound of my voice take you to a place in your body that's calling out to you. It may be a place where you've long had pain. It may be an organ that was once troubled and ill, or one that you're curious about. It may be a place that, to your utter surprise, attracts you in this moment.

Allow yourself to move with the sound of the music, the sound of my voice, the flow of blood in your body, and the oxygen moving in the blood. Your consciousness is moving with your oxygen and your blood to that place in your body that's calling to you, that's saying, "Come here. Come now."

Once you're there, look around. Become aware of what it's like to be in this place. What does it look like? What does it feel like? Are there sounds there? Are there smells?

Make yourself comfortable, and begin to ask: "What am I doing here?" "Why did you call me?" "What do you have to tell me?" Each time you ask a question, wait for the answer. And then, after the answer comes, continue to ask questions.

Perhaps your liver is saying, as it did to Suzanne, the nurse who felt trapped in an abusive marriage, "I need you to take better care of me. I need your help. I'm hurting." And then you may want to say, as Suzanne did, "Am I hurting you?" And then your liver may say, "You're drinking too much beer" or "You're eating too much fatty food" or "You have anger that's hurting me." And then you may want to ask it, "What do I do?" And the first answer may be very simple: "Don't drink beer every night." And when you ask what else you need to know, your liver may go on as it did to Suzanne. "Your anger is there because you won't express it. You always act like everything's okay, but inside you're hurting so much. You drink to drown your anger. You need to write your emotions in your Journal. You need to pound your anger out on pillows. You need to leave your husband."

Whatever the messages are, pay attention to them and keep asking the questions. Challenge the answers if you need to. Suzanne did. "I don't like writing in my Journal." And your liver may turn the question back to you, as it did for her. "Well, what do you want to do? What do you propose?" And an answer may come. "Well, maybe I should tell my husband that I'm angry because he throws his clothes all over the house and doesn't clean up the kitchen. And he reminds me of how little my father cared and how he disrespected me, and how hurt and angry I was. And maybe I'll need to tell him that unless he changes—I'll have to leave him."

"Hmm . . . that's an idea," your liver might say, as Suzanne's did. "That makes sense."

Continue the Dialogue, asking whatever questions you need to ask, becoming aware of the responses, asking again. And after you feel satisfied with what you've found out, thank your liver, thank your body, which is so wise, for helping you. Know, too, that you can always return if you are called again.

Now allow the sound of the music and the sound of my voice, and the flow of blood and the oxygen moving through the blood, to bring you once again back to your heart. Relax here for a few moments, being aware of yourself in your heart, breathing, relaxing, feeling the warmth and strength, the life-giving spirit of your breath and your heartbeat.

Now, let the sound of the music and the sound of my voice, and the flow of the blood and the oxygen moving through the blood, bring you to another part of your body that may be calling to you. Let yourself go wherever you're taken. This is not a matter of thinking, only allowing it to happen.

Perhaps you'll find yourself near the base of your tailbone, in your sacrum, on your right buttock. Look around. Notice that there's tightness here and that you feel confined and constrained.

Now you might say, "What's going on here?" And the answer might come back, as it sometimes does, in a humorous way. "I'm a pain in your ass."

And then you want to ask, "What are you doing there?"

And the answer comes back, "You know very well what I'm doing here!"

And you say, "No, I don't. Really, I need help!"

And the pain in your ass says to you, "Okay, relax a little more."

"Oh," you realize, "I need to let go, I'm holding on too tight. Do you think that's what tight ass means?"

And then your butt says to you, "I certainly do."

"Well what am I holding on to?"

"You're holding on to sadness. There's so much grief you have that you don't let out. You think you have to be so strong."

"Well, how do I let it out?"

"Ask again," says your tight butt.

"How do I let it out?"

"Remember to relax with Soft Belly breathing. Each time you do the Soft Belly breathing, remember that your buttocks need to relax, as well as your belly. Maybe then tears will come, maybe then you won't be protecting yourself."

"Is there anything else?"

"Yes, when people say something to you that you find critical, and you tense up to protect yourself—relax. Open your whole body, including your butt and your belly, and open your heart. Perhaps they're saying something to you that you need to know. Perhaps it's out of concern and caring, not cruelty and criticism, as it was in your childhood. Relax. Open yourself to what you need to learn from your friends and family."

When you've heard and learned what you need to hear and learn from this second part of your body, allow the sound of the music and the sound of my voice, and the flow of blood and the life-giving, healing oxygen in the breath that's flowing in the blood, to bring you back to your heart.

Become aware now of yourself in your heart and of your heart beating. Relaxing here for a few moments. Now let the sound of the music and the sound of my voice, and the flow of blood, and the movement of breath bring you back through your bloodstream to your lungs.

Become aware of the breath in your alveoli, those little sacks in your lungs. Now become aware of your breath, rising from the alveoli through the branching bronchioles, which get wider and wider as they ascend to and join with the bronchi; through the bronchi as they connect to your trachea. As you exhale, feel yourself flowing with your breath from your trachea into your throat and mouth, and out into the air.

Become aware of yourself now, sitting or lying or standing, breathing in through your nose and out through your mouth, with your belly soft and relaxed. Become aware of the air inside your body flowing out, the air outside flowing in. Become aware now of yourself sitting in your chair, lying down, or standing.

Breathe in through your nose and out through your mouth for a minute or two. Slowly now, open your eyes and become aware of yourself, aware of this moment.

Now write in your Journal what happened, all that you saw and felt, all that you learned.

THE ORDER OF this chapter is intentional. As we use expressive meditations like Chaotic Breathing to break free of long-held, habitual constraints, we begin to make a direct connection to parts of our body that can speak to us of disordered functioning, unmet needs, and unattended trauma. As we continue to pay attention, our organs and cells tell us what physical, emotional, and spiritual medicine will heal them and make us whole.

This life-affirming exploration can be critical to detoxifying and learning from the triggering events we'll discuss in chapter 12. It will help resolve the sexual trauma that we'll focus on in chapter 13.

12
Taming Trauma's Triggers

THE OTHER DAY, Emily told me she blew up at her ex-husband. He had told her that he wanted to take three of "my books" from the hundreds that still sat on her bookshelves. "What do you mean," the retired teacher demanded, "by using that singular possessive pronoun 'my' books?" She is shouting to make me hear how furious she was. "I screamed like a maniac, 'Why do you always hurt me?' My heart was racing. I was literally seeing red. Yes, people do that. I couldn't get my breath, and I thought I was going to fall down. It felt like the only reason he was coming over to take me to dinner, the only reason he saw me or said he cared about me, was to get those books. And I couldn't find the words to say what was happening or explain why it was so awful.

"My ex was reduced to stammering. He said he thought he'd been sensitive and kind by warning me several days in advance that he needed the books. And he reminded me that these were books that he'd read and marked up long before he met me. He couldn't understand why I was so enraged. Actually, he didn't know what hit him. And I didn't know what hit me till I thought about it later.

"After a couple of days, I realized how insane I was. How I was acting just as if it were the day he left the house and the day he asked for a divorce all rolled into one. No matter that he's been a good friend to me all these years, supported me financially, taken care of me. No matter that he calls me every day and I love him and I know he loves me. It all went out the window. Those three books blew up into all the pain, all the rejection and hurt of the breakup twenty-five years ago and, if I'm honest about it, all those years when I was a kid and my parents couldn't have cared less about me."

TRIGGERS ARE EVENTS—words, actions, or perceptions—that in some way resemble a past trauma and reawaken it. "They are," the novelist Neil Gaiman has written, "images or words or ideas that drop like trapdoors beneath us, throwing us out of our safe, sane world into a place much more dark and less welcoming. The past," Gaiman goes on, "is not dead . . . triggers have been waiting there in the darkness, working out, practicing their most vicious blows, their sharp hard thoughtless punches into the gut, killing time until we came back that way."

Trigger is such an evocative, appropriate word. Once the trigger is pulled, the consequences burst open in us like a fragmenting bullet, bringing back all the physical feelings, all the emotions of earlier trauma. This is so even if the trigger is only the palest copy of the original, as it was with Emily. Our brain and the rest of our body respond as if it were in brightest technicolor, as if it were all happening, in every terrible detail, right now.

An inadvertent brush of an arm in a bar, and a vet returning from deployment in Iraq pulls back his fist, primed to kill or maim. A woman who, years before, was raped in a dark alley approaches another alley and feels her head spinning, her gut clenching, her feet anchored to the cement. A friend who neglects to respond to our email brings back the stomach-dropping emptiness of early childhood neglect or abandonment.

As you can see, triggers shift our fight-or-flight response into high gear, or perhaps numb and freeze us when the ancient, life-preserving branch of the vagus nerve takes over. Meanwhile, the rest of our brain amplifies the effect. Our dorsolateral prefrontal cortex is deactivated, causing us to lose the context of present experience. Our right hemisphere is on fire with remembered sensations, and our medial prefrontal cortex is unable to evaluate the quality or even the reality of the threat, or modulate the intensity of the fight or flight produced by our aroused amygdala. And our rational, problem-solving, verbalizing left brain, turned off by reawakened trauma, cannot make sense of what is happening or speak of it.

It really does feel as if the present trigger were the actual past trauma. We are as out of control as we were in a battle or when rape or loss or a dear one's death first occurred.

TRIGGERS, AS GAIMAN'S observations suggest, are primitive and aggressive. The fear and agitation and numbing are almost always more extreme than the situation requires, the physical and emotional reaction untethered to any thoughtful evaluation of the actual danger. When Emily's ex-husband asked to borrow his own books, he was not re-divorcing himself from Emily or threatening the abandonment she had experienced as a child. But she reacted as if he were.

We can understand this as a still poorly integrated evolutionary response. An animal seems to learn, without conscious thought, to mount a whole-body reaction to anything that might threaten her survival. And she stores the information so that it is easily and quickly retrievable. The next time she reacts even more quickly to similar, possibly threatening sights or smells—far better to be safe than sorry.

Our far more complex human brain works by analogy as well as similarity. A borrowed book equals a life-disturbing loss. Moreover, the anxiety and anger or numbness and withdrawal that overtake us present an additional challenge. We feel ourselves forced to react, and feel frustrated by and fearful of that reaction—retraumatized by both the trigger and our inability to control our own response to the trigger.

The more often this happens, the more vulnerable we become to this trigger—and the more easily we are triggered.

And to make matters even more disturbing, any significant stress can produce the same emotional and physical phenomena as the trigger that resembles the original trauma: in laboratory experiments, loud noises or stimulant drugs that activate the fight-or-flight response also evoke visual and auditory flashbacks of specific and completely unrelated traumas—a beating, a rape, early loss, the death of a spouse.

To begin to tame these triggers, we need to know what they are. We need then to release the blast of emotions they have provoked, to relax in the center of their storm. As we do, we can begin to reestablish context and perspective: that was then, and this is now. Then we need to move on, using imaginative tools and techniques to encourage our triggers to become our teachers. As we do, they will tell us what is still traumatizing us and offer arrows that point to freedom.

THERE ARE FIVE stages to this liberating, trigger-taming process.

Become aware that you are triggered. First you have to know it's happening, to feel your racing heart and cold hands, to notice that you're looking all around, checking the street for danger, or spacing out in the middle of a conversation that a minute before had been of compelling interest. You have to know you're being triggered before you can do something about it.

Sometimes we catch on fast. Many women understand right away that their sweaty-palmed nighttime fear of open spaces and deserted streets is related to a previous rape or assault.

Sometimes becoming aware of a trigger is more difficult. It took Emily a couple of days to see that harmless book borrowing was triggering long-ago feelings of loss and deprivation. Some of us live at such a high level of arousal, we hardly notice a trigger that raises only a small bump in our agitation. Moira needed weeks and some friendly questions to see the connection linking her fear of open spaces, challenges at work, and harsh words to the helpless vulnerability of her car accident.

Others, like Angie, manage for years to dissociate themselves from their trauma, to look as well as feel pretty "normal." When a trigger is pulled, however, their bodies feel horribly out of control and their thoughts disordered. They're suffused with dread and have no idea why.

As a child, Angie believed that her "yellow skin" was a "mistake." She'd been abandoned as an infant by her mother in China and adopted at six months by caucasians from the US Midwest. "From the time I was a little kid, I felt totally isolated, all wrong, like a tropical flower in the Arctic." Still, she did everything she could to ward off "a tremendous undercurrent of grief," to deny her difference. When other kids called her "chink" or "gook," it was as if they were speaking to someone else. "I didn't feel like that was who I was."

When Angie went away to college, her self-protective illusion shattered. Innocently and accurately classified as a "person of Asian descent" on the invitations from Asian student groups, she was plunged into despair by the deeply buried but intense pain of her biological parents' abandonment. Later that semester, reading about discrimination in books by Asian Americans, she felt crushing chest pain.

Triggers can be even more dramatic and less comprehensible to our conscious minds. They can have Manchurian candidate automaticity. This is how it was, not long ago, for Todd. Without warning, he disappeared. His girlfriend was sure he was going to fulfill a threat he had made a day before to kill himself. In fact he came close, swallowing a handful of painkillers after he'd bought enough heroin and a needle and syringe to finish the job.

When Todd came to my office a day later, he told a long story about the frustrations of being a convicted felon working at menial jobs and living in a slum, hassled by cops who treated him like dirt, ashamed of the crimes he'd committed and despairing that things would ever change. Still, none of this explained why he'd suddenly become suicidal. He'd lived with these challenging, frustrating, and humiliating conditions for years and had never wanted to kill himself. What had changed? What was different?

His girlfriend, who'd called me when she couldn't find him, had told me about a recent phone call with his mother. Todd had asked her for money for a lawyer, and she'd greeted him with a storm of invective. Todd had told me that from the time he was little, she'd beaten him and called him "worthless trash." It was pretty clear to me that his mother had once again made him feel as ashamed, angry, guilty, small, and desperate to disappear as he had felt at four and five and ten years old.

"It was the call to your mother," I said.

"Oh," he looked at me, blank faced at first, "I'd forgotten."

"That's what happened," I persisted. "You heard your mother saying how worthless you were. It triggered all the old pain. You believed her, and you were also furious at her. If you killed yourself, maybe then she'd be sorry. Maybe then she'd care."

"Yeah," he said, his eyes brightening like an archeologist coming across precious, buried bones, "yeah, I think you're right."

AS WE AGE, many of us who were traumatized early in life are more easily triggered. This is likely related to the increasing vulnerability that comes with illness and frailty, as well as the marginal role of the elderly in our modern world, and the too-frequent callousness or indifference of medical care.

Over many years, Diana had dealt courageously and lovingly with physical illnesses, economic challenges, and more than her share of personal loss. Then, in her late sixties, botched surgeries and the chronic pain that followed set her up for triggers. During a day of bad pain or in the face of a doctor's dismissiveness, it is, she told me, "like the foreground disappears and I'm a kid back in my family, and one of them is doing or saying something incredibly hurtful. I have this terrible feeling, and it's too dangerous to put into language, because I know their reaction will only make it worse."

It is, of course, painful to become aware of our triggers, but it's necessary, instructive, focusing. "Pay attention," they are telling us. "Something's wrong. . . . You've got to do something."

You need to tune in when your pulse begins to race and your thoughts grow muddled; when your vision clouds, or you see red without knowing why, or you have the urge to run; or you feel like you're bound to a chair or bed; or when you cannot speak or can only stammer. This is a kind of Biofeedback—your disordered body and mind signaling, speaking to you. If you pay attention, you realize that you have been triggered and you need to find the cause and treat the problem.

Quieting our body, calming our mind. Soft Belly breathing, caring for and bringing balance to ourselves, is often the first step in taming our triggers. As we breathe slowly and deeply with our belly soft and relaxed, we quiet the biological storm. The fear and fury in the amygdala abate, and so does the chest-shaking tachycardia they've provoked. The knots in our gut begin to loosen. The ice in our hands melts. Self-awareness, memory, and judgment begin to come back online. Chaos subsides, and we begin to gain perspective on what has happened to us.

A pattern may emerge: "It was those words or that facial expression or this place or that person who did X or looked like Y" that brought on these feelings. And as we relax, we may realize that those words, gestures, tones, faces, and places evoked others from another part of our lives that had once disturbed, threatened, or indeed, devastated us.

The sooner we are able to relax after a trigger, the better. However, there is no fixed timetable. It took Emily a distraught couple of days, Todd a near-death twenty-four hours, Moira a few weeks, and Angie many years to become aware of what was happening and understand they were being triggered.

And even when we know, as Emily surely did, we may, at least at first, recruit reason to justify our reactions: "How can a person just expect to borrow books whenever he wants?" After a while, though, relaxation allows our perspective to enlarge.

Now Soft Belly breathing "flips the switch" for Angie. "It brings me back into my body." Ever since she learned it, she's been doing it several times a day for several minutes. Now whenever she feels tight or tense, whenever her hands are cold, she does it for another few minutes. "Soft Belly brings me back from the insanity of my thoughts . . . lets me look at what's thrown me off."

Shaking loose the tension. Sometimes when you're triggered, it may feel impossible to sit still, far more natural to shake off the blows, to let out the pain. Go right to Shaking and Dancing then, or one of the other expressive techniques, like Chaotic Breathing or pounding pillows.

That's what Angie does when, on occasion, a nephew's threats or her husband's anger, or the coming of Christmas with its memories of not belonging, or her young son's tantrums reawaken childhood terrors that breathing cannot calm. She does Shaking and Dancing for fifteen minutes. Afterward she feels energized and able to speak and stand up for herself. Sometimes, after her son's tantrums, she puts on music and Shakes and Dances with him. Tears come, and then laughter. They hug each other, and he tells her how scared he was, and she understands.

Angie's a good teacher here. Here's a CliffsNotes version. Make Soft Belly a regular part of every day. It will be reliably there for you when you feel the physical signs of being triggered. Then you, too, can flip the switch. As you breathe slowly and deeply, relax your body, and quiet your mind, the terror of the trigger often subsides. You'll regain a sense of control, gain perspective, see the trigger for what it is: the ghost, not the reality, of past trauma. When Soft Belly breathing doesn't do the job, Shaking and Dancing will usually break the spell and loosen the chains. It will return you, more relaxed and secure, to your present self.

And you can do either or both as prevention as well as treatment: before family gatherings that may reawaken memories of conflict, cruelty, or indifference; or meetings where you expect present challenges to remind you of past condemnation; or when you anticipate any situation—a car, a plane, an unfamiliar neighborhood, a party filled with strangers—where you may feel vulnerable.

Look and learn. If you've quieted yourself with Soft Belly breathing and used expressive meditations to release tension and bring up what's been buried, you're in a good place to look closely at your trigger and learn from it. Any of the techniques that mobilizes your imagination and intuition can help you do it.

Angie likes to use Drawings to explore and learn from her triggers. After a family quarrel that triggered her feelings of isolation, the Drawing of her biggest problem showed walls. A fiery one on her left protected her from her angry husband; on her right, a wall weeping tears separated her from her kids. "I saw so clearly the barriers that made me freeze. My husband's rage and the memories of anger it brought up in me, and my own old loneliness keeping me from being close to my children." In the third Drawing, the "solution to the problem," she has extended her arms to either side—one hand firmly holding her son's hand, the other almost touching her husband's.

A lunch with several young moms triggered Nora—who, at forty and after several miscarriages, is still childless—plunged her into a "black funk." She used the Body Scan to help her understand and heal.

"The scan took me to my uterus, where I really didn't want to be. And while I was asking what the fuck I was doing there, my uterus changed shape. It became a circle and floated up to my head, and I realized it was a crown. And I felt then, for the first time in my life—my parents had always wanted a boy, and now they're hounding me about an heir—that it was beautiful to be a woman. I felt such love for myself and knew I could bring my love into my husband's life and into the lives of many others."

My Wise Guide is my go-to source for clarifying triggers and directing me. When a too-quiet Sunday evening opened into intense longing for the child I'd lost, a hummingbird appeared. "Treasure the love you have for her," I was told. When I asked for more, the bird advised me to "make sure you give your son just as much love . . . and reach out to your sweet godchildren, too."

Taking the next steps. Next comes taking what our triggers are teaching us into our lives and moving ahead.

For Angie, more Drawings were the way. She gathered her family together to do them and asked her husband and kids to share the need and hurt that appeared on their pages; as they did, she felt her own relief as well as theirs.

Nora laughed with pleasure at the image of her "uterus crown," walked around the room with what she playfully imagined to be queenly grace, and found herself "getting romantic" that evening with her happy husband.

I did what my Wise Guide told me to. I wrote in my Journal to my little girl about the trees and animals I'd recently seen that she had loved. I called my son and texted a godson. On the street later that day, I found myself smiling at kids running home from school and babies in strollers.

Once again, here are the steps to take.

- Become aware that you've been triggered.
- Balance your body and mind, quiet yourself with Soft Belly.
- Release tension and emotion, raise your energy with Shaking and Dancing or Chaotic Breathing or another expressive meditation.
- Then pick a way to confront and contemplate and learn from your trigger: Drawings or the Body Scan, the Wise Guide, or the Dialogue with a Symptom (or, after you learn how to create it in chapter 17, your Genogram, your family tree). Work with it till it tells you what you need to understand and feel, and what you need to do with what you're learning.
- Then do it.

If you're triggered again days or weeks later, the pain may still be there, but your reaction is likely to be far less overwhelming. You now know what to do and how to do it. You'll be able to move through the five stages more quickly, with less effort. Afterward, you may feel a bit like you've worked out and showered: stronger, more flexible, and also more relaxed.

A COUPLE OF days of breathing deeply, Shaking and Dancing, and pounding pillows allowed Emily to grieve her losses—of her marriage and in her childhood—loud and long. When she consulted her Guide—a red fox—he was quick to help her appreciate the love and friendship she still had with her ex. "He ain't so bad," the fox confided with a foxy smile before he slipped away. Now she found herself amused at her extreme reaction to her trigger. A few days later, Emily told her ex she had overreacted and happily handed him his books.

13
Make Love, Not War

IT'S A BEAUTIFUL motto but far easier said than done, when you're suffering the aftereffects of any trauma, and much more difficult if the trauma is sexual, as it is for the one in five Americans who were sexually molested as children and for the hundreds of thousands who are raped or sexually assaulted each year as adults.

All trauma takes a toll on our sex and love lives. This is partly because the fight-or-flight response inhibits sexual desire and functioning. It makes sense. If you are in a life-or-death situation, stopping to savor sex could be lethal. When fight or flight persists, it can continue to undermine sexual responsiveness, interfering with existing relationships and discouraging us from forming new bonds.

When the trauma is explicitly sexual, the effect is heightened by memories that now overwhelm desire and make intimacy terrifying. When the trauma is inescapable, as it is with childhood sexual abuse or rape at any age, the damage is far greater and more challenging to repair.

Survivors of sexual abuse are swamped with toxic, terrified agitation and recurrent, unpredictable flashbacks and nightmares that shove them into numbed withdrawal. This withdrawal is biologically, as well as psychologically, induced. The endorphins that are released during overwhelming trauma reduce the physical pain of violation, even as they remove us—"dissociate" us—from the horror that's happening to us.

Over time, however, what was self-protective during a brutal and inescapable assault can become a chronic and terrible liability. We may feel cut off from intimate contact with our own bodies, terrified of other people's, and without hope of ever connecting.

Surgery on breasts and genitals can be traumatic and may evoke the same kind of numbed withdrawal. If a partner is repelled or made anxious by our physical change, the damage is compounded.

Sometimes, if we've lost a lover or spouse, and particularly if he or she has left us, the situation can be similar. The rejection feels physical as well as emotional. We used to feel vibrant and appealing, and now, after our loss, our bodies seem inert, alien. We're sure we're undesirable and unlovable.

Rushing to remedy any of these situations is likely to be counter-productive and even dangerous. If you're not ready for physical and emotional intimacy, the pain of the original traumatic events—the horrors of violation—will return to heighten your fear and deepen your frozen withdrawal. You'll likely find yourself more discouraged about having a healthy romantic or sexual relationship.

It is possible, however, to put your fears in perspective, reclaim your body, and live as a fully sensual and sexual being. This chapter tells Sally's story of violation and reclamation, of emotional, intellectual, spiritual, and sexual rebirth.

SALLY LIGHTS UP the room. I know it's a cliché, but she does seem surrounded by a welcoming glow. She moves and laughs easily and was eager, when we met recently, to hear my news and share her tears at the death of an old friend, as well as her joy in the mind-body program for kids that she's leading.

Sally is fifty but looks ten years younger. She is blond and blue eyed, and her body is strong beneath the kind of softness you might see in a painting of a goddess of mirth or dance, or love. She's a good wife and a doting mom, and is now a sought-after teacher, coach, and counselor.

Sally is a devoted, celebratory user of all the tools you are learning, a living, loving embodiment of *The Transformation*. She is also the survivor of a rural Texas childhood scarred and stunted by poverty, neglect, and violent, incestuous sexual abuse.

In the next few pages, she'll give you glimpses of her childhood and then trace some of the most important steps in her later growth, development, and healing. As she does, I'll highlight how she healed herself with the same techniques and tools I've been sharing with you.

"FOR AS LONG as I can remember," Sally begins, "my mother was trying to leave my father, but she never felt that there was any other place to go. She'd grown up with her own angry, alcoholic family. My father's violence, his sexual abuse of her and me, didn't seem abnormal. She knew she hated it, but she thought it was just how life was lived.

"He'd slap and punch her, and once he broke her jaw. She never knew if he would like the food she made him or throw it on the floor. He sexually tortured her—had her strip and pulled her onto her tiptoes by her pubic hairs. He hit her in the face while he had sex with her.

"From the time I was three, he would hit me with objects like frying pans and throw me against the wall. When he was drinking, he touched and fondled me and kissed me like a lover. At night he would lie on top of me. I felt like he was suffocating me, and I'd smell his breath and feel the bed going up and down and hear the creaking of the springs.

"Sometimes I was happy in the kitchen with my mother, but I grew up tense and tight everywhere in my body, holding my breath whenever my father was around, looking away, not wanting to make a sound, wanting to be invisible. I remember at eight sobbing while he yelled that my mother was a slut and told me that he wasn't sure he was my father.

"When I was nine or ten, he started telling me I was fat and ugly and stupid. I felt crushed and heartbroken. I did think I was stupid and completely worthless. I kept asking, 'Why am I here?'

"And as soon as I hit puberty, he'd leer at me and say, 'Look at that rack on her.' I was sick all the time with bronchitis, asthma, ear infections, strep throat. My teeth got gray from all the antibiotics. I did poorly in school.

"I was conflicted. I wanted so much for my mother to leave him, but divorce seemed so shameful. And like my mother, I didn't know if we could survive without him. When she was finally ready to leave, I had a grand mal seizure."

When I asked Sally how she survived this ongoing horror, she said she found solace in her dog. "She saved my life. I would hold her close in bed and use her floppy ears to wipe away my tears. Dancing was crucial, too. As a teenager, I covered and hid my body, but I needed to move, and I did, in dance classes with other girls and alone in my room."

Sally "craved warmth and kisses and someone putting his arms around me," but she mistrusted, feared, and avoided boys and men. "I was sure they were like my father. They only wanted to have sex and hurt me." She drank alcohol and used drugs to "quiet my fears and disgust," and wound up exploited by abusive boys and men who were very much like her father.

Sally did poorly in high school and avoided college, which was for "rich, smart people." Still, after four years of low-paying post high school jobs, she was desperate enough, and smart enough, to summon the courage to go: "I thought, 'I can't be a cashier in a gas station for the rest of my life.'"

Sally did her best to look and act like a college student, but inside she continued "to crumble." She was depressed and anxious all the time. "The simplest thing required energy I didn't have—studying, walking down the street, sometimes even getting out of bed."

She had the kind of dissociative episodes that often follow severe sexual trauma. "One day, I got off the bus realizing I had no idea how I'd gotten to campus. I would often feel separated from my body, lose track of time and space." She flunked all her courses. "I fell asleep crying and woke up crying. I thought, 'My father's right. Maybe I should kill myself.'"

Sally saw a psychiatrist and a therapist. The pills the doctor prescribed for her anxiety and depression made her feel calmer, but they did little or nothing for her depressed mood or suicidal thoughts. Sally often lost track of what her therapist was saying, but one thing did make a difference. "'Do something you like to do,' my therapist told me." And Sally heard her and did. Tentative and scared, she started country dancing.

"'I'm depressed and suicidal,'" she warned a man who kept asking her to dance. "'I don't like men, but I do like dancing.' He just smiled and kept dancing. A year and a half later, we got married."

Marriage brought some stability, affection, and companionship, but also terror. "My husband wanted to be my savior, and that drove me crazy. I liked cuddling but not the sex. Penises hurt. It was just like I was eight years old again, and my father was lying on top of me and the bed was squeaking, and I was suffocating and going to die. After sex with my husband, I'd run into the bathroom, vomit, curl up on the floor in a fetal position, and press my cheek against the cool tiles."

Sally joined a group for incest survivors. "I realized I was actually abused and I wasn't crazy, and there were other women who'd had the same experience." She felt "a little less ashamed, a little less guilty." Still, she was sure she was inadequate as a mother and in her job as a teacher's assistant.

In bed with her husband or on her way to work, or in moments of reflection, she felt herself sliding back and down, crushed by memories, unable to move or breathe. "I couldn't figure out why I was still so depressed, so suicidal. I thought, 'What's the big deal? Why can't I get over it?'"

The Healing Begins

Sally was a long way from feeling whole and healthy, but she had made progress. I want to highlight four steps she'd already taken to heal her trauma, steps that you can also take.

Reaching out. Sexual abuse intimidates, shames, and isolates those who are being abused. It flourishes in secrecy. Violence or threats of it, fear of exposure, and blame and guilt all compound the isolation and loneliness. This is most complete and devastating when, as it did for Sally, it happens to us as children, when we are imprisoned by the abuse of a parent or other adult on whom we depend. But it's also true for us as adults, when we're assaulted or harassed by people who have power over us.

Reaching beyond the circle of complicity—of compliant, willfully ignorant family members or rationalizing fellow employees—is, in and of itself, an act of healing. Sally did it first with a therapist, but you can also do it with a spouse, a partner, friends, or a family member you feel will understand—and now perhaps with others whom you might meet through #MeToo. The connection may be imperfect, the understanding less than complete, but you have begun to reestablish the capacity for social bonding that trauma ruptured.

This relationship begins to confirm the reality of an experience that you, as well as others, may have denied or repressed. You've been diminished and degraded by shame. Now you feel accepted and affirmed as you are.

Share what you've kept inside with someone you feel you can trust.

Find a way to feel good about yourself. This piece of therapeutic advice was simple and vitally important to Sally, like a rope thrown to her when she was drowning. She had—just about all of us have—the will and wisdom to grab on to it.

When we feel devalued by abuse, we often cease to value what had once given us satisfaction and pleasure. Doing something that makes us feel better is an obvious antidote. It removes us, at least temporarily, from despair, and allows us to embrace part of a recovered and renewed life.

When the pleasurable activity is physical, it's doubly beneficial. As we move our body, we're reclaiming it from our tormentor. It's our own. We're enjoying it. Dancing was Sally's way; Shaking and Dancing saved Darcy, the firefighter; weight lifting did the job for Jenna.

Many people who've been raped or sexually abused gravitate to martial arts. I encourage them. Here, pleasure in movement and physical discipline are enhanced by the knowledge that we are able to defend ourselves against future attacks. Working out and sparring focus us and also release suppressed rage.

Find a physical activity that suits you. Do it. Notice how you feel. Your own increased energy and confidence will encourage repeat practice.

Connecting with others who have suffered similarly. Joining the incest survivors group was another step away from the loneliness that abuse had enforced and a more intentional, focused kind of reaching out. These group members knew what Sally had been through and the toll it had taken. Listening to them, she understood that others shared her feelings and thoughts, as well as her experience, and that perhaps she wasn't as painfully different as she had believed. Sally began to shed the debilitating role of victim and to see herself as an active, strong survivor.

This validating peer experience was central to the consciousness-raising groups of the 1970s women's movement and to Vietnam veterans' "rap groups." It is a vital ingredient of support groups for people with cancer and other illnesses, for family members of those who died in the military, for adult men and women who were abused by parents, and for participants in twelve-step programs for alcoholics and addicts.

Check out the appropriate support group—for women or men who've been abused or raped. Go to a couple of meetings. If it feels right, keep going.

Find a partner who genuinely cares. Sally's attempts at adolescent sexual experimentation repeated her father's exploitation and justified and deepened her fears of emotional and sexual intimacy. This is what so often happens when we've been sexually abused. We are drawn to people who resemble those who hurt us and naively, hopefully, mistake sexual attention for true appreciation, lust for love, and possessiveness for caring. The drugs and alcohol we may use to quiet our anxiety and loosen our inhibitions plunge us into exploitative encounters that may have initially terrified and will later shame us.

Years later, as Sally began to appreciate herself, she could choose more wisely. When a man was persistent and affectionate but not manipulative and punishing, she was able, at least tentatively, to recognize that he was offering the possibility of a real relationship and a safe place for overcoming her anxiety. Though a loving sexual partnership was still beyond Sally's capacity, it was a beginning.

Be open to relationships. Be respectful of your own limitations, and make sure your partner is, too.

Embracing Mind-Body Medicine— and Transformation

Joining one of our Mind-Body Skills Groups. Seven years before Sally and I spoke, she came to a Texas Center for Mind-Body Medicine training, hardly daring to be hopeful but wanting so much to be able to feel at ease, to think clearly, and to enjoy or at least not dread sex with her husband. Soon everything began to change.

The small group was a revelation. Other incest survivors had welcomed, understood, and accepted her. But in a Mind-Body Skills Group (we'll visit one of the MBSGs in chapter 18), she felt something else, something I hope you feel as you read these pages: "Love and acceptance at a deep, caring level. I wasn't just an 'incest survivor,' I was a human being, and *best of all, nobody tried to fix me.*" Sally felt—as I want you to—unhurried, unpressured, safe. She could share her terror and panic, pain, rage, and shame, the shadow that memories cast over her present life, her stumbling ineptitude and lost time, and for the first time ever, the details of her abuse. "It was a paradox. I was PTSD, and I was not. I was so much more."

For Sally, the group was like going to a school where "learning was life-giving." Each self-care technique—each of the ones you are also learning—was like a new step in her very own dance of healing, a dance that she could enter whenever she wanted or needed to.

Learning to quiet her anxiety and find freedom. Soft Belly breathing quickly became Sally's reliable source of strength, as well as relief. Sexual abuse had made her feel powerless. Breathing slowly and deeply, she discovered she could safely, slowly release physical tension and enjoy her relaxing, softening body. "I could quiet my anxiety and stay present, even when I felt my eight-year-old's terror." She could move through rather than be imprisoned by her memories.

Doing Shaking and Dancing with her eyes closed, "I felt something more than social dancing had ever given me, like I could move my body freely for the first time, without it being sexualized. I was actually in my body—not numb, just enjoying it." Emotions—sadness and anger as well as fear—could arise, pass through her and go, leaving her feeling joy, tasting freedom. In all the years since, "when I can't sit still to breathe and feel so angry I could burn a city down," she finds release and relief in Shaking and Dancing.

Accessing her imagination and intuition. Sally and others who have been sexually abused have had their trust betrayed, their self-confidence undermined. They may have little faith in their own judgment and continually second-guess routine decisions, as well as romantic choices.

Now Sally used techniques that mobilized her imagination, like Guided Imagery, Drawings, and Dialogues, to explore and answer the kinds of questions that for years had utterly bewildered and regularly disabled her: "Am I too dumb to understand this concept or do this job?" "Does this person care about me, or is he planning to exploit me?" "Am I thinking clearly about a career decision?" "What kind of sexual contact is comfortable for me this evening?"

Slowly, she built up her muscles of intuition. Each realization increased her confidence, and each decision that felt right reinforced her belief in herself. As she discriminated and judged more wisely, she also found it easier to let go of paralyzing self-consciousness and cruel self-judgment.

Now, when memories threaten to overwhelm her, Sally no longer feels like a "victim" or even a "survivor." She's "a student with questions—'What can I learn? What am I supposed to do?'—and tools to find answers" to social and intellectual challenges and sexual fears.

Sexual recovery. Sally began to share what she was learning with her husband, accepting her own limitations and having the confidence to ask him to do the same. "Go slow," she was now able to tell him. "My Wise Guide is telling me we have to meditate before we touch each other. Let's do it before we take our clothes off. Let's do everything mindfully." Clothes off, they began by holding hands and looking at one another. Then they cuddled and fondled one another slowly, enjoying the contact and connection, creating a respectful, safe intimacy in which Sally, now controlling the pace, could welcome and savor arousal.

For weeks this is what they did and where they stopped. Then, only when she felt both ready and safe, did she allow him slowly, tenderly, to enter her. When fear came up, they breathed together and relaxed. Slowly, slowly, Sally was able to accept and enjoy intercourse and embrace orgasm and release, to feel, for the first time, that she was "actually making love."

Understanding her abusers. The Genogram—the family tree we'll discuss in detail in chapter 17—was a revelation for Sally. As she drew her many-generational diagram, she began to find explanations for what had previously been incomprehensible. She realized that the parents who had inflicted so much suffering on her had themselves been abused by their parents and other relatives. Their models for caretaking were, she realized, murderers, rapists, and alcoholics whose own fears and rage had blinded them to the humanity of those they'd harmed.

Seeing the patterns of her family tree on the page helped Sally relax with the reality of her past. She understood, for the first time, that she truly was not responsible for, or deserving of, her own abuse. And with safety and emotional distance, she was, to her surprise, even able to feel some compassion for those who, having been so badly hurt, visited such pain on her.

Sally's Genogram also offered glimpses of ancestors—refugees from famine and persecution—who brought with them examples of post-traumatic resiliency she could call on for inspiration. And as she drew symbols representing members of her new, chosen family, she recognized friends and teachers, Mind-Body Skills Group members and pets, all of whom she could call on for comfort, support, and guidance.

Finding Meaning and Purpose. Sally's story doesn't end with recovery. It continues. As she embraced her trauma-healing lessons, an alchemical process began to take place. Her mind cleared, her heart opened, and her motivation began to soar. As she found the courage to face what had once terrified her, she began to feel compassion for others who had suffered in similar ways and to realize that helping them was her mission and also an ongoing part of her own healing. She finished college, got advanced degrees in teaching and counseling, and began to lead Mind-Body Skills Groups.

The horror of incestuous abuse had opened a door of understanding for Sally, and she had walked through it, learning to love herself and her life, embracing her new generous Purpose.

Sally continues to share what she keeps on discovering and living with children and adults who have been sexually abused and also with those who abused them. The clinicians in her community gratefully refer patients to her.

Sally is a teacher by profession, but it is her life story, and Sally herself, who gives the greatest lessons. Her courageous commitment calls to me when I resist the path of self-discovery and self-care that will help me find my own way forward. If you, lost in present turmoil or imprisoned and hobbled by your history, ever feel despair, you may want to read her story again. Let her hold the light of Hope for you. If she can do it, so can you.

14

Nature Heals

THE FIRST FEW times I saw images of the natural world in the third Drawings I prescribed—the ones that showed people with their biggest problems solved—I was surprised and curious. In their first Drawings, of "Yourself," the artists had often appeared bent to a task, usually isolated and alone but occasionally in a stiff formal portrait with a family member or a friend. In the second Drawings, of "You with your biggest problem," they were sometimes hemmed in by prison bars representing family or work constraints, or, like Azhaar, tiny, barely visible in the corner of the page. Sometimes they were being menaced by domestic predators or armed soldiers, stalked by images of medical procedures, or intimidated by implacable clocks.

The third Drawings were, however, quite different. I kept seeing the unmistakable shapes of trees, flowers, mountains, and rivers. Usually the bodies in these third Drawings were more substantial, the faces more expressive, the clothes brighter. Imagining being in Nature seemed to have brought more life to the artists. And far more often than in the first two Drawings, there were others with them—people and animals of all kinds—as if hope for a solved problem was repopulating the natural world, as well as the mind of the artist.

Pretty soon I was noticing that a significant number of third Drawings—maybe even a majority—featured people, happily, even joyously, in Nature. Whatever their problem was, Nature was part of its solution.

It seemed reasonable for someone like Hervé, the security guard who lived in Haiti and loved to garden. I could easily understand why he drew his renewal, after his wife's death in the earthquake, as plants and flowers coming back to life. But I also saw Nature in the Drawings of Gaza's children and adults—trees with birds circling them emerging from landscapes of rubble, women covered in abayas, holding hands and looking out to sea.

When I started to pay attention, I found it was the same here in the US, and for city dwellers as well as rural people. The solution for an executive suffering through cancer chemotherapy was a climb on a nearby green mountain under a blue sky. A girl coming to terms with the betrayal and humiliation of her father's sexual assault was happily walking in her city park.

These Drawings remind us that Nature heals. We are a part of her (and, yes, I do think of Nature as primarily feminine, our nourishing, sustaining Mother). When we feel connected to her, we can relax, like a tree with deep roots. Our tight shoulders drop. Our breathing deepens. I remember these feelings from childhood, running and laughing as I embraced the freedom of New York's Central Park, or leaning on a railing contentedly watching the East River flow by. When we are close to Nature, our feet fall more happily on the ground. We feel once again that, like Nature herself, we, too, can grow and change.

THE SCIENTIFIC LITERATURE has begun to urge us to do what the intuition of traumatized people has grasped and our broken connection to Nature requires. Thirty-five years ago, researchers observed that hospitalized patients whose rooms looked out on trees were significantly "less upset and tearful" than those whose windows faced alleys or brick walls. Feeling better, recovering faster from their medical trauma, they left the hospital earlier.

In the years since then, researchers around the world have explored the variety of ways we can reconnect with Nature and the gifts she brings to our mental and emotional life and our health. People who look at pictures of rural scenes recover faster from stress and are more resilient than those who watch films of urban settings. Women dealing with the trauma of surgery for breast cancer are able to focus better when they spend time in Nature. Depressed people who stroll in green places have significantly better moods than those who walk city streets.

Recently, Gregory Bratman and his Stanford colleagues have shown that city dwellers who walk in Nature for only ninety minutes decrease activity in the subgenual prefrontal cortex, an area of the brain associated with morbid rumination, the repetitive, unproductive chewing over of negative thoughts about our lives and ourselves—exactly the kind of self-defeating mental activity that hobbles the brains of traumatized and depressed people.

This is a worldwide phenomenon. Research in England shows that people living among farms, fields, and meadows are less stressed and depressed, and they live longer than those in less green areas. One study suggests that the *mycobacteria vaccae* organisms that live in the soil contribute to this therapeutic effect by increasing levels of the calming, mood-enhancing neurotransmitter serotonin.

In Japan, research on *Shinrin-yoku*, "forest bathing," has shown the therapeutic power of walking in the woods, enjoying the sights, and breathing in air perfumed by leaves and bark with medicinal properties. Forest bathers in two dozen locations have demonstrated decreased cortisol, lower blood pressure, and increased vagus nerve activity—just the kinds of changes that are likely to benefit us when we're traumatized or chronically stressed.

We know now that Nature really does help us heal. So, what to do? Where? For how long? And how to get started?

SHARON HAS LESSONS to share. She grew up more at home in the wilderness than in her often neglectful, combative family—roaming the plains and climbing mountains in Wyoming, just like the Lakota people a hundred years before. Much later in life, isolated and crippled by car accidents and surgeries, and saddened by loss, she has maintained an instructive life- and meaning-giving connection to the natural world.

She renews it most intimately as she touches her body in those long, daily baths. She cooks deliberately, creatively for herself and a few close friends. She also enjoys the good fortune of living on a street with trees, in a house with a small yard. She pays close attention to the tug of the moon's phases on her joints and mood, and looks up nightly to wish on the first star. She delights in the faces and moods of the natural world around her, appreciates subtle changes in temperature and humidity, the warmth of the spring sun, the first blossoms on the tree outside her window, and fall's bracing winds. Sharon tends a tiny herb garden and uses her body to make angels in the first winter snow.

Most of what nourishes Sharon is available to all of us. Those of us who live in viewless apartments on treeless streets have to put out more energy to see and smell the natural world, have to tune in more consciously to its natural rhythms, but it's possible—and worth the effort. Over the last twenty-five years, I've come to know a number of HIV-positive former heroin addicts in New York City, many of whom were long confined to prisons. Traumatized in childhood and by the adult life they lived, they've told me about the joys of morning and evening pilgrimages to parks; deep salt-flavored breathing as they emerge from subways onto the sands of a public beach; and the thrill of floating, almost weightless, on waves. They speak with wonder about the joys of tending a plant on a roof, a fire escape, or even a windowsill.

TAKE TIME WHENEVER and however you can to be in Nature—an hour, an afternoon, a day, a weekend, or longer, to renew and heal yourself, to honor Nature and learn her lessons.

A twenty-minute mindful walk will get you started and give you the benefits promised by the research. Sometimes now I walk on my own street very slowly, noticing and saying to myself what I notice: the leaves on the trees, the reach and twists of the branches, little birds hopping and calling, insects buzzing and gliding around my head, the plants and flowers that flourish over several seasons in my neighbors' yards.

If your street is Nature deficient, go to the country or to a park. Even a small one will reward your effort and your awareness. Your eyes and mind will move up to leaves and branches. Your feet will feel the texture of dirt and rocks, your ears record the running water of streams.

Feeling Nature's rhythms, participating in her ever-cycling birth and growth, death and rebirth, we're reminded that change is also always happening in us—in our inner world of thoughts and feelings, organs and cells.

In Nature we may feel—without effort or warning—that trauma's burdens are slipping from our shoulders. We know then in our bones the truth that the studies tell us: that Nature relaxes and focuses us, lowers our stress hormones, and lightens our step. We get the message: the trauma that once overwhelmed us is not forever fixed.

Here, as always, our breath is a great teacher. As we breathe slowly and deeply, we can feel the connection between the natural world outside us and the one within us. We may recall, too, that the connection is both intimate and universal: trees provide the oxygen we inhale, and the carbon dioxide we exhale in turn feeds the trees. Breathe deeply, relax, and be aware that you are a part of Nature, that she is always caring for you, sustaining you.

MANY YEARS AGO, Shyam suggested some experiments that significantly enhanced my appreciation of Nature and of myself.

Here is one of them:

> Set aside twenty minutes or half an hour to look closely at a dozen leaves from a tree. Observe the size and color of each one, noting the great or slight differences in their shapes and contours. Look slowly, carefully, at a dozen more, or two dozen. You'll be surprised and pleased by the differences in each leaf.

You are as much a part of Nature as the leaves on a tree. And as you come to appreciate Nature's variety, you will also grow in appreciation of your own uniqueness. You'll get the message: differences between you and other people that may have made you uncomfortable can be opportunities for appreciation, reasons for celebration.

Planting a tree or flowers or a garden is an ancient and wise way to deal with the inevitable trauma of loss and death. Not long ago, at a meeting of families of men and women who had killed themselves while in the military, sponsored by TAPS, the Tragedy Assistance Program for Survivors, I had coffee with a farm-equipment salesman from a southern town. Richard spoke slowly, with a hint of a drawl, and offered me cream and sugar with formal courtesy.

"I sometimes see pictures of these TAPS families in my mind," he told me as we sipped our coffee. "All six hundred or eight hundred people from last year's meeting or the year before's—we've all been through the same thing. There's comfort and support, and I learn things, too."

He told me that the Soft Belly breathing I'd taught him in my afternoon workshop had quieted his preoccupied mind; Shaking and Dancing had helped him cry for the loss of his son, an army sergeant who had shot himself in the head after a quarrel with his wife. After the dancing, he felt the joy of his son's life. "Nothing makes the hurt go away," he explained. But he thought that these new techniques would "add something important" to what he has learned over the years about dealing with grief and commemorating and honoring his son's life.

There was one form of honor for his son—and healing for him—that he particularly wanted to tell me about, something he thought I might want to share with the people I worked with.

Several years before, he had planted a tree in a spot that was special to both him and his son. Since then he had regularly watered and weeded around the tree, watched it grow, and sat by it. Often, he came to the tree exhausted and dispirited. After he sat for some time crying, he felt renewed with wonder at the new life that was rising in the tree, at the hard-to-explain sense that this new life was somehow connected to his son.

RICHARD'S SON, the army sergeant who killed himself, had never had the healing immersion in Nature that should be the right of returning warriors. Indigenous people around the world understand that a cleansing of blood and rage, loss and guilt, is a necessary prelude to warriors being able to return to a peacetime community; that this purification and reunification needs to take place in Nature, in ceremonies where the weight of male aggression is balanced by female nurturing. In a number of North American Indian tribes, women elders used to bathe warriors and attend to their psychological as well as physical wounds.

Modern veterans, poorly served by perfunctory discharges, deprived of ritual reintegration into our society, have created their own rites of passage and repatriation that reaffirm this healing connection with Nature and their reunion with communities to which they're returning. What they have done can teach and inspire the rest of us.

The first man to walk the entire Appalachian Trail from Georgia to Maine was a World War II veteran named Earl Shaffer, who had decided to "walk the army out of my system, both mentally and physically." Sixty years later, significant numbers of veterans are hiking the Appalachian Trail or walking from one coast to the other.

Heath Lanctot, a former reconnaissance marine with two tours in Iraq, was offered eight different drugs by Veterans Administration doctors but "didn't want any pills." He decided instead to walk through the snow and desert on the Continental Divide, "to think about my past actions and clean things up."

And of course, it's not just veterans who understand the need for wilderness trauma cleansing. Cheryl Strayed's account of healing loss and addiction by trekking the Pacific Crest Trail was recently a huge bestseller. Many thousands of modern women and men are now walking "the Camino," the road in northern Spain where two thousand years ago James, Jesus's brother, is said to have made his pilgrimage.

Walking for weeks or days in the wilderness wears away old habits, wears down old fears, and extinguishes the guilt that has burned us. But occasional days or even hours in Nature can also help us let go of a trauma-heavy burden we no longer need, allowing us to move into the ever-renewing life of the present moment. "In wilderness," Thoreau observed in his essay "Walking," "is the preservation of the world, the one in which we live, and the one inside us."

Bending to Nature, bonding with her, we are pulled out of trauma's doomed loop, back into the ordinary, ever-flowing current of life and of our lives, of life and death and rebirth. We are reminded, too, that we are a part of something so much larger than ourselves, a world of wonder and awe and renewal that can calm our tense, trauma-fueled efforts to defend against past hurt and ward off future wounds.

Take the time. Make the effort to visit with Nature.

15
Animal Therapy

ANIMALS OFTEN APPEAR as our Wise Guides, as well as companions in our hopeful third Drawings. Over the years, hummingbirds, crows, and dragonflies have been my Wise Guides more frequently than ancestors, mentors, or gods, and as often as the beloved children who are my great teachers.

All of Nature can be healing, but our close cousins the animals offer us something special. They speak to us without words. They allow us physical closeness and offer undemanding affection. They listen to the pain we confide in them without questioning or judging. They are friends with feelings. And we can show them affection. This can make them especially important to us after we've been hurt by others or lost someone we love, when close human contact may seem dangerous or raise the specter of yet another loss.

After the twenty children were murdered in the elementary school in Sandy Hook, Connecticut, in 2012, many of the surviving kids were afraid or unable to share their terrible memories and ongoing nightmares with concerned parents or competent professionals. On the other hand, they flocked to events with therapy dogs and spent long, comforting hours holding and talking to them.

Children facing potentially fatal cancer and vets returning from combat often rate the companionship of horses—equine therapy—highest on their lists of healing experiences. Petting, feeding, and caring for rabbits sustained me as a lonely six-year-old away at summer camp. My youngest brother, Jeff, who bore the full force of our parents' escalating conflict, told me that he couldn't have survived the nights of shouts, tears, and blows without the sweet puppy who slept with him. Remember Sally, sexually abused by her father, wiping away her tears with her dog's floppy ears.

FOR MORE THAN two hundred years, sensitive clinicians have recorded and embraced the healing power of animals. At the end of the eighteenth century, psychiatric patients at the York Retreat in England were encouraged to spend time with farm animals. Benjamin Rush, known as the father of American psychiatry, patterned his Pennsylvania hospital program on York's. In the late nineteenth century, Florence Nightingale observed that visiting with small animals decreased the anxiety of hospitalized children and adults. And not long afterward, stern Sigmund Freud noted that his psychoanalytic patients lay more comfortably and happily on the couch and shared their painful memories more freely when his little dog Jofi moved close to them.

Over the last forty years, a number of researchers have measured this therapeutic effect. Several studies on healthy adults and those with hypertension have demonstrated that brief sessions with animals can decrease blood pressure.

One small study published in the *Journal of Psychosomatic Research* showed that this positive change was accompanied by decreases in the stress hormone cortisol, along with increases in mood-elevating beta endorphin, energizing dopamine, and oxytocin, the hormone responsible for bonding. And the experience was also a happy one for the dogs involved. Their levels of endorphins and oxytocin also increased. Interestingly, these hormonal increases occurred in the dogs as well as the humans *after only five to twenty-four minutes of interspecies interaction.*

Several years ago, Erika Friedmann and her colleagues published a particularly dramatic study of successful animal therapy. Pet-owning people who had been hospitalized with heart attacks or angina pectoris—heart-related chest pain—had significantly greater one-year survival rates than petless patients: "Of the thirty-nine patients who did not own pets, 11 died. Whereas only 3 of the 53 pet owners died within one year"—28 percent versus 6 percent. The difference was highly significant statistically and lifesaving for the pet owners.

Studies also indicate that people who have even brief contact with animals enhance their connections to other people. After three ten-minute play sessions with guinea pigs, autistic children smiled and laughed, and they talked to and touched other people significantly more than when they played with toys. These latter findings are especially important. Trauma may make us withdrawn, fearful, and suspicious. Our connection with animals, our sense of being known and accepted by them, and of caring for them, can be a living bridge bringing us back to caring for and connecting with other people.

Recent observations of bonds that form between people and parrots (yes, parrots) are particularly amazing. There are as yet no controlled studies, but the anecdotes and testimonials that are often the first stage of scientific exploration give us a gorgeous, moving picture of animal-human healing possibilities.

Early in 2016, a half-dozen friends forwarded me an article from the *New York Times*: "What Does a Parrot Know about PTSD?" by Charles Siebert, a writer for the *Times Magazine*. It brought me to tears, even as it raised my spirits in praise and hope.

Here is the gist of it. Several severely traumatized US veterans, disordered and disabled by the horrors they had seen and the ones they had perpetrated, had found redemption and recovery in caring for and connecting with parrots who themselves had been twice devastated by trauma.

The men and women, some previously suicidal and confined in psychiatric hospitals, came into the parrots' lives as emotional cripples, sleepless and enraged, mostly mute, often hopeless. The parrots they met had first been stolen from the wild flocks to which they belonged and had then, through death or desertion, lost the human owners who had given them a second secure home.

Rescued and arriving in sanctuaries, these disheveled, distracted birds exhibited many of the same symptoms as the traumatized vets they would meet. In Siebert's words, they were "ceaselessly pacing, rocking and screaming, cowering in corners, self-plucking, and screaming with broken-record remembrances."

Empathy—feeling with and for one another—bound vets and birds together. Fifty-four-year-old Lily Love, a coast guard helicopter rescue swimmer whose mind was fractured by guilt over dear friends' deaths, had been poorly served by prescribed medications that left her seeing "little green men and spiders jumping out of trees." Caring for the birds and cleaning their cages, Lily began to put herself back together. She is keenly aware of "the mutual trauma that I suffered and these birds have suffered, and my heart just wants to go out and nurture and feed and take care of them. And doing that helps me deal with my trauma."

During his time in the navy, forty-three-year-old Matt Simons, a brilliant student and former college football quarterback, "saw a lot of killing and things I wish I hadn't." Discharged, he became a heroin addict, almost killed someone in a bar fight, and wound up in jail. VA psychiatric medication and psychotherapy hardly helped, but meeting Joey, a yellow-headed Amazon parrot, made all the difference. "I was shy, burned by humans, isolated, angry. Joey had what seemed to me the same attitude. So we bonded. He let me touch him. Only me."

Parrots have brain centers that are highly specialized for the fellow feeling that permits them to fly in flocks and tune in to human speech and emotions. But the capacity for empathy is widely distributed in the animal kingdom. And all animals seem to have the capacity to evoke human compassion.

THOUGH THE SANCTUARIES where vets and parrots come together are exemplary, they are not necessary for bonding and healing. Here in much more ordinary and accessible circumstances is Lucy, a thirty-year-old artist who was cleaning a house where, not long ago, I was staying.

Lucy had struggled with depression since adolescence. A year before I met her, her boyfriend died in an accident. After he died, she resumed taking antidepressant medication, but she soon stopped it. "The pills cut off all my creativity. . . . I need to have a way to express myself, a reason to live."

Like many people who suspect they have experienced childhood trauma, Lucy still can't remember it. She does know that she always felt "alone and abandoned." Psychotherapy was helpful—she, like all of us, "needs someone to share my story with"—but animals, particularly since her boyfriend's death, have made all the difference.

"My most important therapist," she told me, "is my dog." When I asked why, she smiled, a bit puzzled by a question whose answer seemed so obvious to her. "Well, it's unconditional love, of course. No matter what you're doing or what you look like, or how bad you smell, she loves you.

"And then there is—I guess the best word for it is *presence*. I don't, of course, know what my dog is thinking, but it feels like she's just here now, with me, not obsessing about the past the way I sometimes do, no worry about the future. So she brings me into the present, too. I guess she sets an example for me.

"I take care of her and I love her, and that gives me meaning. It also reminds me to take care of and love myself.

"And also, it's so simple for my dog. All she needs is food and shelter and love. And when I worry about fitting into some social box, or what's going to happen in the future, I realize that's all I really need, too—food and shelter and love.

"Of course, sitting beside her, petting her"—she shows me how, stroking the air lovingly—"that's the best.

"And to expand the possibilities," she reminds me, "it doesn't have to be a dog or a horse; it can be goats and sheep, too, even pigs."

YOU DON'T HAVE to have animals with you on your trauma-healing journey, but they clearly can and do make the way easier. As they keep you company, they invite you to recover or enhance your capacity for trust, empathy, and generosity, lowering your levels of stress, soothing and comforting you. Little by little, they make it easier and safer to enjoy other people, to trust in and come close to them.

If you have a pet—and a remarkable 50 percent of US households do—take a little extra time so that you can fully enjoy the connection and appreciate the care and joy you give and receive. If you don't have a pet, visits with animals are a good place to start. There have been times throughout my life when an afternoon at the zoo, or even minutes of watching a squirrel hopping on a branch, a dog playing with a ball, or ants walking in a line, have quieted my agitated mind and opened my tension-closed heart.

You can also spend brief periods with someone else's pet. When, after a family death, my then ten-year-old son grew anxious, he had the wisdom to ask his godparents to let him "borrow" their golden retriever for quiet conversations and cuddling sleepovers.

And yes, if you are in the market for a pet, as Lucy suggested, get one who suits you and your lifestyle. As I write this, I remember that at different times in my life, I've found comfort and companionship from dogs and cats, as well as rabbits, horses and ponies, chickens and pigs, a goat, and even a goldfish.

You can also go someplace where you can spend time with animals: a friend's house, a zoo, the woods, or the seashore—or, for that matter, pretty much any patch of grass. As you sit near animals, silently watching, you may find yourself recovering a childlike innocence and wonder that has survived all your life's traumas.

A few final words:

Consider volunteering in a shelter or adopting a rescue animal, like Lily's and Matt's parrots or Lucy's dog. Their special needs seem to confer special blessings, allowing us to safely feel and have compassion for our own pain and sorrow, calling us beyond the fear and isolation that have followed in trauma's wake, to the caring and kindness that help restore us to our own best selves.

16
Laughter Breaks Trauma's Spell

READER'S DIGEST USED to tell us each month that "laughter is the best medicine." Drawing on folk wisdom, *The Digest* was reminding us that laughter could help us through the ordinary, daily unhappiness that might come into our lives.

In 1976, Norman Cousins, the revered editor of the *Saturday Review*, wrote a piece that signaled the arrival of laughter in the precincts of science. It was called "Anatomy of an Illness (as Perceived by the Patient)" and appeared in the *New England Journal of Medicine*, the United States' most prestigious medical publication.

When the best conventional care failed to improve his ankylosing spondylitis—a crippling autoimmune spinal arthritis—Cousins took matters into his own hands. He checked himself out of the hospital and into a hotel, took megadoses of anti-inflammatory vitamin C, and watched long hours of Marx Brothers movies and TV sitcoms. He laughed and kept on laughing. He noticed that as he did, his pain diminished. He felt stronger and better. As good an observer as any of his first-rate doctors, he developed his own dose-response curve: ten minutes of belly laughter gave him two hours of pain-free sleep. Soon enough, he became more mobile.

Cousins's report is what scientists describe as "an n of 1 experiment," one with a single subject. There is a cynical medical saying that when another physician describes a positive result in a single patient, it's an "anecdote." When, however, you see that kind of change in your patient, and especially in yourself, it takes on the dignity of an n of 1 experiment, an experiment with one subject.

This particular n of 1 struck a sympathetic chord. Cousins's doctors were as impressed as he was. The book based on his article, *Anatomy of an Illness*, became a bestseller that is still widely read.

ONCE THE HEALING power of laughter was on the medical map, researchers began to systematically explore its stress-reducing, health-promoting, pain-relieving potential. Laughter has now been shown to decrease stress levels and improve mood in cancer patients receiving chemotherapy, to decrease hostility in patients in mental hospitals, and to lower heart rate and blood pressure and enhance mood and performance in generally healthy IT professionals. In numerous experiments, people with every imaginable diagnosis have reduced their pain by laughing.

Laughter stimulates the dome-shaped diaphragmatic muscle that separates our chest from our abdomen, as well as our abdominal, back, leg, and facial muscles. After we laugh for a few minutes, these muscles relax. Then our blood pressure and stress hormone levels decrease; pain-relieving and mood-elevating endorphins increase, as do levels of calming serotonin and energizing dopamine. Our immune functioning—probably a factor in Cousins's eventual recovery—improves. If we are diabetic, our blood sugar goes down. Laughter is good exercise. It's definitely healthy. And it's first-rate for relieving stress.

Laughter also has a transforming power that transcends physiological enhancement and stress reduction. Laughter can break the spell of the fixed, counterproductive, self-condemning thinking that is so pervasive and so devastating to us after we've been traumatized. It can free us from the feelings of victimization that may shadow our lives and blind us to each moment's pleasures and the future's possibilities.

After you finish laughing, you'll likely feel more relaxed, more energized, more present. Often, you'll have some perspective on what's been making you miserable. Laughter, after all, is an expressive meditation, like Shaking and Dancing. It helps soften and melt the body that trauma has frozen. Its goofiness and its physical force help to dispel the excessive worry and seriousness that haunt our lives after we've been traumatized. Laughter challenges and breaks up the crippling shame and self-criticism that trauma brings with it.

You can heighten the effect by laughing at yourself in a mirror. As you do it, you'll become even more aware of the absurdity of holding on to outworn, self-defeating ideas about yourself and your identity as a victim.

One more thing about laughter: it's contagious. Do it with your family or friends. Afterward, de-stressed, you may find yourself relaxing with them and enjoying each other more—perhaps more than you have since you were traumatized, maybe even more than you ever have. What I see when I do it with some of the most traumatized people on the planet is that my laughter sets theirs off. Then, laughing together, we feel more in harmony with one another, more compassionate toward each other.

THE MARX BROTHERS movies that Norman Cousins watched give hints about the varieties of laughter's power. At its most basic level— the gloomy philosopher Nietzsche called it the "herd level"—we laugh at others. This has its virtues. The Marxes' targets of choice were the pretentious and pompous, the rich and powerful. The brothers delighted in bringing chaos into arenas of order, on ocean liners and in department stores, at parties of tuxedoed "swells," and at the opera, and in other temples of high culture. This skewering can be deeply satisfying and also democratizing. We realize the swells are no better than the rest of us.

And there's another, more subtle benefit. As we watch the Marxes making monkeys out of the powerful, we begin to realize that we, too, however poor and unfortunate, can be just as stuffy and self-important, and that, at least from time to time, we all take ourselves far too seriously. By gleefully puncturing their own as well as others' self-inflation, the Marxes hold up a mirror to us and make sure we get the message. Remember one of Groucho's most famous quips about never joining a club that would have him as a member. And remember, too, that Groucho was Jewish, and that for people who are oppressed and marginalized and traumatized by it, laughter has long been a way to lighten the load of their pain, as well as to level the social playing field.

MY OWN GREAT teachers—Bob Coles and Bill Alfred, Shyam and Sharon—have invited me or pushed and prodded and nagged me to laugh at myself, "to stop," as Shyam would say, "taking yourself so bloody seriously."

Over time, and not without effort, I've learned. When I'm tempted to engage in herd laughter at someone else's foibles, I notice my own similar ones—my own vanity and foolishness. I flip the laughter in my direction and laugh at my own unlovely pretentions. I become more aware of speaking inauthentically—with self-importance and pomposity or flattery; of acting selfish or getting frustrated; of worrying about what anyone else is thinking of me or how they may be judging me. And as I become aware, I laugh louder and no longer feel so burdened.

I've also learned to notice that even my real grief and genuine concern can start clotting in self-defeating thoughts and self-indulgent self-pity. And that awareness brings laughter and breaks the spell.

Sometimes I'll laugh out loud. When it seems too disruptive to make sounds, I let the laughter rise inside. All you might see is a smile broadening my face and crinkling my eyes, my shoulders relaxing, and my breathing slowing and deepening.

THE WISDOM TRADITIONS of the East extend laughter's lessons. Zen Buddhism surprises us with thunderclaps of laughter to wake us from mental habits that have brought unnecessary, self-inflicted suffering. Sufi stories do the same job but more slyly. Over the years, I watched as Shyam, himself a consummate joker, punctured the self-protectiveness, pomposities, and posturing that kept his patients and students—including, of course, me—from being at ease and natural, joyous in each moment of our lives. The stories he told from India, China, and the Middle East brought the point home: seriousness is a disease. Sorrow is real and to be honored, but obsessively dwelling on losses and pain only adds to our sickness. Laughter at ourselves and all our circumstances is our healing birthright.

A story I first heard from Shyam about the Three Laughing Monks is apropos.

It is said that long ago, there were three monks who walked the length and breadth of China, laughing great, belly-shaking laughs as they went. They brought joy to each village they visited, laughing as they entered, laughing for the hours or days they stayed, and laughing as they left. No words. And it's said that after a while everyone in the villages—the poorest and most put-upon and also the most privileged and pompous—got the message. They, too, lost their pained seriousness, laughed with the monks, and found relief and joy.

One day, after many years, one of the monks died. The two remaining monks continued to laugh. This time when villagers asked why, they responded, "We are laughing because we have always wondered who would die first, and he did and therefore he won. We're laughing at his victory and our defeat, and with memories of all the good times we have had together." Still, the villagers were sad for their loss.

Then came the funeral. The dead monk had asked that he not be bathed, as was customary, or have his clothes changed. He had told his brother monks that he was never unclean, because laughter had kept all impurities from him. They respected his wishes, put his still-clothed, unwashed body on a pile of wood, and lit it.

As the flames rose, there were sudden loud, banging noises. The living monks realized that their brother, knowing he was going to die, had hidden fireworks in his clothes. They laughed and laughed and laughed. "You have defeated us a second time and made a joke even of death." Now they laughed even louder. And it is said that the whole village began to laugh with them.

This is the laughter that shakes off all concerns, all worries, all holding on to anything that troubles our mind or heart, anything that keeps us from fully living in the present moment.

Writing this now, knowing it, I cannot help thinking of Viktor Frankl, who in the midst of unimaginable tragedy and "in spite of everything," was "saying 'yes' to life."

RESEARCHERS AND CLINICIANS may lack the total commitment to laughter of the three monks, but they are beginning to explore and make use of its power. Working together in various institutions, they've developed a variety of therapeutic protocols that may include interactions with clowns and instruction in performing stand-up comedy. "Laughter yoga," which has most often been studied, combines inspirational talks, hand clapping, arm swinging, chanting "ho, ho" and "ha, ha," deep breathing, and brief periods of intentional laughter; it often concludes with positive statements about happiness.

I agree that funny movies and jokes and games of all kinds can be useful tools to pry us loose from crippling seriousness. Still, I prefer to begin with a simple, direct approach: three to five minutes of straight-out, straight-ahead, intentional belly laughter. It's very easy to learn and easy to practice. I'll teach it to you.

I do it with patients individually or in groups, when the atmosphere is thick with smothering self-importance or self-defeating, progress-impeding self-pity. It's not a panacea, a cure-all. But, again and again, I've seen it get energetic juices flowing, rebalance agitation-driven minds, melt trauma-frozen bodies, dispel clouds of doubt and doom, and let in the light of Hope.

This laughter needs to begin with effort. It must force its way through forests of self-consciousness and self-pity, crack physical and emotional walls erected by remembered hurt and present pain.

Once you decide to do it, the process is simple. You stand with your knees slightly bent, arms loose, and begin, forcing the laughter up from your belly, feeling it contract, pushing out the sounds—barks, chuckles, giggles. You keep going, summoning the will and energy to churn sound up and out. Start with three or four minutes and increase when you feel more is needed.

You can laugh anytime you feel yourself tightening up with tension, pumping yourself up with self-importance, or freezing with fear. And the more intense those feelings are, the more shut-down and self-righteous, the more pained and lost and hopeless you are, the more important laughter is. Then laughter may even be lifesaving. After a few minutes of forced laughter, effort may dissolve, and the laughter itself may take charge. Now each unwilled, involuntary, body-shaking, belly-aching jolt provokes the next in a waterfall of laughter.

Laughter can be contagious. Other people will want to laugh with you.

And after laughing, as you become relaxed and less serious, you may find that people relate to you differently. Sensing the change in you, they may greet you or smile at you on the street. And you may find that you're happy to see them and that you enjoy the warmth of this new connection. Don't take my word for any of this. Do the experiment with daily laughter and see.

SOMETIMES, WHEN LAUGHTER seems most improbable, even inappropriate, it is most healing. Several years ago, I was in Jordan, at the UN's Zaatari camp, where almost one hundred thousand Syrian refugees were living cramped together in rows of tiny tents. I was there at the invitation of CMBM's Jordanian partner, the Noor Al Hussein Foundation, to learn about the refugees' lives and needs, to plan and find funding for a program for healing their population-wide psychological trauma. Five hundred thousand Syrians have died in that country's war, and one million are now living in Jordan, in camps like Zaatari and among the general population.

As I walked through the medical tents, men pulled up their pant legs to show me bullet wounds. Women raised listless children toward me, squeezed their mouths open to reveal tonsils swollen with pus. They gestured at little ones who hid their faces in the skirts of their coats. "She does not sleep and wets herself," one mother says. "He cries every time he hears a man's voice, thinking it's a soldier," another tells me. "This one, who has lost his father," says another, gesturing to an eight-year-old boy, "will not leave me, even for a minute."

A young man, I'll call him Hamid, stands apart from a group in the Noor Al Hussein tent. He is tall and slim, honey-colored, handsome, his nose a bit flat against his face. His short hair is carefully combed, and his shirt and pants are creased, as if they had just emerged from a box.

"I do not find rest at night," he answers when I ask why he has come to the tent. His sleep, it turns out, is broken by nightmares that replay his ten months of torture in Syrian prisons. He raises his arms to demonstrate how he was strung up before being beaten; he nods toward his nipples and genitals to show where the electric current was attached.

"I do not want to be around anyone," he says, as if the torture sessions were removing him now, as well as then, from human contact, as if he believed, as many who have been tortured do, that he should be ashamed, that he was somehow complicit in what he had to endure.

"Once," Hamid adds, as if it were another life, "I was studying to work in the hospitality industry." When I ask what used to give him most pleasure, his face opens just a little bit: "I loved cooking."

Ordinarily, when I begin work with an individual like Hamid, or a group, or in our training programs, I start simply, by teaching Soft Belly breathing. And I will do it half a dozen times on this visit—in tents with families, standing outside clinics, and in meetings in offices with aid workers.

Right now, I only have a few minutes, and I'm searching for any possible way to loosen the hold of Hamid's torturers—to let him see that it may be possible to find moments of freedom from the pain and humiliation they have visited on him.

Perhaps laughter could help. It's not really a thought—more an intuition, born of so many years of being with people who have suffered terribly, of seeing what's possible when I pay attention to the person in front of me and my own inner knowing. I do worry that Hamid will feel that I'm not taking his suffering seriously. Still, laughter feels right.

"You're a cook," I begin, feeling my way forward. "That means you must like experimenting with food." Hamid nods. "I have another kind of experiment, one that might help you with your nightmares." He looks skeptical but says he is willing to do the experiment. A dozen older men lean toward us, unasked but curious and hopeful.

"I want you to laugh like this." I show him, laughing in explosive barks, my stomach muscles contracting. He looks at me as if I were mad. "I am a bit crazy," I assure him, "but it's an experiment. Will you try?"

"Nothing is funny to me anymore. How can I do this? And why?"

"Force it," I say. "The torturers had you for ten months, and they still have you now, every night and during the day, too. You have to see that you can break the chains."

"Yes," he says, "it's true." The men around him murmur agreement and prepare themselves to accompany us.

We begin together, bent at the waist, our contracting bellies forcing the laughter through our throats. "More," I shout, "push it." And they do. Men who smoke too much to "quiet nerves" are coughing as much as laughing.

After three minutes we stop, but many continue to laugh, surprised at it but laughing naturally, easily now. When everyone has stopped, I ask Hamid, "How do you feel now?"

"More relaxed," he says, "at this moment," smiling a little.

This is no "cure" for Hamid's suffering, no enduring barrier to the flood of terrible memories. But now he knows that he can bring himself a small measure of relief and overcome, at least for a few moments, the feelings of helplessness and hopelessness.

"Do this laughing every day," I say to Hamid as I write it on a piece of paper. "I believe that every day you will find some moments of relaxation."

Hamid is smiling more broadly now, saying he will. The chorus of men around us nods in agreement, "Insha'Allah," they say. "God willing."

SOMETIMES WHEN MY spirit is shadowed by longing and pain or the world around me looks especially unpromising, I think of Hamid, or the Marx Brothers, or the Laughing Buddhas, or Shyam, and the surprising sound and sudden brightness of laughter rises inside of me. It breaks the spell of grief and grimness, lightens my spirit, gives me less clouded eyes, and opens my heart. "Why not laugh?" I say to myself.

Why don't you, my reader, try it?

17

Reading the Leaves on Your Family Tree

NOT LONG AGO at The Center for Mind-Body Medicine's Advanced Training, I led a "fishbowl"—a ninety-minute demonstration Mind-Body Skills Group.

I do this in every Advanced Training to give participants an example of how to teach the techniques they've been learning—the same ones I've been teaching you—and how to lead the groups I'll describe in the next chapter. I want our trainees to see and feel how to use our check-in process—each person speaking in turn, no one interrupted or analyzed. I want to show them how to help group members name the trauma that may still be torturing them, and how to use the techniques we're teaching to begin to undo the knots in which trauma has tied them. And I want them to see how group members can hear and learn from one another.

The participants—doctors, therapists, teachers, clergy, first responders, and community activists—volunteer for the group, each one explaining in front of all of us why he or she wants to join. The problems they present reflect the everyday trauma that might bring anyone to a therapist: "I can't be intimate with my husband." "I'm facing surgery for cancer and I'm scared." "My girlfriend left me." "My husband killed himself and I can't get back on my feet." "I'm fed up with my job." "I feel so alone." "I can't get my childhood abuse out of my mind." And always there are several people who are "terrified to get up and share my feelings" but don't know why and want to fight through their fears.

For this group, I invite people to volunteer whom I don't know and haven't worked with before. We call it a "fishbowl" for an obvious reason: the hundred and fifty participants who sit in concentric circles around us can watch us sharing and being with one another, meditating, crying and laughing, and Shaking and Dancing, just the way we watch fish swimming in a glass bowl.

Those who watch us are quiet and respectful. At my invitation, they will join us when we meditate or do Guided Imagery or move our bodies.

In this recent fishbowl, after our opening meditation, a young, Mexican-born social worker speaks. She is small, her voice muffled by her bowed head. "When I came in this circle, I was scared of exposing myself, scared of everyone thinking I'm crazy because of my fears and nightmares. Now sitting here, I know everybody is kind, but I can't help being nervous. I feel like I'm back home, where people who look like me"—she opens her hands and slowly looks around our small circle—"like an Indian, are treated like dirt. 'Why do they need schools?' the white people ask. The same white people whose ancestors killed my people. 'Healthcare is wasted on them. They don't take care of themselves.' When my parents go into town, even if they're dressed nicely and have money, they walk like they're ashamed, heads down and afraid, never looking at anyone. And that fear and shame, that's there in me, too. That's what I'm realizing as I sit here. And this is the first time I've ever shared these feelings with anyone.

"I guess," she goes on, "this is the historical trauma that people talk about. I never realized I had it."

The members of our group listen respectfully, tenderly, as we have to everyone who has spoken. When we go around our circle for a second time, it feels like each of us is shaking loose from a burden we didn't know had weighed us down. A doctor speaks of the rage he feels when, returning home late from his hospital, police stop him for "driving while Black." He is "furious" now at his parents, who continually worried about him "getting in trouble" or offending "just about anyone on the planet." A nurse from South Carolina, facing cancer surgery, wonders if generations of "social inferiority—I'm a typical redneck"—have undermined her immunity. A psychologist curses "the WASP uptightness, the goddamn greedy need for control" that make him afraid of leaving a safe but unsatisfying government job to work with the homeless kids whose loneliness calls to him.

And so it goes, around the circle, each of us revealing, beginning to peel away the legacy of generations of being oppressed, or indeed, oppressing others, of fear and pain and constraint. Speaking, listening to one another, we become more aware of how trauma in the lives of previous generations has been limiting us, distorting how we see the world, constraining what we are allowed to feel and whether and how we can speak about it.

And when it's my turn, I find, to my surprise and embarrassment—it seems so small next to the legacies of slavery and genocide—that I'm also speaking of this historical trauma. In this circle of sharing, I'm more aware than I've ever been—even after all those years of therapy, analysis, interpretation, and meditation—

that I am the grandchild of eastern European Jews, and of how it has shaped me. I can taste the self-hate of shtetl dwellers, bowing to their gentile "betters." I feel the terrors of ancestors who heard the hoofbeats of Cossack horses and escaped the slaughters of pogroms. I'm acutely aware of my grandparents' need, once in America, "to fit in" and their deep unadmitted conviction that we Jews would always be "the other" and "less than."

I imagine these painful, shameful emotions still running, like small, neurotic animals, through my nerves. And I feel, too, stove-hot anger—inexpressible in the old country, or in the holds of ships that brought my ancestors here, or the businesses, schools, and professions that offered my grandparents and parents tunnels up to the generous spaces of the American gentile world.

HISTORICAL TRAUMA IS indeed a disturbing reality. A pregnant mother's suffering produces a cascade of stress hormones that may make her unborn child far more susceptible to stress and trauma, and their physical, emotional, and social consequences—anxiety, depression, chronic illness, drug addiction, and antisocial behavior.

In recent years, a number of studies have shown how trauma can be transmitted not just in utero but from one generation to the next. Stress can bring about changes in our chromosomes that can be inherited. These epigenetic changes—the ones I described in chapter 2—are not in the genes themselves but in the structure of the DNA and in the RNA. Still, they have the same power to create psychological and biological changes in the children and even the grandchildren of those who have been traumatized as do the mutations we learned about in high school biology.

Studies on animals have clearly and repeatedly shown the correlation between specific epigenetic changes and increased susceptibility to stress. And these changes have also been observed in the descendants of Holocaust survivors—in studies by Rachel Yehuda and her colleagues at New York's Mount Sinai Hospital. The bottom line is painfully biblical: the sufferings of the fathers—and mothers—are transmitted for at least two generations. And the children who carry these altered genes usually have no idea that these genes have altered their attitudes and behavior. Ignorant of the origins of their fears and constraints, they are even more vulnerable to stress, anxiety, depression, and chronic illness.

Knowing that what has happened to our ancestors is still affecting us allows us to understand feelings and behavior that had seemed inexplicable: we may see why we are so fearful of intimacy or anxious about a new situation or unable to deal with criticism. And understanding the source of our distress can help us free ourselves from the terrible powerlessness, shame, and guilt that are often the most intractable features of historical trauma.

As we make these discoveries, it feels, as it did to all of us in the fishbowl, as if a light is shining into long-feared, previously unknown dark places. As we come to know what has happened and why we feel the way we do, we can begin to do something about it. Using the techniques we've learned, we can mitigate or even reverse the epigenetic changes of our ancestors' trauma and the biological and psychological consequences we're experiencing. We can shed our ancestors' burdens.

As we do, we'll discover that family misfortune can instruct us, as well as hobble us; it can show us vulnerabilities and tendencies that we can anticipate, learn from, and address.

We can also look to our family and its history for inspiration, support, and guidance, for the example of people who have overcome challenges similar to ours, for the wisdom that moves, together with trauma, through the trunk and along the branches of our family tree.

We will likely find, too, that even the most disordered of our families has members who can help us discover who we are and how we are meant to live in and through the challenges that life brings to us. If we learn how to ask, our ancestors and relatives, dead as well as living, can help us address both current crises and historical trauma. And of course, families can be great sources of practical assistance and emotional support and reassurance.

Genograms

Over the years, my colleagues and I have used Genograms—three-, four-, or five-generational diagrams of our family—to make these discoveries, to help us come to terms with past hurt and harm, and to find our way forward.

I've seen these Genograms help people all over the world gain perspective on and begin to free themselves from historical trauma; deal with present, often overwhelming challenges; and find enduring sources of strength and wisdom. This has been so for those who fled ethnic cleansing in the Balkans; for Holocaust survivors in Israel and their children and grandchildren; for Palestinians who were driven out of their family homes and have lived under occupation; for Native Americans demoralized by a history of genocide, forced confinement, brutal boarding schools, and reservation life; and also for mainstream Americans, groaning under the burden of neglect and abuse, insecurity, and loss that mark the lives of so many families, including those of my fishbowl colleagues and my own.

It's now your turn to create a Genogram and to learn the life lessons it has to offer. Don't worry, I know you'll be able to do it. Our CMBM program graduates have done it with hundreds of thousands of adults all over the world, many of whom have never finished high school, as well as with children Azhaar's age. Just approach your Genogram playfully, with curiosity.

After I've taught you how to construct a basic Genogram (there's more guidance in the McGoldrick text listed in the Notes), my friend and colleague Sabrina N'Diaye is going to share hers with you. Sabrina is a fifty-two-year-old African American Muslim woman, a social worker and psychologist. I'll ask her questions about her Genogram, encouraging her to explain when and how it has guided her in resolving past trauma, learning from and dealing with present challenges, and moving ahead with her rich, complex, and loving life. From time to time, I'll pause to let a few other people share stories of what they've learned from their Genogram.

OKAY, LET'S GET STARTED. You'll need a blank piece of paper—ideally 11" x 14", with enough room even for a big family. Actually, you may want two sheets, so you can redraw a rough version more neatly.

You'll want to use a pencil with an eraser, so you can correct and modify as you go along. You'll use the symbols on page 239 to create this schematic picture of your family—your Genogram.

Begin by folding the paper in half horizontally. Now fold it in half again. This will give you three creases and four distinct compartments, like this:

In the topmost compartment on the left, you'll draw your father's parents and their siblings and the connections among them. You'll use appropriate symbols for each person (squares for men, circles for women), and draw lines to indicate the relationship between spouses, parents, and siblings. Make double lines to show close connections. As you'll see in the symbols below, you use broken, interrupted, and jagged lines to indicate different kinds of disruption in relationships. You'll repeat this process with your mother's family in the top right compartment.

If you know little or nothing about these ancestors or other relatives, that's okay. You can still draw the symbols for them and fill in the picture. The ones you don't know and what you don't know about them are also parts of who you are—perhaps they're also reminders of deprivation or longing or Hope.

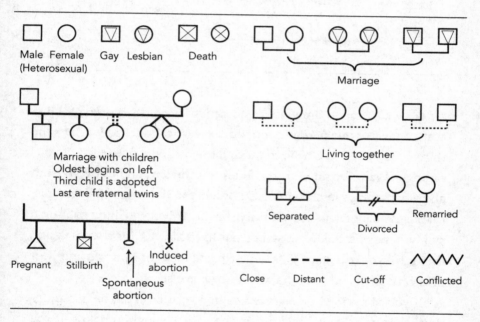

Vertical lines of connection will take you to the next compartment below, where you'll locate your parents and their siblings. You'll draw them in order, going from the oldest on the left side to the youngest on the right. In this same compartment, you'll show the connections between your parents and any other spouses or partners, and your aunts and uncles, and their important relationships. Here is Sabrina's Genogram so far.

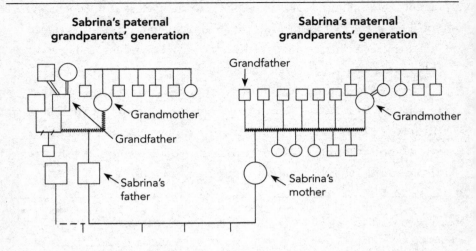

Sabrina's paternal grandparents' generation

Sabrina's maternal grandparents' generation

Grandfather

Grandmother

Grandfather

Grandmother

Sabrina's father

Sabrina's mother

Now it's time to draw your generation. From the horizontal line that connects your parents, you'll draw vertical lines down into the third compartment. One is connected to you and one to each of your siblings. Again, begin with the eldest on the left, and draw yourself and your siblings in chronological order. You'll want to indicate miscarriages or abortions as well as live births. When you draw your own symbol, make it bold so it stands out like this: **O** for a woman and this **☐** if you're a man. This will help you focus on yourself and your connections to and conflicts with everyone else.

If you're married or divorced or in a relationship, you'll want to draw that, as Sabrina has done, in the basic Genogram below. If you and your spouse/partner have children, they'll take their place in the fourth compartment. You can put your children's spouses and partners there, too, and your grandchildren.

Sabrina's basic Genogram is on the next page.

When Sabrina looks at it, this is what she sees:

First, her parents: "The most unlikely pair. . . ." She points to her "super smart" father, growing up and out of his own hardship. Com-

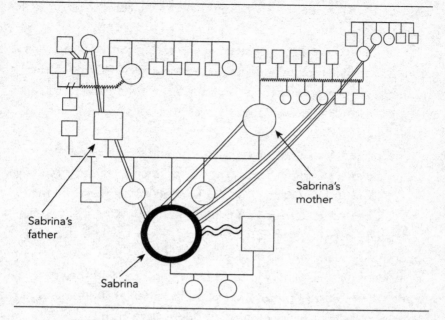

mitted from childhood to a "scientific approach to life," he became the first Black man in his pharmacy school. And then her mother, "just as smart" but because of the educational system's ignorance, her color, and her wandering attention, "siloed" into special ed classes. She failed to graduate from high school.

Sabrina traces her father's path ever upward—a "commitment to stability, the first or second Black in his Fortune 500 company." She taps on the circle representing her mother and describes the red-hot rage she has maintained against the white world of money, power, and bureaucracy—a world that had threatened to separate her from her own mother, brothers, and sisters, a world that had kept her down and feeling down on herself.

Now, as Sabrina takes a longer look at previous generations, "I see the severity of the life of poor Black folks, and also the strength that came from that life." She also sees generations of men and women whose lives were damaged and shortened by alcoholism and addiction, a history both Sabrina and her parents have had to come to terms with and struggle against.

And then there's the mystery of repeating patterns. Sabrina's grandmother and mother both pregnant at seventeen. Sabrina's father's mother not wanting him to marry Sabrina's mother, and he in turn resisting Sabrina's future husband, Serigne, for the same reasons: "Too poor, too Black."

"I continue to struggle with the pattern and then break it. Before I met my husband, Serigne, I was with a lot of men who drank like my mother's family. I wasn't an alcoholic, but I definitely was drinking."

Looking at the Genogram for more understanding, Sabrina can see herself "between two different worlds." On the left, the white, upper middle-class, suburban neighborhood where her father's talent and drive took their family. And on the right, the South Bronx tenements where most of her mother's family still lives. Looking at her Genogram, Sabrina feels heir to both, appreciates both.

The double lines she draws show her the sources of her own strength, in her always supportive, "super-attached" father and her mother's fierce pride: "She let me know that I was gonna be better than any white girl."

Already, the Genogram is revealing powerful life-shaping patterns to Sabrina, and perhaps to you, as you draw yours. And there is much more to draw and learn.

Give names now, and current ages, to the people who've been most important to you. Put Xs in the circles and squares of those who've died, adding their ages at death. As you do this slowly, you may become aware of feelings connected to the people and the relationships you're describing, the deaths you're noting. Already you are well on your way to constructing and recovering the story of your family, to seeing where you come from, how you fit in, and how it feels. Remember, don't worry if you don't know all the details.

Here is Sabrina's evolving Genogram.

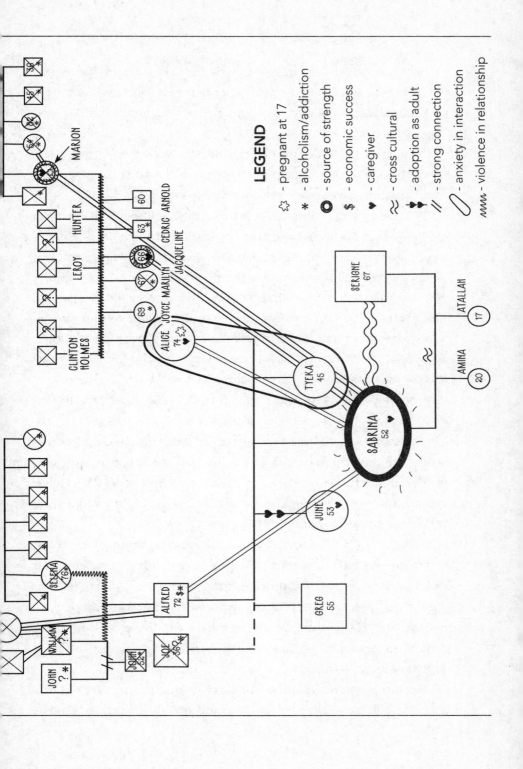

LEGEND

☆ - pregnant at 17

* - alcoholism/addiction

◎ - source of strength

$ - economic success

♥ - caregiver

≋ - cross cultural

➤➤ - adoption as adult

∥ - strong connection

∿ - anxiety in interaction

⬭ - violence in relationship

Sabrina observes and has given symbols to challenges that repeat, like "alcoholism/addiction" and "violence in relationships," as well as the multigenerational virtues of "caregivers," "economic success," and "strong connection."

Now take a few deep Soft Belly breaths with your eyes closed. Open them and look at the big picture of your own family. Here are some questions to help you see what you're looking at.

What are the most important patterns in your family? For example, of illness and health, character and occupation, ethnicity and religion, wealth and poverty, etc. These patterns, and the importance you and your family attach to them, are the form and color of your family portrait. You could be noting three generations of doctors or lawyers, firefighters, nurses, or soldiers; cancer or depression running in the family; several generations in which siblings don't speak to each other. You might want to create, as Sabrina has, symbols for these character-istics or patterns and put them inside or next to the circles and squares that represent the appropriate family members. Previously unattended patterns of tragedy or talent may also emerge.

Now ask yourself if there are others who belong in the Genogram— people who are not biologically kin but have been particularly sup-portive or hurtful or inspirational. I always put Bill Alfred, Bob Coles, and Shyam in my Genogram, as well as my godchildren and their children, and my closest friends.

What about pets? Many of us, like Lucy and my brother Jeff, whom you've already met, have relationships with animals that may be even closer than with kin. If appropriate, put pictures of four-leggeds on your page—perhaps signifying them with ears and paws, or hooves.

Ask, too, if there are family members who have been ignored, denied, or shunned—a disabled child hidden in an institution, a wayward father banished as a pariah.

Because we humans are so wonderfully unique, there are remark-able one-offs. Several years ago, I found myself looking at David's

Genogram with mounting distress. The mother that this kind, wise, but worried middle-aged minister pointed to had been a prostitute who had abandoned him days after his birth. His father was then in prison. He described the grandmother who raised him as "an indifferent caregiver."

"How," I finally had to ask, "did you get to be who you are?" And then, "Who in this Genogram gave you the strength?"

David paused for a moment's thought, then broke into a big grin. "It's not there . . . yet." He drew and then pointed to an unmistakable form with its label, "Starship Enterprise."

"Star Trek," he said. "That was my world." The Enterprise rescued him, just as it had other survivors on endangered planets. Its crew provided a model of caring and cooperation, a source of inspiration and a family for a sad and lonely boy. Its humanitarian missions showed him heroic possibilities and provided him with an ethical compass to navigate childhood chaos. And then, as a still young boy, he was able to join the real, live, worldwide community of Trekkie communication and gatherings.

WHEN YOU LOOK at your own Genogram now, what do you see? What people or pictures or patterns seem most important to you? Write them down. What lessons does your Genogram have for you now?

When Sabrina consults her Genogram for perspective on her marriage, which has, in recent years, gone through "low times," she realizes that she and her husband are just as different from one another as her parents are. "He's an African man, an immigrant, comfortable with having his job and his wife and his kids. And I'm fiery and on a mission."

When she looks more closely, she realizes that Serigne has her father's commitment to stability, to marriage and family, and "a deep respect for women." "Even in low times" she knows he is "forever family. I think, 'How could I leave him?' It makes no sense. It would be like breaking up with my thumb."

When Sabrina looks to her Genogram for further guidance—about her life as well as her relationship to Serigne—she focuses on her connection to her mother's mother. It's a loving bond—stronger than even the bolded double line can show. It continues to sustain her, years after her grandmother's death.

"I'm so connected to my grandmother, despite the fact she couldn't talk, perhaps because she couldn't. A white cop had apparently put a gun to her head, and the next day she had a terrible stroke. She never had the rehab she needed, maybe because she was too poor and Black.

"My grandmom taught me to listen without words. I had to figure out what she was telling me. When everyone else was avoiding her, I let her play with me and bathe me.

"Now I'm a therapist, and I listen for a living. I sit with people who don't even speak my language. I look past the external drooling, the diapers that have to be changed, to see their heart.

"And when I get really fed up with my husband, I look at my Genogram for guidance, and turn to my grandmother, and do a dialogue with her. 'Grandmother,' I said the other day, 'he's a pain in the ass.'

"My grandmother says, 'So was I.' That makes me pause. And she goes on, 'I was a pain in the ass, and you wiped my ass.'"

GIVE YOURSELF SOME time now, and do as Sabrina did: consult your Genogram.

Breathe deeply for a few minutes with your eyes closed. Think of a challenge that's appearing in your life, an issue you're struggling with that would benefit from some perspective and wisdom like Sabrina's relationship with her husband. Now open your eyes and take a look at your Genogram. First, for a while, at the big picture, the patterns.

Now ask what your Genogram can tell you about the challenge or issue that's come to your mind. What patterns can help you understand it better? What family strengths can you draw on? What connections—to ancestors, siblings, children, friends, or pets—can sustain and support you? Who or what can help you discover what you need to see and know and do?

When my physician-colleague Rita came to the US from Brazil, she asked her Genogram how she could fit into an academic medical department that had no other people of color and few women. Her eyes drifted to her great-grandmother, a *bruja*, a traditional healing witch. She was an outsider, a strange but wise and kind woman who was universally respected. Rita realized this woman could be a model and an inspiration, encouraging her to bring her own particularly Brazilian wisdom and compassion to an academic world that needed and might well welcome them.

Whenever she feels loss and loneliness, Maya now goes to her Genogram to "fill in the gaps," to reconnect with the love and support of "the angels with skin" who have been part of her life, to imagine and draw connections to new ones who might come calling with needed wisdom and comfort.

Not long ago, looking at my own Genogram, I saw and appreciated the commitment to excellence and service that I've inherited from my parents. And I find, surprisingly, amid my family's fears and constraints, a model for creativity and joy. My father's father, I'd once been told, used to stop in the evening, after long, tedious days painting houses, to play the fiddle in cafés. His music brought light notes into his somber life. As I look at my Genogram and picture it, it graces mine.

Take some time now to write down the answers that come to you. Don't worry about grammar or punctuation or even logic.

Take a look at what you've written. See if you still have questions. If you do, look again at the Genogram. You may well get additional guidance. If you're still puzzled, put it away for a day or a week. Return and ask again. And if there's information you feel you need—about ancestors who've died or your parents' childhood—ask your relatives. They often know stories that can help you get a bigger and more nuanced picture of where you came from and who you are. Add what you learn to your Genogram. It's a living, evolving document and guide.

Just about everyone who does the Genogram, like Sabrina and Rita and Maya and me, holds on to it, keeps checking it out, continues to find it helpful.

18
The Healing Circle

S MALL GROUPS—anthropologists call them "bands"—are the social unit in which, over hundreds of thousands of years, our species evolved. These bands nourished our ancestors and continue to sustain our aboriginal brothers and sisters. They shaped the genetic code we carry and were shaped by it. It makes sense, then, that small groups can bring healing to all of us who continue to carry these genes.

Indigenous people everywhere understand the power of the group. When a tribal person has a minor problem or illness—a cold or sprained ankle, mild anxiety, or depression—he asks his "granny"—his grandmother or someone else's—for help. She knows the community's physical and emotional first aid and offers it, with maternal comfort and confidence. When the problem is more severe, more traumatic—a life-threatening illness or injury, a poisonous snakebite, a compound fracture or serious infection, a child or adult tormented by psychosis or suicidal depression, a warrior returning from combat—the tribal member consults the officially recognized healer.

These authorities are known by different names in different cultures: shaman, wise woman, witch doctor. In parts of Latin America traditional healers are called *curanderos,* in southern Africa, *sangomas.* These official healers have mastered the local pharmacopeia and the rituals that summon the aid of healing powers and deities. This can be a prodigious task. Credo Mutwa, perhaps the most respected *sangoma* in South Africa, told me that he knew the names, songs, and therapeutic properties of some three thousand plants, animal products, and minerals. I remember thinking that his repertoire dwarfed my own Harvard training in pharmacology.

When traditional healers take on a case, they most often bring together members of the patient's extended family—or indeed, her entire community. They understand that though a condition may exist in one individual's body and mind, it also signals a rupture between the ill or troubled person and the social, natural, and spiritual world in which she lives.

The group assembled by the healer participates in processes of confession and care, of prayer and ritual, and these help restore the balance in the body and mind of the affected individual, as well as between her and her community. The healer, whose task is far more inclusive than a modern doctor's, also leads rituals that strengthen the connections between the community and the natural world that sustains it, and the spiritual world that gives meaning to illness and health and everyone's life.

UNTIL RECENTLY, modern medicine had neglected the healing power of groups. In the last sixty years, we've begun to rediscover it. We've learned that simply creating a safe place for people to come together to share the fears that have debilitated them, without the threat of criticism, is itself healing for many people—including alcoholics and addicts, Vietnam veterans, women sharing histories of abuse and discovering sisterhood and their own authority, and people with eating disorders, depression, and cancer. Millions of people have benefited from, and many physicians now speak respectfully of, twelve-step and support groups.

Recent research by UCLA psychologist Shelly Taylor helps shed light on why these and other groups may be so powerful in reducing stress and healing trauma.

Synthesizing data from studies on animals and humans, Taylor and her co-workers concluded that a female's response to stress is significantly different from a male's. When a threat arises, male animals—and men—fight or run. Females under threat—from natural disasters or predators—often gather together to care for and protect one another and their young, a response that Taylor calls "tend and befriend."

The male's response is driven, as we've seen, by adrenaline and testosterone. These hormones are also crucial to the female response, but her biology is more nuanced. Oxytocin, the hormone that promotes bonding between adults, as well as mothers and infants, rises, along with adrenaline and testosterone, modifying their effects. The female hormone estrogen and pain-relieving endorphins also increase more than in men.

THE SHARED CONFIDENCES and feelings of safety in many groups probably mobilize the tend-and-befriend response. It's likely that the intimacy, mutual respect, and compassion of The Center for Mind-Body Medicine's small Mind-Body Skills Groups amplify and deepen this response.

People of every age and educational level and cultural and religious background, even those who forcefully assert they are "not group people," benefit from these MBSGs. They soon feel safe enough to experience and admit to their past pain and present confusion, and calm and free enough to learn and use the self-care techniques that I've been teaching you. They also become comfortable enough to share with one another what they're discovering about themselves.

Many who've previously participated in multiple therapies and even other groups have appreciated MBSGs—which combine timeless wisdom and modern science with self-expression and an appealing education in self-care—and found them powerfully effective. "I learned so many possible ways to help myself," they say. "I felt such love and respect." There is, as one observed, a "continual invitation to authenticity, to be just the way you are." "And best of all," as Sally, the incest survivor who had participated in many other therapies, concluded, "it was the first time nobody tried to *fix* me."

Over the past twenty years, we've repeatedly demonstrated the power of a series of ten Mind-Body Skills Groups to reduce PTSD in war-traumatized children and adults (in Kosovo and Gaza) by 80 percent or more, significantly improving their mood and restoring their hope.

These groups have also been shown to enhance the well-being and biology of stressed-out health professionals and workers, and of medical students—at Georgetown, where I teach, the University of Washington, and Duke.

Students who participated in our groups had significantly lower levels of stress and felt happier. They studied more efficiently and slept better, were more hopeful about becoming physicians, and—most interestingly to me—exhibited the tend-and-befriend response of greater compassion toward one another. When their Georgetown classmates studied for crucial examinations, their testosterone levels soared. Not so our group members. There was no comparable increase in male or female students, and both genders didn't have the expected exam-driven increase in the stress hormone cortisol.

In this chapter, I'll show you how a Mind-Body Skills Group unfolds and give you some snapshots of its members' sadness and struggles, their triumphs and revelations. You'll see group members growing in understanding and in compassion for themselves and one another. And you'll observe the unforced intimacy and sustaining support that the group provides.

I invite you to feel a tender connection to these group members, a connection that can inform your own healing journey. I believe the ways they use individual tools and techniques and begin to put together their programs of self-discovery and self-care will encourage you in developing your own program for ongoing self-care. And I hope that glimpses of the power of coming together may inspire you to invite family and friends to participate in the healing journey with you, to share what you're learning with them, and to learn and grow as they share themselves with you.

Also, I'd like you to consider this chapter an invitation to join a Mind-Body Skills Group led by someone we've trained, in person or virtually (you can find them on our website), or, indeed, to come to one of our trainings. The six thousand people CMBM has trained—Azhaar's teacher in Gaza, Sally's group leader in Texas, Sabrina in Baltimore, Maya in the Midwest—all use the same basic structure and sequence for their small groups.

WHAT FOLLOWS ARE glimpses of an eight-session group I led. You'll see that these group members are using the same techniques I've been teaching you and then sharing what they're learning with one another. It took place a few years ago during a training. This group is as unique as the individuals in it, but the meaningful learning, the sharing, and the surprising connections happen just about every time, no matter who's leading the group or where it takes place.

The first group begins with members—there are usually eight to ten—sitting in a circle with a leader. It's the same here in a training program—where each of twenty small groups periodically breaks out from the two hundred who are enrolled in the program—as it is in the Mind-Body Skills Groups in your community, the ones led by doctors, therapists, teachers, and peer counselors whom we've trained, and those CMBM offers online.

We begin always with "the group ground rules," making sure everyone understands and agrees to follow them. These ground rules are designed to ensure safety and establish order; to create a climate of respect that encourages self-discovery and self-disclosure to make it possible for you to safely share what you're learning as you practice self-care techniques and to learn from the discoveries others are making about themselves.

Confidentiality is the crucial first ground rule. Everyone in the group needs to feel safe to share whatever she is feeling or thinking without fear that it will be retold to friends or colleagues, family members, or a neighborhood.

I ask each person to speak or nod his head in understanding and agreement. Remarkably, confidentiality is almost never breached, even in the gossip-ridden confines of refugee camps or the gossip-filled corridors of hospitals and prisons, schools and businesses.

Next are rules about structure and procedure. Groups begin and end on time. If a group member can't come or is going to be late, I ask her to let me know. It's respectful and will keep all of us from anxiously wondering about how and where she is.

I explain that this is a different kind of group, that each person is there to make discoveries about herself, to share what she wants, when and if she wants to. No one, including me, analyzes, interprets, or interrupts anyone else. Everyone speaks in turn.

Many leaders pass an object around the circle from the person who is speaking to the one who will speak next. Some use talking sticks, as tribal societies do, others a felt or wooden heart, to remind each group member to "speak from the heart." Everyone is encouraged to share as she wishes; no one is required to. You can say, "I pass," and the leader will return to you later. There is no pressure to speak, and there is unconditional respect. I explain that as each of us shares the lessons we're learning and the discoveries we're making, all of us can learn. We are all each other's teachers.

I tell the group members that I'm the leader. My job is to ensure that the group begins and ends on time, that no one interrupts or analyzes anyone else, that everyone has a chance to speak, and that nobody monopolizes the time. And I'm also a participant, sharing my own experiences and feelings, doing the techniques I'm teaching—the Soft Belly breathing, the Drawings and Dialogues, the Guided Imagery—along with everyone else. I'll share what I've seen and felt, written and drawn, just as all the other group members will.

All this can be a bit of a shock for therapists who've been taught to "remain a blank screen"—to stand apart and analyze but not share—and for people accustomed to such therapies. After some resistance, which I and all our leaders acknowledge but don't argue with, just about everyone appreciates or is at least interested in the model. Many professionals find they enjoy the freedom from constraints that have become customary in the therapeutic professions. They feel that in these groups they are able to more fully embody the desire to care and share that originally brought them to their professions. They find themselves happy to be companions, as well as guides, on a healing journey.

WHEN WE DO Soft Belly breathing at the beginning of the first group, I explain, as I did in chapter 3, the physiology of meditation: how it quiets our body, reduces agitation, decreases stress, and allows us to be more aware, more compassionate, more connected to ourselves and others. I explain that Soft Belly creates the calm and self-awareness that make it possible for us to learn and use all the techniques I'll be teaching.

Now comes the check-in—each person responding to the four questions that signal participation in and commitment to the group, questions that may also be useful to you as you develop your own program of Transformation: "Who are you?" "Why are you here?" "What do you want to get out of this experience?" "How are you doing right now?"

The last question is an important one, which I and all leaders keep coming back to. In other kinds of groups, there may be long periods spent recalling past events, as well as discussions of and debates about the meaning of each person's words and questions about their thoughts and feelings about them. In these groups, my job is to help group members focus on staying in or returning to present experiences and on developing a relaxed, meditative view of their story, a moment-to-moment awareness of how it makes them feel *right now*. It's a way of being that I also want to keep encouraging in you.

When a group member is lost in a maze of story or speculation, I'll gently recall her to the present: "How are you feeling now?" Relaxed and aware in this moment, group members gain perspective on and feel less burdened by remembered pain, agitation, and fear of what hurt them, and less worried about harm that might come again. I explain that every moment of present awareness is an antidote to the stress and trauma that plague our memory and shadow our future.

Usually the first round of introductions is factual, cautious, low key. In a weekly group in a community setting, participants may lead with their diagnosis or description of a trouble: "I've got hypertension." "I've been depressed for years and can't sleep at night." "I'm anxious about my relationship." "My husband died two months ago, and it feels unspeakable. I'm completely alone." They may mention the treatments they're receiving and the shortcomings of what they've done so far. "The antidepressant medication stopped helping; now it just makes me feel numb." Usually we go around the circle twice.

In a training program, where this group is taking place, participants often open with professional titles, hopes for helping others, or admissions of burnout. Dot, a trim fifty-year-old in pressed jeans and a cashmere sweater, with a neat cap of gray hair, presents herself and her credentials crisply. She's a primary care physician and leads a community clinic, is "feeling fine," and is "interested in learning." Asa is a graying retired engineer who volunteers in a church support group and tells us he has trouble speaking publicly. Farima, a psychiatrist who fled from Iran after the revolution, is overwhelmed by the rigidity of her profession in the US, as well as in Iran. She speaks sadly of her US home, which was recently destroyed in a fire, and of her concerns for her elderly, ill parents, her children, and the stream of refugees who flood her office.

Small, bald, and rumpled Matt is a businessman and minister. He's eager to report that after Soft Belly, his "vagus nerve is very happy." Della, a social worker, leans forward to tell us how frustrated she is. She wants to use mind-body skills to address her community's ongoing epidemic of poverty and violence. Jose, a teacher, wants "new tools and techniques," to help the low-income, minority children in his classes. Shauna, who is a nursing school dean, worries about her own as well as her students' vulnerability to stress, but feels "relaxed" after Soft Belly.

Toward the end of the second round of check-in, Clara, intense, shaky, and sixtyish, breaks the chain of decorous sharing and tentative hopefulness. "I'm not sure," she announces, "if I should be here or in a psychiatric emergency room. I once ministered to a parish, now I'm almost a homeless person." I assure her she's welcome in our group.

Toward the end of the first group, we do the three Drawings that you'll remember from chapter 4: "Yourself," "Yourself with your biggest problem," and "Yourself with your problem solved." Della laughs at the oversize head she has given herself in her first Drawing, and the symbols of demand and signs of stress that dominate her second Drawing: a clock, a dollar sign, the outstretched hands of clients, the open mouths of family members. Just about everyone nods in recognition. Della tells us she longs for a little peace, for a place on the tree-shaded country road of her third Drawing.

In all his Drawings, Matt is close to the bottom of the page, even smaller than he is in person. In the second one, he's on his knees praying for guidance in dealing with a thorny parish problem. In the third, he's rising with open-armed gratitude for the problem solved.

Shauna draws herself as a stick figure. In the Drawing of her biggest problem, other stick figures are scattered on the ground, cut down by the gun violence that is devastating her nursing school neighborhood. In her solution, she "connects the dots": her figures are now in a circle holding hands, creating a community. She looks around, recognizing the model for it in the circle of our group.

Jose stands on one side of his second picture, looking anxious. He draws his elderly, ill dog in the other corner. He's worried that she'll die alone. His third Drawing shows him with his other puppies and his loving partner. "Maybe," he says, "I can survive what I can't change."

"I don't like talking about myself," says Dot, who's one of the last to show her Drawings. "But look at me there." She's laughing now. It's all out there. The capital letters ME dominate her second Drawing, with thick arrows emerging in every direction. "I feel responsible for everything, want to cure everyone." In the third Drawing, there's a rainbow and a heart. "I'm smiling, loving myself, trusting," she says, hardly believing it. "Wouldn't that be nice."

A few of us have to wait our turns and show our Drawings in the next group meeting. In his second Drawing, Asa's throat is covered in a blur of blackness. "I was stabbed there," he tells us. "I had a cancerous cyst as an infant. I had to have surgery. It's my weak spot. I've never been able to speak up for myself about anything important." The black area is smaller in his third Drawing, more blemish than giant bruise. Looking at the Drawings, Asa "can see that it's up to me to decide how big my fear is."

Even before she shares her Drawings, Clara's shaking is more pronounced. She tells us that, like Asa, her bright and kind grandson has trouble speaking; he's a stammerer. When he was a boy, his father, Clara's son-in-law, used to force his penis down his throat.

The circle grows heavy with Clara's pain, and with knowing the terrible things that adults can do to children.

Now Clara shows her Drawings. In the first she is "a professional woman, wife, and mother," confident, carrying her "heart of healing" in one hand and a "sword of righteous advocacy" in the other. "This is how I look to the world." In the second Drawing, her mouth is a slash of mute, red rage. She tells us that it wasn't just her grandson who was sexually abused. As a young woman, she was raped by the minister who was her mentor. Neither the minister who abused her nor his superiors had ever apologized or even acknowledged what had happened. Confronted, they had suggested she was exaggerating, misunderstanding, mistaken, maybe even deluded. "I was twice victimized. The rape was terrible, and the way the system treated me, even worse. All that pain, all that anger, has been burrowing deeper for forty years."

We sit for a few minutes in stricken, silent communion with Clara, several of us crying, others close to tears. And then, rumpled, kindly Matt leans forward. "It breaks my heart to hear you. As a minister of your faith, I want to tell you how ashamed I am of our religion's actions. How sorry I am."

And now, after forty years of stuffing her feelings, Clara is crying. "You are the first man of the cloth who has even said, 'I'm sorry.' If only someone had said it forty years ago, maybe healing could have happened. Now, for the first time, I believe it can begin."

When I ask at the end of the group if it's okay if all of us stand to do Soft Belly breathing with our arms around one another, everybody nods yes. Matt's tears are flowing now. "That's what I wanted, too," he says. As we file out of the room, Clara, like a priest at the end of a Sunday morning service, shakes hands with each of us, gravely, appreciatively.

THIS IS ONLY the second group, but already we are sensing something surprising, even wondrous. What are the odds of a woman who has been raped by a minister in a faraway city being in a small group with a minister from the same denomination who comes from a different state? And of that man being so immediately empathetic and whole-heartedly compassionate?

And yet, this kind of improbable connection happens in many of our groups. Not long after 9/11, a New York City firefighter listened in one of the groups, open mouthed as the devastated and depressed widow of a buddy who'd died at the World Trade Center described a dream in which her husband spoke to her. "Yeah," the firefighter said, "I saw him, too, in my own dream, and I heard what he said to you." Then he was speaking, and she was silently mouthing the exact same words. "Babe, get your ass off the couch and take care of business."

There's no logical explanation for this. The woman who assigned people to groups had no idea about Clara's abuse by a cleric or that Matt was a minister of the same denomination. The firefighter and his friend's widow had had no previous discussion about her depression or their dream lives.

Carl Jung described these meaningful but not cause-and-effect connections as forms of "synchronicity." When people come together in the safe, exploratory, meditative meetings of our groups, these otherwise inexplicable synchronicities multiply.

IN THE THIRD group, we find our Safe Places and meet our Wise Guides. Now even those who were most reluctant to share are eager to say what they have seen and heard and learned. One begins, and others, like tentative jumpers from a high bridge into water, note the lack of harm, the group's welcome, and the great relief—and find the courage to follow.

Dot, sitting in the garden of her Safe Place, asks a butterfly named Hope why she has such a hard time with the way things are. To her relief, she is reminded that she doesn't have to have an answer, that she can enjoy everything.

Clara finds her Safe Place near a flowing river, sitting on a boulder, among trees and shrubs. Her Guide has no words, but sitting on a nearby boulder, he is an immensely comforting presence. His name is Emmanuel, which Clara remembers means, "God is with us."

Farima, who is struggling with the conflicting demands of parents, small children, and patients, finds herself in the rebuilt kitchen of her destroyed home; she is contentedly cooking her culture's traditional foods. A comforting figure remembered from childhood study, Ali, the prophet Muhammad's son-in-law, appears. "Don't fight," he tells her. "Be here now, loving and present. You are doing everything you can."

Matt meets Jesus near a pond on the land where he grew up, and hears that Jesus is pleased with Clara and with Matt, too.

Jose finds himself on a rough, snowy path to a log cabin where his unlikely Guide—he blushes as he tells us it's Macaulay Culkin—tells him he need not fear his dog's death or marrying his partner. "Life changes, like the weather," little Macaulay reminds him. "The sun always rises."

Shauna finds herself sitting by a mountain lake where she used to fish with her grandmother. Three Guides come, older women for whom she'd cared as a hospice nurse. "We're your guardian angels," they tell her. "We're here to help you grieve your losses. You've never grieved the loss of your grandmother or us, or the loss of your own innocence. It's beautiful to grieve. Do Shaking and Dancing. It will keep the feelings coming." Shauna is crying.

IN THE FOURTH group we are eager explorers as we do the Dialogue with a Symptom, Problem, or Issue.

Asa asks Emptiness what he needs to feel more fulfilled and hears that he has to "open up," to let the words and feelings he has kept to himself up and out of his wounded throat.

For a while, Dot's Dialogue is like a boxer, circling the Insomnia that has plagued her. Then Insomnia lands several jabs: "Start forgiving yourself," "You've given me too much power," and most insistently and tellingly, "Why do you need to have problems?" Dot laughs and laughs at the truthful blows.

When Shauna's turn comes, she speaks "to the Pain in my right side," the one that has eluded the diagnostic efforts of excellent doctors. "I want you," her pained side tells her, "to feel something that you have a right to feel. I want you to know that you are just as important as anyone else." And here Shauna looks up from the page of her written Dialogue and tells the story that only her husband knows.

"When I was twenty years old, I had to fly back to Alabama for my father's birthday. The night before, I was at a party with football players. The guys were drinking. I was drinking. And then the next thing I knew, it was morning, and my vagina hurt and I had a black eye and bruises. I felt beaten all over, and I knew I'd been raped and thought I'd been drugged. I went to the campus police. They took my statement but didn't seem interested. After all, I was drinking, and these were football players."

She felt terrible physically, and ashamed and alone. At home later that day, "my mother said it was my fault." Back at school, the football players yelled insults at her as she walked across the quad.

"I had loved school," she said, crying, "but I couldn't complete the semester." She felt "totally violated," exposed, bewildered, out of touch with and unable to enjoy the body that had previously given her pleasure. Self-inflicted calamities followed, along with life-threatening injuries.

After several years, Shauna began to find peace and purpose in helping people who were deeply hurt and dying, including the women in hospice care who had come as Wise Guides to embrace and counsel her. But she had never healed from the rape and the ridicule and shame that followed it. And until Clara had spoken, she couldn't identify with other women in similar situations, couldn't imagine speaking about her rape, exposing herself to the public condemnation she feared would follow. Only now, here, in this group, did she feel safe enough to mourn the innocent self-confidence and hope she'd lost, to believe that she might somehow recover a full measure of self-respect and self-love.

IN THE FIFTH GROUP, we construct our Genograms, just as Sabrina did. Over the next three sessions, each of us, in turn, will put the Genogram in the center of our circle and trace the four or five generational patterns of connection and conflict. Until now, we've been focused on present exploration and discovery. Now we're looking to the past to inform our present.

I ask each person—as I asked you in the previous chapter—to focus on a challenge that she or he is facing right now, to see who in the Genogram has faced similar challenges, and who can now provide useful guidance and support. I ask the others to sit quietly, noticing what they see and feel as they look and listen, as they become sensitive to the resonance between the Genogram we're looking at and the structure and dynamics of the personalities and challenges in their own families.

"Why," Dot asks as she spreads out her Genogram, "do I have to worry so much?" Almost immediately, answers leap off the page. Her great-grandfather lost the family fortune and killed himself. His daughter, Dot's grandmother, never spoke of what had happened, but she always worried about what *could* happen. Her son, Dot's father, who is also a worrier, worried even more after he lost his own business. Worry, it now seemed to Dot, was an understandable multigenerational dysfunctional strategy—a debilitating reaction but also an attempt to control the uncontrollable. She wonders if this ancient, agitated worry had contributed to the eating disorder which had shamed her, her chronic, global uneasiness, and of course, the insomnia that plagues her. As she speaks, Dot looks stunned and stymied. "Is there any way out?" she asks.

"Look in the Genogram," I suggest. "See if there's someone there who can help you." After a moment, Dot starts tapping her pencil on the square that represents her son. "He's not a worrier," Dot says. "He's broken the cycle. Maybe I can learn from him." And now, in a rush, "I can also do Soft Belly and Shaking and Dancing. They're already helping."

Her Genogram shows Farima how to cut through the confusion about her future. The light of love that lived obscured in her father's family—she's drawn faint lines radiating from them—is here now, in her love for her father-in-law as well as her father. And as she sits in this group, she is seeing the light in herself, feeling the desire and the strength she needs to bring the light to those who fill the page of her Genogram: her family, her patients, and the whole community of refugees she so generously serves. And as she keeps looking, Farima also sees that her desire to serve those most in need is not, as she had feared, a miscalculation or an indulgence. It had once been, she now remembers, her mother's childhood aspiration, the mission to which she had called Farima.

Della, who had felt trapped in her big head in the first group, sees that her own great joy comes not only from intellectual achievement but also from the double lines that make a "loving connection" to so many family members and friends. Looking at her Genogram, the possibilities for fulfillment multiply.

To show their powerful connection, Shauna colors her paternal grandmother's circle and her own deep purple. "When I was six or seven, she said to me, 'Honey, I'm going to die soon,' and then she walked me through her dying days, let me feel proud and loving as I sat and played with her." As she tells us, Shauna feels able to honor the caretaking role that had always been hers. And without willing it, she looks with softer eyes at the circle representing her own mother, now accepting and loving this woman whose rejection and blame, years ago, had hurt her so much.

IN THE FINAL GROUP—the eighth one here, the tenth or twelfth of a series that our graduates lead in their communities—we do a second set of three Drawings and a closing Ritual. I'll share this group with you in the final chapter of this book, when you'll also do the Drawings. Then we'll compare them to the first set we did in chapter 4, mindfully exploring similarities and differences. Like my group members, you're likely to see all the ways you've changed. After we work together on our own Drawings, we'll do our own closing Ritual.

I WANT TO close this chapter by calling your attention to three more blessings that this group and other MBSGs confer on group members, and perhaps on you as you read about it.

Without anyone pushing for it, these groups invite us to question and reevaluate our preconceptions and prejudices, the ways we judge others and ourselves. Perhaps we began, in the first group, by envying Dot's accomplished perfection or distancing ourselves from it and her.

As she met her Guide and did the Dialogue, we saw the anxiety that compelled her to shield herself, the pain that fueled her perfectionism. Then, as she showed her Genogram, we felt Dot's vulnerability and the sweetness of her connection to her son. Perhaps, as we appreciated all this, we became aware of our own strained efforts at social presentation, our own self-defeating perfectionism and our own need to let down our guard and come close to those we love. Clara's rage and disorganization may initially have put us off, but Matt's embrace and Clara's grateful yielding set an example of kind attention and showed us the possibility of profound change.

As we participate in or even read about an MBSG, we also realize that all of us truly are, as the Lakota people say, "related" to one another, that we are each other's teachers. Each of us gives the others a mirror in which we can more easily see our own challenges, a mirror that may show us unexpected ways to meet those challenges.

Finally, a number of us become an ongoing part of each other's lives. On the third day of the training, my group members began to have lunch together. On the last evening they went out dancing. In the years since, a number of us have continued to connect, to work together and become friends.

19
Gratitude Changes Everything

G RATITUDE IS THANKFUL appreciation for whatever we receive or experience. This chapter invites you to swim in the current of Gratitude. It teaches you how to ride its waves.

When we've been hurt terribly or lost what is most dear to us, we feel anxious, fearful, and unhappy. Understandably, we wonder why we should be grateful. Brother David Steindl-Rast, a Benedictine monk who has devoted many years to helping people live in Gratitude, turns the question on its head. "It's not happiness that makes one grateful," Brother David says, "but gratefulness that makes us happy."

Some people seem more inclined to feel grateful. Recent scientific studies show that these grateful people more easily decrease their levels of physical pain, generally feel better, exercise more, and spend less time in doctors' offices. Grateful people who have had one heart attack are less likely to have a second one. Sleep, so often interrupted after trauma and when we're under stress, is significantly easier for those who can experience and express Gratitude; they're less likely to dwell on the negative, worrying thoughts that make it hard to fall asleep, thoughts that might also startle them awake in the middle of the night.

And research is now demonstrating that gratefulness can decrease the symptoms of post-traumatic stress disorder and improve the mood of those who've been traumatized. In fact, one Israeli study shows that Gratitude (happiness with life as it is) was highly effective in preventing trauma-exposed children from developing post-traumatic stress disorder.

Some of us are naturally grateful. However, the rest of us can learn to be more grateful. We can nurture our capacity for Gratitude and reap these and other benefits.

GRATITUDE REQUIRES A shift in attitude. It sometimes happens in the midst of trauma or just after it's over—a burst of appreciation for being alive, for having survived. It's certainly worth remembering a moment like this, savoring it, keeping it as a touchstone. But if we're to move among trauma's contending claims of fear, grief, anger, agitation, guilt, and shame to live with Gratitude, we must cultivate and tend to it.

I've seen many people do this. The appreciation with which so many cancer survivors, like Jane, come over time to assess their terrifying diagnosis and debilitating treatment is an ongoing source of wonder and inspiration. "I would not wish to have had cancer," Jane said, "and it has been the most valuable experience of my life. I now know what's important to me. For the first time I'm really alive."

For Jane and so many others, meditation was the starting point. That's not surprising. Meditation is itself a form of Gratitude. When we do Soft Belly breathing regularly, day after day, we become aware of what is happening in each moment, of all our thoughts, feelings, and sensations. This awareness matures, little by little, to appreciation, which is simply Gratitude for whatever is happening. All you need to do is breathe, look, and listen.

Ismail, a tall, bearded, slightly stooped, forty-year-old Palestinian middle-school teacher, felt this shift. On the fourth morning of one of our Gaza trainings, he paused at the door of the room where our small group was meeting. "I have something to tell you before I come in," he announced. "Something I am ashamed of and something I am proud of.

"For six months, ever since the end of the last war, I've been very irritable. I sleep poorly, and I seem to be dissatisfied with everything. Many days I come home, pick up a stick, and beat my children. I'm a teacher and I know I shouldn't, but their arguments and their noise make me so angry I cannot help myself.

"Yesterday evening, I came home and saw them wrestling and heard their music and shouting. But this time I stood there, just as I'm standing here in this doorway, and I did Soft Belly breathing for five or ten minutes, just as we learned it here a few days ago. And I relaxed.

"And when I opened my eyes, I saw the same scene that got me so angry every other day, but it looked different. 'These are my children,' I said to myself. 'They're adolescents. This is the way adolescents act.' And it made me smile, and I felt love for them."

AFTER A WHILE, we may even find ourselves, like Jane, grateful for our pain and hurt. It's not that these are pleasant feelings; it's simply that as our capacity to let uncomfortable thoughts and feelings come and go increases, we realize that pain and hurt are part of us, that we can learn from as well as endure. And we also know that they are *only* a part of us, that we are more than our distress. And we feel grateful to know it.

Sometimes, after I've done Soft Belly for a few minutes, I find myself spontaneously smiling, appreciating, thoroughly enjoying the experience of breathing. Sometimes before I begin, I remind myself to smile with Gratitude as I exhale. Five or ten minutes later, after I finish, it feels like I've put on a pair of glasses that make everything I see softer, more inviting, more hopeful. I suggest you do this now. Take five minutes to consciously appreciate the process of breathing that gives you life and keeps you alive, that connects you with all of Nature. Smile with pleasure in it.

YOU CAN ALSO consciously focus on those things in your life for which you're grateful. This doesn't mean denying pain or loss. It's simply a matter of encouraging yourself to remember the gratifying part of your life that trauma has not obliterated.

The simplest way to do this is by keeping a Gratitude Journal. Robert Emmons of the University of California at Davis, who is probably the world's leading Gratitude researcher, has published many studies on the benefits of these journals. The numbers of weeks or months that people kept journals varied, but the bottom line was constant: those who kept Gratitude Journals felt better physically and emotionally; they exercised more and had fewer physical symptoms; were less anxious, angry, and ashamed; slept better and were more optimistic. In addition, people who wrote in their journals daily reported that they were significantly more likely to provide emotional support to others; their Gratitude encouraged them to act in ways that gave others reasons to be grateful.

My recommendation, based on Emmons's research and my experience with traumatized people, is simple: **Write down, at the beginning or toward the end of each day, three to five things for which you're grateful.**

Here are a day's entries from Sharon, whose chronic pain had increased exponentially following a fractured femur.

I'M GRATEFUL:
For my goddaughter's phone call.
For my neighbor, Dave, who brought the morning paper to my
    door.
For the fresh basil in my garden that I can sprinkle on my
    tomatoes.

Sharon's days are filled with pain and shuttered by her limited mobility. Her Gratitude Journal reminds her to celebrate what she *does* have. "It doesn't make the pain disappear. But it does ensure that pain is not the center of my existence. Some mornings it's hard to find something to be grateful for. Still, I do it, and it makes me smile and sets me up for the day."

A Gratitude Journal is just a beginning. Every one of the experiments we've done together can be an occasion for Gratitude, for enhancing our enjoyment of our body and mind, our hope for ourselves, and our connections to others. All we need to do is pause, perhaps do Soft Belly breathing for a few minutes, and allow ourselves some moments of Gratitude for what we've done and learned.

Mindful Eating, with its acts of choosing, preparing, and slowly savoring food, is an example. After each bite, we can become aware of our pleasure in taste and texture, appreciate the contribution each mouthful is making to our health and well-being.

The other techniques we've learned provide the same service, offer the same opportunity for us to feel Gratitude: the Wise Guide's helpful words, the insight that emerges from a written Dialogue with a Symptom, the never-before-seen problem-illuminating detail in a Drawing.

OTHER PEOPLE OFFER us many opportunities to grow in Gratitude: friends and family, people we meet in groups and classes, even casual acquaintances or chance encounters. All it takes is relaxing and paying attention, and letting yourself appreciate that this other person is actually there with you, talking to you. As she pauses and speaks and listens, she is affirming that you are worthy of attention, that you are good, or at least good enough to be with.

What these other people do and say can multiply your Gratitude. A few words of kindness or a smile from someone ringing up your purchases in a store, or taking your token on a bus, or pouring coffee, or checking you in at an airport are delicious—if you stop to savor them. And the words and acts of friends are even more valuable—especially when they share themselves with you or ask with genuine interest how you are and what's going on with your family members and mutual friends. If I am relaxed and really paying attention when this happens, I feel so grateful for the sustaining circle of connection, concern, and affection, for this fundamental, life-giving human experience.

IT'S EASY IN the press of daily demands, especially if we're feeling irritated, anxious, or overwhelmed, to neglect to be grateful. That's why it's important to consciously call Gratitude to mind. When I look with Gratitude at the twisting branches of the winter-bare trees outside my window, the brown of the earth, the shape of a hill, what I see seems as gorgeous as a Cézanne painting.

And if I suggest the possibility of Gratitude to others, they often respond with recognition and satisfaction. On the first evening of a weekend workshop titled "Trauma and Transformation," I mentioned that I'd been writing about Gratitude. A woman whose daughter had died of an overdose several years before said she was glad I'd reminded her of Gratitude. It made her realize she was grateful for what she'd learned in a previous workshop with me, and grateful also for our upcoming weekend. "I'm so grateful," she said, "because now I know that the more deeply I go into my sadness, the easier it is for me to find greater joy."

Then several other people who'd been traumatized by loss and illness spoke. They realized that even with their troubles, they were "blessed" to have a weekend to be with themselves, and the money and time to make it possible. Deborah, who'd been feeling adrift and hopeless in the void left by her father's death, smiled dreamily as she recalled her Gratitude for her almost silent bus ride to our retreat, "watching as the snow fell so peacefully, covering the ground and trees."

AND HERE'S ONE more way to invite Gratitude into your life.

Many years ago, near the end of my dear professor Bill Alfred's life, he looked up from the morning eggs he was scrambling, raised his eyebrows, and gave a small smile. "Don't you think it would be a good idea," he asked, "if sometimes, instead of praying or asking for something for ourselves, or even someone else, we just said to God, 'Thank you for a very nice day'?"

These words return to me often. Sometimes I do exactly what Bill suggested—thank God (sometimes I say "Nature" or "the Universe") for the trees outside my window or the sunlight coming through it, or moments with a friend or a patient, or a phone call from someone I love, feeling Gratitude for what I've been given. When I'm feeling "blue," as Bill would say, or frustrated, I remember his words and see his smile and feel my own smile, blessing, even in the middle of distress, each moment, each day.

I'm not someone who prays regularly, and I don't know if you are, but I'd like to suggest Bill's prayer to you: "Thank you, God, for a very nice day." It's simple, unpretentious, and nondenominational. Any of you can do it. As you do, you are experiencing a blessing, Gratitude for all your life's opportunities—for quietly meditating, or sharing food or feelings, or walking down the street, or taking a deep breath.

I THINK OF Gratitude and Forgiveness as subtle but strong currents that can pull us through and beyond the whirlpools of remembered rage and relentless distress that trauma may have left in its wake. Gratitude gives us a progressively smoother, easier passage. Forgiveness, which we'll explore in the next chapter, is trickier, more challenging, but potentially even more rewarding. Gratitude prepares us well for Forgiveness.

20
Forgiveness

FORGIVENESS—LETTING GO OF negative emotions toward whoever or whatever has done us harm, and toward ourselves for the real or imagined damage we have done to ourselves or others—is a powerful ally in trauma recovery. But we need to know when and how to make this alliance.

We also need to understand that Forgiveness and justice are not necessarily opposed. Forgiveness is far easier if we feel justice has been done. A measure of justice—punishment for a murderer or rapist, returned money from a thief, heartfelt apologies from an abuser—helps us overcome our sense of powerlessness and victimization. Ultimately, though, we embrace Forgiveness because it is such a powerful force for healing us and making us whole.

Many aboriginal tribes have regular or periodic rituals of confession and apology, restoration and justice, that free their people and their community from the disruptive and destructive forces of hatred and resentment, as well as the individual and social dangers posed by revenge.

The world's major religions and spiritual traditions celebrate Forgiveness and treasure it as a blessing to the one who forgives. On Yom Kippur, the highest of Jewish holidays, Jews ask for Forgiveness from those they have harmed and then ask God to forgive them. Forgiveness of others is one of Jesus's central teachings and is inextricably linked to finding Forgiveness from God: "And when ye stand praying, forgive, if ye have ought against any: that your Father also which is in heaven may forgive you your trespasses" (Mark 11:25). In Buddhism and Taoism, Forgiveness is treated in an explicitly psychological way. Buddhist texts tells us that anger, and the resentment and hatred to which it gives rise, are poisons that must be drained.

Modern science has confirmed ancient wisdom. Holding grudges, nurturing a desire for revenge, and feeling resentment are all dangerous to us. If we haven't forgiven the hurt and anger, the resentment we feel at who or what has traumatized us takes a biological toll. Our levels of stress and stress hormones rise and reinforce the destructive effects of our trauma. We grow more suspicious and fearful. We may define ourselves by our suffering and live our lives as ongoing victims of our trauma.

Forgiving is therapeutic. It purges us of resentment's emotional and spiritual poison and its high levels of biological stress. When we forgive, regions of the brain that are compromised by trauma, including the prefrontal cortex, become more active. Forgiveness quiets the fear and anger of the amygdala, balances the sympathetic nervous system's hyperarousal with vagal calming, and enhances our capacity for perspective and compassion. A number of scientific studies have shown that in forgiving others we become more relaxed. Chronic pain subsides, and high blood pressure goes down. Our mood improves. We feel more optimistic. Combat veterans who are more capable of Forgiveness have fewer symptoms of post-traumatic stress disorder.

Thinking about Forgiveness we may find ourselves objecting, resisting, asking: "How do you forgive the unforgivable?" "Who would

I be?" we may protest. "How could I respect myself if I forgive X?" And more poignantly, "How can I forgive myself for what I've done—for failing to protect myself against who or what has hurt me, or for provoking, collaborating with, or creating my own or others' trauma?"

The damage that trauma has done to our brains compounds our doubts and our resistance to Forgiveness. Trauma, unresolved, continually activates centers of fear and anger in the emotional brain and inhibits functioning in areas of the frontal cortex that facilitate compassion. Gila, a generous, kind Israeli psychologist who lives not far from the periodic combat with Hamas's Gaza militants, put the dilemma well: "I know the people of Gaza have suffered terribly, but I'm so frightened for my children that I have no room in my heart to care for the adults, or even the children, of Gaza."

IN THE EARLY stages of our work together, I didn't mention the benefits of Forgiveness or encourage you to consider it. If I had, many of you might have wondered why I was even raising the topic. What does Forgiveness have to do with surviving the loss of a loved one or confronting cancer? Those who'd been violated by predators would have been understandably outraged.

I'm discussing it now because we've taken steps that make Forgiveness a possibility: quieting our minds and bodies through meditation; releasing tension, energizing ourselves with movement; learning to accept and let go of fear and rage; balancing our physiology and psychology with diet; mobilizing our imagination and exploring our Genogram to gain perspective on our trauma and its triggers; learning to welcome support from other people and the natural world that will help sustain us as we move beyond our identities as victims.

Feeling Gratitude is particularly important. As we begin to find ourselves grateful for each unfolding moment, for who and what we now are, we will find it harder and harder to bear hatred against who or what has hurt or wronged us. Gratitude opens us naturally to Forgiveness.

There are a few people who have learned to endure hate and hardship without resentment, who have a stunning, Christ-like capacity for forgiving even the most brutal crimes against them. Several days after Israeli soldiers mistakenly shelled and killed three of his daughters and his niece, the Palestinian Muslim gynecologist Izzeldin Abulaish, spoke to me with hard-to-fathom but utterly genuine compassion for the soldiers who had fired the shells, and even for the commanders who had ordered them. Black parishioners at the church in Charleston, South Carolina, prayed for Dylan Roof, the white supremacist who had wantonly gunned down nine of their family and friends.

These people are my teachers, but the bar they set is colossally high. It is painfully hard for many of us to move beyond the hurt and anger caused by far lesser offenses. Still, if we are willing to consider it, to risk it, we too can experience life-giving, spirit-affirming Forgiveness.

THERE ARE COMPREHENSIVE, intensive programs to promote Forgiveness, most often based on a model developed by Robert Enright, an educational psychologist and professor at the University of Wisconsin. Enright's model, which has been used with individuals and in classroom situations, begins with an "uncovering" phase, in which you become aware of the damaging effects of unforgiveness. In the second, "decision" phase, you appreciate the benefits of Forgiveness and commit to it. In the third, "working" phase, you do your best to understand the person who has harmed you and his motives and behaviors in the context of his life; you cultivate empathy and compassion for the offender. In the fourth, "deepening" phase, Enright asks you to look for a higher meaning in your experience.

Children and adults generally finish Enright's months-long programs with lower levels of anxiety, depression, and anger, and higher levels of self-esteem and compassion than matched controls.

The program you and I have created together doesn't focus on or demand Forgiveness; however, it evokes and includes most of the important elements that Enright describes. His approach requires an explicit commitment to Forgiveness; ours comes as a natural consequence of the trauma-healing process. I'm not insisting but instead inviting each of you to embrace Forgiveness, if and when it is right for you.

What follows is a simple, effective way to encounter the obstacles and challenges and explore the possibilities of Forgiveness, and to reap its rewards. Sometimes it quickly yields remarkable results. More often the discoveries come slowly but reliably.

I first learned it many years ago from my friend, the anthropologist and Zen Roshi Joan Halifax, and have modified it slightly. We teach it in our trainings and do it in all of our Mind-Body Skills Groups. I return to it regularly.

Forgiveness Meditation

There are four parts to this meditation, which is also a kind of Guided Imagery. You can do it in silence or while you're listening to a gentle melody. Here it is:

Sit comfortably. Close your eyes. Breathe in through your nose and out through your mouth, allowing your belly to be soft and relaxed. Breathing slowly and deeply, feeling yourself present, here and now, relaxing into your chair with each breath. Breathing in and breathing out.

Allow an image to come of someone toward whom you have anger or resentment. Let yourself see that person now, as if he were sitting across from you in a chair. Choose whomever you like. It doesn't have to be the person who has hurt you the most, just someone toward whom you hold resentment.

Look at that person and say to him, "I forgive you. For whatever you may have done to harm me, intentional or unintentional, I forgive you." Soften toward that person. Imagine him coming into your heart. Breathe in. Hold him there in your heart for a moment, breathing in and breathing out, staying present with him, relaxing, feeling Forgiveness for him, breathing. Allow yourself to be there for a minute or two more. Now let him go, saying, "I forgive you."

BE AWARE OF yourself again, breathing in through your nose and out through your mouth, allowing your belly to be soft, breathing slowly and deeply, feeling yourself present, here and now, relaxing into your chair with each breath, breathing in and out.

Now, imagine someone whom you have harmed in some way. Imagine her as if she were sitting in a chair across from you. Choose whomever you like. It doesn't have to be the person whom you have most harmed. Just someone whom you have hurt and whose name or image comes to you now. Look at that person and say to her, "Forgive me for whatever I may have done to harm you, intentionally or unintentionally. Please forgive me."

Open your heart to this person, and imagine her opening her heart to you. Breathing in and breathing out, imagining your hearts melting together. Hold her in your mind and your heart for a few moments, breathing in and breathing out, staying soft, relaxing, feeling Forgiveness flowing from her toward you, feeling your hearts melting together. Breathe for a few moments more. Now let her go, thanking her for whatever Forgiveness she's offering you, allowing yourself to feel the Forgiveness flowing from her to you, the connection between the two of you.

Breathing slowly and deeply, feeling yourself present here and now, relaxing into your chair with each breath, breathing in and out.

NOW, ALLOW THE image of yourself to come to you. Imagine that you're sitting in a chair across from yourself. Look at yourself and say to yourself, "I forgive you for whatever you've done to hurt me; for however you've let me down, I forgive you." Feel the sensation of opening your heart to yourself, feeling the connection between you and the image of yourself, sitting in a chair across from you, the connection between your hearts. Allow the sensation of opening and softening to spread from you to your image, from your image back to you, uniting you. Breathe in and out, staying soft, relaxing, forgiving yourself, for a few moments more.

Now, allow the feeling of Forgiveness to spread from you, from your heart, to all those on the planet who are in need of Forgiveness. Allow this feeling to grow and expand, breathing in, breathing out, relaxing. Saying to yourself and to everyone on the planet who needs Forgiveness, which is really all of us, "I forgive you. Please also forgive yourself." Breathing in, breathing out, relaxing for a few minutes. Now let that image fade.

Feel yourself now, sitting in your chair, your back against the back of the chair, your seat on the seat of the chair, your feet on the floor, breathing deeply, relaxing.

When you're ready, open your eyes and bring your attention back into the room.

Now write about your experience in your Journal.

FORGIVENESS IS DESIRABLE and possible. This meditation is basic, easy to work with. Over time, you'll grow easier with it, more skillful at it, and the benefits will multiply. Meanwhile, you'll be discovering opportunities for Forgiveness that you can explore with the other techniques you've learned.

If you're prematurely ambitious, the results may be mixed but still interesting. A few months after the war in Kosovo ended, a newspaperman announced that he had found the Forgiveness Meditation "impossible. I cannot forgive the person I saw, the man who killed my brother. On the other hand"—and here he raises his eyebrows in ironic comment—"I decided while sitting here that I did not want to spend the rest of my life seeking revenge."

At first it may be difficult to connect with the person who's hurt you or the one you've hurt. We erect barriers to protect ourselves from repeated injury—and from the pain of knowing what we've done. This resistance, these barriers, may appear in images of our own or another's stiff body, of eyes turned away or flat with rage and suspicion. As you encounter these barriers, you may feel the fear or guilt that created them. That's not pleasant, but it's good. As these emotions emerge from the place where pain-fueled denial and suppression have buried them, they may crack the barriers, soften your posture or the posture of the one who has hurt you or whom you've hurt. You may see facial expressions change, feel Forgiveness emerging.

Forgiveness can't be forced. It's usually gradual and requires patience, a muscle that must be slowly built. Instead of beginning with an abusive parent or treasonous partner, you may want to start with an image of the guy who cut you off in traffic. As you feel the heat of remembered road rage, breathe deeply, relax with it, feel it cool. Next time, or the time after, you may want to invite someone who has hurt you more.

Sometimes, though, particularly if you've been practicing the other techniques you've been learning, you may immediately feel Forgiveness's surprising blessing.

It happened that way for Linda EagleSpeaker, a Blackfeet tribal elder and social worker who was in my group at a training. She, like so many Indian children who grew up in the 1950s, had been forcibly taken from her parents' tribal home. Confined in a state boarding school for years, she'd been demeaned as a "savage," beaten for speaking her native language, kept away from her family. In our first group, the Drawing of her biggest problem had revealed the black outline of a building with four empty, black-framed windows, a place where soul-killing "monsters" brought despair to Native American children.

During the Forgiveness Meditation, Linda saw her Drawing of "that building." She resisted the image, not believing she could ever forgive what went on inside it or the monsters who made it happen. "Then, suddenly, without wanting it or expecting it, I realized that the ones who did all those terrible things to me actually were human and had souls, and I felt a great burden of hatred and fear lifting."

IT'S THE SAME with asking to be forgiven. Don't force the issue. Before you ask your lover or spouse to forgive you for a relationship-wounding betrayal you may have never admitted, you may want to ask Forgiveness for acts of inattention or words of condescension.

NOT INFREQUENTLY, the person you're forgiving and the one from whom you're asking Forgiveness are identical. That's not surprising. Often our most intimate relationships—with life partners and parents, children and siblings—have been fraught with hurt inflicted and received, with hurt unresolved.

For several years, when a former partner of mine appeared in both roles, we both looked as stiff and combative as the terra cotta warriors we had long ago visited in China. Even my most energetic efforts to open my heart and invite her to do the same felt contrived, futile.

Not long ago, after many, many tries, I could see and feel our stiff bodies cracking and opening. Now, as I slowly named each of the hurts I'd inflicted on her, I felt my internal balance shift. My previous dutiful pleas for Forgiveness were yielding to a real, surprisingly humble acknowledgment of all the hurt I had done. And then, as I began to forgive her for hurting me, my cold constriction yielded to images warm with how she had once cared for me and I for her. Wonderful old feelings of attraction, appreciation, and tenderness revived, along with memories of shared adventures and discoveries. I didn't expect that this meditation would change her, but I felt a little easier, more content and expansive, as if a flower were blooming in my being.

FOR MOST PEOPLE, the third part of this meditation is the hardest—sitting across from yourself, forgiving yourself. This is true for those who have been horribly abused, as well as for those of us who have inflicted harm on others and for any of us who regret what we've done to spoil our own lives.

Even as a small child, Maya knew the horror of the way her mother treated her. Still, Maya felt unreasonably responsible for her mother and guilty for the degradation she'd inflicted on Maya and herself—the days of drunken abandonment and the times when she traded her daughter for money or drugs.

Like Maya, many of us feel that what was clearly beyond our control was still our fault. Others of us, like Diana, have been angrily, consistently told that we're responsible for what's been done to us. Any experienced social worker has heard abusing fathers lay this kind of blame on a five- or ten-year-old daughter: "She was coming on to me."

Those of us who've actually inflicted harm on others have also been traumatized by our actions. We, too, need to forgive ourselves. This kind of trauma has been described as "moral injury." It's what soldiers like Jason feel after they've perpetrated, witnessed, or were unable to prevent death and destruction. Partners of parents who abuse their children feel it; so do those of us who, in betraying a loved one, know we are also violating our own values.

Admitting what we've done is the first step in asking for Forgiveness and the necessary precondition for forgiving ourselves. As we sit, at least in our imagination, with those we've harmed, and feel their pain and take responsibility for what we've done, our hearts open to them and also to ourselves. Then, as we humbly ask for their Forgiveness, we feel worthy of it and ready to begin to forgive ourselves.

YOU CAN USE the techniques we've learned and the perspectives we've gained to facilitate, enhance, and deepen Forgiveness.

Here again Soft Belly breathing is fundamental. A meditative mind is crucial to Forgiveness. Remember Ismail, the teacher in Gaza. Instead of once again reacting angrily to his children's noisy behavior and beating them, he stopped, breathed, opened his eyes, and looked. He appreciated, felt Gratitude for them and, yes, forgave them as well.

Chaotic Breathing, pounding pillows, and shouting allowed Howard to release his anger at his ex-wife. Then Forgiveness arose spontaneously.

Guided Imagery pulled Jason through the skeleton-strewn landscape of his buddies' deaths to a place of love for them, to peace with and Forgiveness for his own inability to save them.

Sometimes this is a many-step process. When I ask my Wise Guide why I'm holding on to a grievance or nursing a harm that's been done to me, the butterfly, bird, or child who appears may turn the question back to me: "When did that happen before?" "Whom does that remind you of?" "What are you getting out of staying so hurt and angry?" Each question pushes me to take a larger perspective on the pain and resentment that have been closing my mind and cramping my heart. And as the dialogue unfolds, it really feels like I have someone or some being, at once more tender and tougher and wiser than I am, who is committed to helping me find the Forgiveness that I now know is important to me.

SOMETIMES FORGIVENESS BLOSSOMS suddenly, in mysterious ways. After ten years of work with Soft Belly, Guided Imagery, and Shaking and Dancing, Sally, who had been incestuously abused by her father, went on a retreat. The first night she "woke up with horrible abdominal pain. It felt like labor, but I wondered if it was my PTSD, if I was dissociating? I was crying and crying. And then all of a sudden, I realized, 'My father is here. He's still alive,' though I'd considered him dead for twenty years. He was wearing white, and he was calling every single person in my life who'd hurt me to come together. And all these people gathered in a circle, and they said they were sorry for everything they'd done. And in this image I saw that, here and now, my father had become my Wise Guide. Finally, I felt Forgiveness for him."

Genograms are a particularly powerful tool for forgiving others and ourselves. As you continue to look at them, they offer you an ever-wider perspective—at once comforting and strengthening—on who hurt you and whom you've hurt, how and why it happened, and also what you can do about it now.

When Sabrina's younger sister treated her disdainfully at a family party, her Genogram allowed Sabrina to understand and hang in, rather than condemn and withdraw. "I saw the circle I drew in my Genogram, around my mother and my sister. She was raised with my mother's anxiety and anger in a Black bourgeois community where she never quite fit in. She resents me for being so at ease, but she was with my mother, with her anger, all the time. She never really had a chance to form her own identity. I damn sure don't like how she treats me, but I have to feel compassion."

Until she began to work with her Genogram, Maya "hadn't realized the true horror of my mother's life. When she was just a baby, her father died and her mother—my grandmother—became catatonic." Checking with family members, Maya learned what her mother had never told her: "That she'd been raised by teenage brothers who raped her regularly and 'harnessed her to a plow and beat her like a donkey.'"

Over the years, Maya has returned often to her Genogram. "I had to look, again and again, at that circle in my Genogram that represented the little girl who was me. I had to feel her sad belief that she controlled her life and was responsible for her mother's suffering and her own. I had to realize how utterly vulnerable and powerless she had been. Then I could cry for her and how hard she tried and how unfair it all was. Then I could forgive her—and myself."

21
Love, Meaning, and Purpose

Trauma shows us who we can be, as well as who we really are. And trauma makes it possible for us to become that person.

People struggling to survive trauma, and therapists who work with them, often cite Nietzsche's famous aphorism "That which does not kill us, makes us stronger." Nietzsche's words can be encouraging in dark times, but they're also limiting and even misleading. We do gain strength as we move through our traumas, and the effort and will we mobilize can energize us. Still, trauma's greatest gift is Love.

Love is, as Viktor Frankl learned in the concentration camp, the "ultimate good" that carries us through and beyond trauma's terrors. It shapes and blesses the Meaning and Purpose that we subsequently find. Love lights up the Drawings that Azhaar, once heartbroken and despairing, did at the end of her Mind-Body Skills Groups—the tiny stick figure with the downturned mouth has become a big girl, solidly planted on the earth, pleased with her brown curls, loving Nature, devoting herself to healing the hurt hearts of her fellow Gazans.

Jason, a leader in a war that took away his soul, becomes whole again as he welcomes a mission to heal soldiers undone by traumatic brain injury. Diana was "crushed" when she was young, degraded and emotionally crippled; every day she devotes herself to a disabled child, and becomes the mother she wishes she had had.

Once lonely and suicidal, Howard the entrepreneur sheds his shame and discovers his gifts; he finds joy and satisfaction in coaching and mentoring others who are as conflicted and isolated as he once was. Sally, profoundly depressed and disorganized after her father's physical and sexual abuse, discovers pleasure in her own mind and body, and fulfillment in sharing what she's learning with others who've also been hurt.

As we use the tools I've shared with you, we progress from self-awareness and self-acceptance to self-love and compassion, and to Love for others who are suffering similarly. We open up to, soften with, colleagues, family, and friends for whom we had believed we needed only to be cool and competent. There is a new resonance between us and those whom we might have previously avoided or ignored, or even feared or condemned. After her diagnosis of stage IV cancer, Jane, a fastidious, conservative suburban housewife, joins a new church and goes on a mission to El Salvador. She lives in a poor family's shack and cares for the war-orphaned children whose suffering now speaks to her.

This is a progression that I've seen over and over again, which you can find in just about everyone I've introduced you to. And it's not that I or anyone else is saying this is how you *should* feel or what you *have to* do. It's what people are discovering for themselves, a possibility of bonding with and caring for others that is built into our biology. It seems as natural as seeds growing into plants and plants flowering. It is a little like what Bill, my old professor, called the "duty of delight." It's humans becoming whole.

This process can be described as a "spiritual awakening," one that can come outside of, as well as within, established religious traditions. It is one that shamanic healers have known and nourished for millennia. It is embodied in the rites of passage they preside over, the consciously chosen, tradition-sanctioned trauma that separates young people from childhood and brings them into alignment with adult roles that demand responsibility and wisdom, into harmony with the natural world and their own natures. Understanding that this awakening is possible and natural, shamans treat the wounds of those who suffer from wars, diseases, and loss as opportunities for them to heal themselves and, eventually drawing on their own experience, to heal others.

EACH OF THE techniques you've learned helps lay the biological and psychological foundation for this flowering of Love and the Meaning and Purpose it animates. Breath, which is synonymous with spirit in so many languages (Sanskrit, Hebrew, Arabic, and Greek), is the starting place and provides the enduring connection. Soft Belly breathing quiets the amygdala-based fear and anger that are Love's enemies, enhances the frontal cortex's capacity for compassion, as well as judgment, and encourages us to bond with others. Remember once again the agitated teacher in Gaza who had been beating his children, now standing in the doorway of his home doing Soft Belly breathing and opening his eyes to see that those same unruly children are "only adolescents." Biofeedback and Autogenics, and all the other quieting techniques, deepen the experience.

Expressive meditations release the tension that fear and anger have buried in our bodies. They allow you to relax, to feel more at home in yourself, less defended against—more open to—other people and the world. Darcy the firefighter, Howard the entrepreneur, and the Kosovar Man of Sorrow all felt this. Jane, dancing daily, falls in love with her own cancer-filled body and opens her heart to orphaned Salvadoran children.

Keeping a Journal nurtures this growth. A 2008 study published by psychologist Joshua Smyth showed that men and women with severe PTSD—Vietnam veterans and survivors of sexual assault—who wrote about their emotional reactions felt significantly greater "personal strength and appreciation of life . . . and greater hope for new life possibilities."

Drawings, Wise Guide Imagery, Dialogues, Body Scans, and the Forgiveness Meditation all allow us to discover and explore possibilities for caring and connection outside the box of traumatized thinking. Jason's Wise Guide showed him why his life had been spared and what his life work would be. In Nora's Body Scan, her uterus, emblem of her long-disparaged femaleness, became her crown and reconnected her to her husband. Linda EagleSpeaker, the Blackfeet elder who, to her astonishment, felt compassion for those who had brutalized her, lovingly shares what she has learned with trafficked girls and homeless women.

The Genogram offers examples, guides, and inspires. As Sabrina returns over and over to talk to her disabled, long-dead grandmother, she grows in appreciation of her own vulnerability, and in her dedication to communicating with and caring for the lost and lonely. Maya, locating long-forgotten "angels with skin," is confirmed in her commitment to being a human angel for other children, to bringing light and comfort to their lives.

This compassion for others and the gifts it prompts us to give are a continually renewed source of well-being for us, as well as a sign of our healing. Recent research on this altruistic activity confirms our experience. Those who reach out to help others—volunteering to serve strangers as well as aiding family and friends—feel less depressed, less anxious and angry, less constrained by trauma's psychological troubles and hobbling biology. They have fewer symptoms of physical illness and feel more fulfilled. And these benefits encourage them to give and share more. It's a virtuous cycle of joy and fulfillment. Altruistic people live longer.

We see and hear it every day in our Mind-Body Skills Groups. "It was so great to feel everyone's love and support," people say. "And it was even more amazing to discover that my story, my struggles, what I was learning, could help somebody else."

AT FIRST, WHEN you're moved to reach out or help or share with others, you may feel uncertain, vulnerable, or foolish. It makes sense. You're exposing yourself, bringing into the open a tender part that's been growing inside you. This is the kind of unaccustomed generosity against which we may have been warned, the chance-taking that parents or peers may have mistrusted or mocked as naive or "soft" or self-destructive. After we've been traumatized, hurt, or betrayed, we're likely to be even more reluctant to risk our hearts.

It makes sense that you're fearful, and it's actually okay if you feel foolish. Fools in many cultures are understood as agents of awakening and change. I know that just about everything important I've done in my adult life—from falling in love, to caring for children, to admitting the hurt I've done, to exploring the new ways of helping people that I've been sharing with you—seemed at first risky and foolish, and was often enough dismissed by others as outrageous or even deluded. Still, when I've responded with generosity, however imperfectly, I've felt good and at ease. When I've resisted or second-guessed myself, I've regretted it, felt constricted, and remained preoccupied with what I hadn't done.

I suggest you treat your loving, generous impulses as experiments.

If it suddenly occurs to you to call a family member or friend from whom you've been distant or estranged, don't wait. Do it. If it seems right, volunteer at a homeless shelter. See and feel what it's like while you're doing it and afterward. And take these steps lightly, expecting nothing other than the satisfaction of knowing you've done what it feels right to do.

Afterward, you'll likely be a little more relaxed and at home in your body, perhaps pleased with the courage it's taken. If it turns out to be awkward and you're rejected—if your brother is twice as cranky and critical and unwelcoming as you remembered—you've still done what felt right. Perhaps sometime later he'll remember and respond differently.

IF THIS GROWTH into Love, Meaning, and Purpose seems familiar, it's not surprising. It is the psychobiological infrastructure for the Golden Rule, which is the essential common denominator of the world's religions.

About two thousand years ago, so the story goes, a "pagan" challenged Rabbi Hillel to teach him the entire Torah—the Bible of the Jewish people—while standing on one foot. "If you do," said the pagan, "I'll become a Jew."

Rabbi Hillel replied: "What is hateful to yourself, do not to your fellow man. That is the whole of the Torah. The rest is commentary. Go and learn it."

What a moment that must have been: the rabbi pulling up his gown as he raised one foot, speaking without hesitation, the pagan stunned.

It's a moment that seems to have occurred, a teaching that emerged, in all the great religions. Sometimes it's stated, as Hillel did, with an emphasis on not doing what is hurtful. Sometimes the focus is on what we *should* do. Here's Jesus in Matthew 7:12: "Therefore, all things whatsoever you would that men should do to you, do you even so to them, for this is the law and the prophets."

The Golden Rule reminds us of how intimately connected we are to one another. It tells us how to fulfill ourselves, that we find Meaning and Purpose in acts of Love. Moving toward the light of this Golden Rule, we continually, peacefully, move beyond trauma's crushing grip.

This sense of trauma being transformed is what makes great souls, like the Dalai Lama and Archbishop Desmond Tutu, such compelling and inspiring models. In their presence we feel that fear and anger have melted in the warmth of compassion. Still, it is a process for them as well as us. Living this everyday miracle—staying true to the Love that's growing in us and the Meaning and Purpose toward which we're moving—is ongoing and requires reminders. Here are some perspectives I've found helpful and some specific tools to help you stay true to Love, Meaning, and Purpose:

- Keep your mind experimental and open. It has allowed you to do the (sometimes strange) techniques in this book. It allowed you to open the book in the first place.

- Stay in the present moment. Pay attention to what attracts you now. Don't dismiss a person or activity because she wasn't your "type" before or you "never did that." That was then. That's your history. Remember, you're always changing. This is now.

- Life is a mystery to be explored and lived. Check out the person or opportunity. As long as there's no obvious and irrevocable danger—walking between men who are shooting at each other, leaving a happy twenty-year marriage because of a passing attraction—see what happens. You never know. An interviewer once asked the great trumpeter Miles Davis what he did about playing "wrong notes." "There's no such thing as a 'wrong note,'" Miles replied. "It's the next note you play that tells you if it's right or wrong."

- Use the techniques for mobilizing your imagination and intuition—Drawings, Wise Guide Imagery, Dialogue with a Symptom, the Body Scan, etc.—to check out the relationship or activity you're experimenting with. Stay tuned in. Listen to the answers you get.

- Relax into and enjoy what you're doing. Don't force it. Finding and fulfilling your Meaning and Purpose requires work, but it's not about being a good boy or girl and piling up virtue points. That's a recipe for self-righteousness, for souring generosity. Perhaps you can, as my friend Marc Raskin once said, "follow the music of your heart."

- Be patient with yourself and others. Opportunities for Love, Meaning, and Purpose will arise. I find the old Eastern saying to be true: when I am ready to learn or change—when I've paid enough dues and am receptive enough—the right teacher, the right life-fulfilling opportunity does appear. Sometimes it's simple, ordinary: a homeless woman needs money and a little conversation, and I'm in the mood for it. Sometimes, as with Clara, who was violated by one minister and disparaged by his superior, the surprising connection—to another minister who believes and values her—is miraculous, life changing.

- Make Laughter your friend. It will relieve your tension and raise your mood, give you perspective on your obsessive concerns, and relax the need to control that cramps generosity and foils freedom. A couple of minutes a day can make a big difference.

- When it feels right, share what you've learned, what's made your life better, with others. You might suggest Soft Belly breathing to a family member who's nervous about a medical procedure or to co-workers before a staff meeting. Explain that it may help decrease your relative's pain or help everyone at work listen better, be less tense, think more clearly. But don't be a bully about it. It's an experiment. It's great if your husband or colleagues want to do it, but don't take it personally if they don't.

- Do your best to be humble. You may well be doing a remarkable job of transforming your trauma, and that's wonderful. Enjoy it. But if you start patting yourself on the back or insisting that others do as you're doing, you lose the rhythm and fall out of step on the next part of your journey.

- Check in with friends. Not for approval. It's not, as Sally observed, about needing to be fixed by their advice or good opinion. But do look for the wisdom that helps you see yourself more clearly. Welcome the compassion that warms the circle of Love.

- Be generous. Don't hold back as you give and grow. And this is not, as Shyam would remind me, just about giving more. What's needed is what he called "emperor giving"—giving spontaneously without thought, motive, or expectation, so that the right hand does not know what the left hand is doing.

- Read and reread the stories in this book. Let yourself take in the example and inspiration that these very real people offer. Look as well at research on post-traumatic growth. It confirms what you've read in *The Transformation*. Again and again, the terrible trauma of the widows and disabled people studied by the researchers turned out to offer them access to great gifts: increased inner strength, openness to new life possibilities, closer and deeper relationships with friends and families, life-defining commitments to others who have suffered similar losses and disabilities, and stronger religious faith. Remember Azhaar opening her broken heart in Love, committed to healing other hurt hearts.

At the end of our trainings, our faculty sings songs to the people who have come to learn from us. After the first phase of our training—the one where they learn to use the same skills you've been practicing—it's often Kate Wolf's "Give Yourself to Love." Kate was a friend of my college roommate and dear friend, Rick deLone. Kate died very young of cancer. Rick, who died not so long after, also of cancer, used to play the song on his guitar.

My faculty and I sing it because Love is, after all, the goal of our work, the most important opportunity we're offering, the great lesson we're learning and teaching.

I cry every time I hear the song, thinking of Rick, missing him, and also for all my losses and loneliness. And then, without willing it, I find myself wiping away the tears and relaxing, remembering, feeling my Love for Rick, and Laughter and dance come. You should listen to Kate sing the song. But, until you do, here are the verses:

Kind friends all gathered 'round, there's something I would say:
That what brings us together here has blessed us all today.
Love has made a circle that holds us all inside.
Where strangers are as family, loneliness can't hide.
You must give yourself to love if love is what you're after;
Open up your hearts to the tears and laughter
And give yourself to love, give yourself to love.

I've walked these mountains in the rain and learned to love the wind;
I've been up before the sunrise to watch the day begin.
I always knew I'd find you, though I never did know how;
Like sunshine on a cloudy day (you) stand before me now.

So give yourself to love if love is what you're after;
Open up your hearts to the tears and laughter
And give yourself to love, give yourself to love.

Love is born in fire; it's planted like a seed.
Love can't give you everything, but it gives you what you need.
And love comes when you're ready, love comes when you're afraid;
It'll be your greatest teacher, the best friend you have made.
So give yourself to love if love is what you're after;
Open up your hearts to the tears and laughter
And give yourself to love, give yourself to love.

Many times after our Advanced Training—the one where our program graduates learn to teach to others what they have been learned—we sing "This Little Light of Mine." The message is clear: they, we, all of us, are going to take out into the world the light of Love, the healing virtue of the techniques we've learned, the brightness of our Hope. We're going to share the best of ourselves—all of ourselves—with others.

This is what I want for myself, what I wish for all of you, as we keep on practicing what we're learning. Take every opportunity to give yourself to Love. Let your light shine.

22
Next Steps

THIS LAST CHAPTER is a summing up of where we've been and what we've been through, and an opening to the future—to where and how we want to be, physically, emotionally, socially, and spiritually. It will also help us see how to get where we hope to go. As in our concluding Mind-Body Skills Group, we'll begin with a second set of Drawings and conclude with a brief Ritual of affirmation—a rite of passage, of farewell to what we no longer need and preparation for our future.

Before we do the Drawings, check in with yourself. Are you aware of any changes from when you first opened this book? Changes in what's on your mind and in your heart? Are fewer thoughts racing through your brain or happier ones occupying it? Your shoulders might feel less tense, and you might find yourself breathing more slowly and deeply. Perhaps you've been comforted, reassured, and inspired by the stories you've read and by some changes you feel in yourself. Perhaps you're recognizing what still needs to change. Take a look at yourself in a mirror. Who and what do you see? Maybe your eyes are a little brighter or you find that you're smiling.

Take some time to appreciate everything you've learned, how you've changed, what you still need to address, and how you are— right now. Write down what you've noticed, what you've learned.

NOW IT'S TIME for the second set of Drawings.

They will give you more information about who and how you are, now, after the weeks or months you've spent with your trauma-healing program of self-awareness and self-care. They will help you discover and take the next steps in your journey through and beyond trauma.

When you compare these Drawings with the ones you did early in this book, while you read chapter 4, "Embracing Hope," you'll see some similarities and likely many differences. They may well show you how far you've come, how and how much you've changed. They will give you Hope and guidance, and may well energize you as you move ahead in your life.

Let me invite you, now, to join all the people you've met in *The Transformation* and everyone who is reading this book, and me, to create a second set of Drawings. Before you do, make sure you have the first set nearby. Don't look at them. I don't want you to be thinking about "then," just focusing on "now." Afterward, I'll ask you to compare the Drawings you're doing with the ones you did at the beginning of our journey together, as you staked your claim on Hope.

HERE ARE YOUR INSTRUCTIONS.

Once again, there are three Drawings, and you'll need three sheets of blank paper—8½" by 11" is fine—and crayons or magic markers. Do the Drawings quickly, about five minutes for each. Remember, "first thought, best thought." Don't control. Let it come, let the inner wisdom with which you've become more familiar guide your hand. That way the Drawings will be uncensored, authentic, surprising, revealing. Afterward, you'll see how they can play a creative, guiding role in your life.

Okay. Let's get started.

Begin by doing two or three minutes of slow, deep Soft Belly breathing with your eyes closed. Relax. Repeat "Soft" as you breathe in and "Belly" as you breathe out, noticing your thoughts, feelings, and sensations come and go, and gently bringing your mind back to "Soft Belly."

Now open your eyes and do the first Drawing. Once again, it's "Yourself." Don't think about what you drew before. That was then, this is now. Just let it come. Do it. Once you've done Drawing #1, put it aside.

The second Drawing is "Who or how you would like to be." Again, take some deep breaths before your begin. You don't have to think about this. Let your intuition pick your colors; let your inner wisdom guide your hand. Let it all unfold on the page. Once again, take about five minutes.

Put aside this Drawing, then close your eyes and breathe slowly and deeply for several minutes more.

Now the third Drawing. Draw "How you're going to get from Drawing #1 to Drawing #2—from where you are now to how or where or who you want to be." Once again, let your imagination and intuition guide you. No second-guessing. Trust what appears on the page. After five minutes, put aside this Drawing.

ONCE YOU'VE FINISHED, you'll put these three Drawings and the three you did before on a table or desk. There will be two rows. The Drawings you did at the beginning of this book in chapter 4 will be in a row below those you've just done.

Before you look at these two sets of Drawings, go back to the opening scene in the first chapter, to Azhaar sharing her Drawings of death and rebirth in that cold, rainy Gaza ruin. Hear and feel once again what she is saying.

Now take some slow, deep breaths, perhaps five minutes of Soft Belly breathing. When you've finished, open your eyes.

Look now at the two sets of your Drawings. What's your general impression? Look at the size of the figures, the content, and the colors you chose. What are your feelings as you look at each set?

Now look at your Drawings one by one, slowly, closely.

Begin by comparing the first Drawing in each set, the ones of yourself as you are now. What's similar? What's different? What are your feelings as you look at each? How do you look? Check out the details.

Azhaar was a tiny stick figure in the corner of her first Drawing. Her mouth was turned down in sadness. In the first Drawing of the second set, she is a substantial girl, standing proudly, filling one side of the page. Curls frame her face. Her features are distinct and visible, carefully drawn. Eyes open, mouth turned up in a smile. There is a heart in the middle of the page, an arrow that flies from her chest and pierces it. The words inside the heart are "I Love Nature." They tell us she's connected, joyous. The tree toward which the arrow heads is lush with green life.

The differences in your #1 Drawings may be less dramatic, but they're likely to be there. In my Mind-Body Skills Group, Della's oversize head is now proportional to a well-formed, graceful body. Farima thought she looked "nice" in her first Drawing, but she was alone. Now she has drawn "all of me . . . myself, my husband, children, my religion, me cooking at the stove, my patients, all in a circle around me." Shauna, who hadn't yet shared the pain and shame of her rape, was a stick figure in the first set. Now she says, "It's amazing. I have a body and light in my heart."

Sometimes the differences bring smiles to all of us. Asa points to his throat, now bright with the color that streams from his mouth and he tells us, with a resonant voice we've never heard before, that he has energy where there'd been deadness, and confidence to speak. Matt, a tiny bald man in his first pictures, is now large, full of energy, and long-haired.

Write down everything you see and feel as you continue to look. It will likely bring back memories of where you were, give you a feeling for how far you've traveled, as well as where you are now.

Now, take a look at Drawing #2 in the first set. This was "You with your biggest problem." Remember what it felt like when you drew it. Take some time to feel the feelings—the pain, fear, frustration, constriction, discouragement, hopelessness, despair. How do you feel now as you look at it again?

Azhaar, you'll remember, was overwhelmed by death and destruction. Her father, uncles, and aunt lay bloody and dead on the ground; stones were falling from her bombed home, the Israeli planes that had brought her loss flying overhead. Della's Drawing was dominated by symbols of demand and signs of stress—a clock, a dollar sign, and the outstretched hands of needy clients—and she was tense. Shauna felt mournful, surrounded by stick figures gunned down by violence.

Now look at Drawing #2 in the second set: "Where or how or who you want to be."

Compare it to Drawing #3 in the first set: "You with your problem solved." Notice the similarities and differences between the solution then and the aspiration now; recall the feelings you had when you did Drawing #3 in the first set and the ones you have as you look at Drawing #2 in this set. They'll tell you a good deal about how you may have changed.

The difference for Azhaar was dramatic. Before she began the Mind-Body Skills Group that transformed her, her "solution" was to die, to join her father in a grave. In the second Drawing of the second set, she became a life-bringing heart doctor. The rectangular form of the grave metamorphosed into her examining table.

In Drawing #3 of her first set, Shauna "connected the dots." She formed the stick figures into a tentative circle. Now in this Drawing of who she wants to be, she is "a butterfly emerging from a cocoon, bringing people together." Farima had solved the problem of temporary homelessness in Drawing #3 of her first set: she was content in her kitchen. Now she aspires to something far larger and more gratifying: to be "my best self, living a meditative life, enjoying every aspect of the process of returning home." Della's previous solution and present aspiration are similar in content, but the feeling and images are quite different. Then, there were people joined in a circle. Now, you see "a radiance coming from my heart and around me, and not just from me, but from everyone in the circle."

Now look at Drawing #3 in the second set. This is something quite new. It's a prescription that you're giving yourself for getting where you want to be. It may be simple, logical, straightforward. Azhaar was sitting at her desk, studying to become the heart doctor she showed us in her second Drawing. In your Drawing #3 you may be returning to school to train for a new, more satisfying career to replace the one that no longer serves you; or stretching on a mat in a yoga class to deal with stress and make connections with other people. Your Drawing may be more symbolic: you're walking on a mountain path, reminding yourself of your need to get away from work, collect yourself, and connect with Nature; you're smiling with your arms around family members who were distant or absent from previous Drawings. It may be more purely aspirational. Shauna draws herself speaking to diverse groups in her neighborhood, inviting them to join her in a program of community-wide understanding and healing.

Now tell the story of each set of Drawings, writing it down in your journal. As you do, become aware of the differences in the stories. And write down what you're discovering. Azhaar might have written that before she began her mind-body group she felt overwhelmed, insignificant, in despair at her beloved father's death, yearning only to die to be with him. After using the same tools and techniques you've been practicing, she saw that she could turn toward life, enjoy the world around her, and imagine herself preparing for a future in which she could care for other people with skill and love. Perhaps she saw herself offering others a professional version of the loving care her father had given her.

If you've been doing these experiments with a partner, tell the stories to her. While she listens, become aware of what you're seeing and feeling as you speak. Then, ask her to show her Drawings to you. Be there as a witness, an appreciative, silent partner, noticing, once again, what is happening with you as you sit with her.

Whether you're doing the Drawings alone or with a partner, write down what you've seen and heard, and the feelings and thoughts you've had.

AT THE VERY end of trainings or a series of our mind-body groups, after we've shared our Drawings, we have our closing Ritual.

Rituals are ceremonies that mark transitions. They're organized to create an experience that is distinct from the ordinary events of our daily lives.

Rituals are as ancient as human society, and they are a part of every culture. All of us in the twenty-first century still participate in Rituals—there are religious ones like the Catholic Mass, Islam's five daily prayers, and Judaism's Sabbath observance. And there are secular ones, like yearly birthdays marked with presents and a cake with the appropriate number of candles, brought ceremoniously to the table and accompanied by singing.

Rituals strengthen the bonds between us and enhance the tend-and-befriend response. Rituals make us feel more secure, giving reliable structure to our lives and reducing anxiety. Rituals are particularly important at times of change and uncertainty. They provide ordered, safe passage for children becoming adolescents and adolescents transitioning into adulthood. They organize, solemnify, and sanctify the marriage commitment, and they can help us deal with the traumatic dissolution of divorce. Rituals are used to celebrate our achievements and mark our retirement from work.

Rituals soften the terrible blow that death's finality inflicts; they help us to express our grief and invite others to share it with us. They can give us a feeling for a continuity and connection that transcends death.

The circle of our Mind-Body Skills Groups provides the structure for a Ritual. When we do Soft Belly meditation at the beginning and end of our groups, we are participating in a Ritual. The check-in after our opening meditation is a Ritual. So, too, is the overall structure of the group, with each person speaking in turn. When we sit together to do Guided Imagery or Drawings, we are also participating in a Ritual. Ritual deepens and celebrates our experience of all the tools and techniques we are using to understand and help ourselves.

When you mindfully, respectfully do each of your experiments in self-care, you are also participating in a Ritual. Reading and absorbing the teaching stories in this book can be done with the respect and have the gravity of Ritual.

These Rituals can all be healing ceremonies, helping us to grow through and beyond trauma.

THE RITUAL YOU and I are now going to participate in marks the end of the time we've spent together. It is an appreciation of what this book has offered you and what you've accepted and embraced. Like the Drawings you've just done, it recognizes and celebrates what you've learned and how you've changed. It also reaffirms our connection to each other and launches all of us onto the next stage of our life's journey.

I've often used the Ritual that follows. Like much of what is important and life changing, it's simple. It invites you to identify and let go of what you now know you no longer need and to take with you all that will serve you well as you move ahead in your life. This Ritual requires two pieces of paper, $8\frac{1}{2}$" by 11" or a little smaller, white or colored, elegant or simple, depending on your preference. Get the paper ready. Now take a few minutes to prepare yourself, breathing slowly and deeply, relaxing. Notice your thoughts, feelings, and sensations. Let them come and go.

Now open your eyes and write down, on one of the pieces of paper, everything this book has helped you learn about and explore that you'd like to leave behind: your anxiety or agitation, your shame at the trauma you've experienced, your fearfulness of triggers, your tendency to interrupt or argue rather than listen, your stubborn self-judgment, your desire for revenge. Whatever comes, just put it down on the paper. Take your time. Let yourself feel what you're writing, and feel yourself willing to let go of it as you write it down.

When you're finished, put this paper down. Take another couple of minutes to breathe deeply, once again noticing and letting go of the thoughts, feelings, and sensations that arise.

Now, on the second sheet of paper, write down everything you want to take with you from reading and working with The Transformation and living your life while you've been doing it: glimpses of Hope and moments of awareness, and the excitement of discovery that goes with them; memories of release in your body and the unexpected joy of Shaking and Dancing; the astonishing tenderness you may have felt toward someone you once feared or disliked; Gratitude for kindnesses and pleasures you had previously ignored, or devalued; the discovery of a family connection that gave you understanding or comfort or courage; images of the people you've met in these pages, and stories of their struggles and triumphs that may have inspired you. As you write down each experience and realization, feel yourself making it a part of you, claiming it as your own. Savor the experience.

READ THE FIRST piece of paper—the one with everything you're letting go. Become aware, again, of what you want to leave behind and how it feels to let go of it. In our Mind-Body Skills Group, these papers were filled with "fear," "ambivalence," "lack of connection to my body," "people who have caused me pain," "numbness," "self-doubt," "loneliness," and "darkness."

Put this paper aside for now, and plan to burn it. Not right away, but perhaps in a day or two, or a week from now, when you can take some quiet time and give this Ritual the respect it deserves.

Please burn the paper in a place that feels good and safe—near a stream or close to a mountain, or in your backyard or a room in your home. Take a little time to choose the place. It will become, like the places that indigenous people have always chosen for Ritual and ceremony, special to you, dedicated to the changes, the Transformation that you're experiencing and will continue to experience.

After you've burned this paper, scatter the feathery gray ashes in water or in the air. Or, if you'd like, bury them, so the death of what you no longer need can feed the growth of what is new, in you and in the earth.

Keep the second piece of paper, the one with everything you're bringing with you. Read what you've written as many times as you'd like. Many people put this paper in a place where they can see it often: on a bulletin board in a study, next to a computer, on the refrigerator, or on the wall of a tent in a refugee camp. These are the touchstones for your Transformation. They will help you know what to do and where to find what you need when your body is tense or your mind triggered, when you feel discouraged, lonely, or overwhelmed.

You may find yourself looking at this paper saying, as I do, "Oh yes, I remember Shaking and Dancing. That's how to free myself from this funk." Or "I need my Wise Guide to show me the way out of this disappointment." Or "It's time for me to connect with my old friend, who will listen to and love me, in spite of my sadness."

TAKE SOME TIME NOW, or in the next few days, to write down anything else that you hope will keep you on the path from where you are now to where you want to be—what will help you stay true to what you've learned and who you are. This includes the attitudes and aspirations, tools and techniques you'll be using and your plan for the weeks and months ahead.

You'll want to note your preferred tools for calming and quieting your mind and body—perhaps Soft Belly, Biofeedback and Autogenic Training, and Mindful Walking—and the kind of regular movement and exercise you're going to do. How you're going to make food your medicine, as well as your joy. What expressive techniques you can choose to break up anger and release tension, and give yourself to Laughter and Love. How and when you're going to stay close to people you care for and celebrate your connection to Nature.

You may make a commitment to staying open when you're challenged and relaxing when you're triggered, to embracing the change that will inevitably come to you. Perhaps you want to put the last set of Drawings or both sets on your wall, so you can look again and again at what your imagination and intuition have told you—at who and where and what you want to be, and how you're going to get there. And hopefully, you'll want to remember—and remind yourself again and again—to give yourself to the Love that makes it all possible.

For me, this list includes less food and wine, eaten and drunk more slowly and with greater pleasure; exercising more; daily tai chi; longer, more appreciative looks at the trees outside my window, the branches with the leaves and birds and squirrels on them; Shaking and Dancing, even before irritation or apprehension overcomes me; regular consultation with my Wise Guide; renewed attention to my Journal; reaching out to friends and family the second, if not the very first time they come into my mind; more patience and more tender, open-hearted listening as I stand by my son Gabe as he grows up, as

I wait to see those I dearly miss and as I work with my colleagues; a total willingness to surrender to the Love that rises in me; and always, always, especially when I'm in physical or emotional pain, Soft Belly breathing, staying aware, feeling everything, relaxing.

YOU MAY WANT, as well, to say and write down a few words to this book, which you've held and read. Words of Gratitude are wonderful, and of course, I appreciate them. But this isn't for me. It's for you to recognize what everyone in these pages has shared, what you've felt and learned as you've read, and everything that's been awakened in you.

I know that I'm grateful for the writing I've done, for meeting the challenges of putting what I'm learning into words; for the new, deeper understanding that comes every time I practice the techniques I'm teaching or explain them; for the inspiration the people in this book continue to give me; and for the satisfaction and joy of writing to and for you.

As you become aware of what you've learned and how far you've come, you'll appreciate who and how you are now. You'll know, too, what still needs to be healed, and how you're going to use your new tools to help the healing go even deeper. Your Transformation is ongoing. It's becoming who you're meant to be. It is the energy and glory of your life.

Appendix: Finding Other Help

I'VE WRITTEN *The Transformation* to give you the hope and the confidence to heal yourself from the trauma life brings to all of us and the tools you need to do the job.

I also know that there are times when all of us—no matter how wise or strong or true to a program of self-care—need help from others.

In chapter 7, I wrote about the critical importance of social support, of family and friends who are "there" for us in challenging times—accepting, listening to, loving us. In chapter 18, "The Healing Circle," you sat in on one of our Mind-Body Skills Groups—a supportive, respectful, safe place to learn to use the tools of self-care and share the discoveries you're making with others who are doing the same. If you look on our website (cmbm.org), you'll find information about joining these healing circles in person or online. You'll also see that many of our 130 faculty and 200 certified practitioners as well as a thousand program graduates (almost all are licensed health professionals) are available to use the tools of *The Transformation* with you, in individual and family sessions as well as MBSGs.

Here in the Appendix, I want to extend the possibilities for therapeutic support. I'll begin by offering you some guidelines for choosing professionals who can work with you to enhance your journey and deepen your experience. Then I'll show you snapshots of some evidence-based therapies you may want to include in your trauma-healing program.

THE APPROACH YOU'VE worked with in *The Transformation* is comprehensive. It's also foundational. It invites you to proceed at your own pace. Other therapies can provide intensive, time-limited, therapist-directed attention to particular aspects of trauma healing. Some make use of perspectives and techniques that I've shared with you. All may augment and deepen what you've been learning and doing and how you've been changing.

Remember that the approach you've been reading about and embracing hasn't just been offering the symptom relief and understanding, as important as they are. You've been walking on a path of Transformation, becoming who you're meant to be.

Remember also when you read the descriptions of these therapies that your program of self-awareness and self-care, of giving yourself to Love and discovering Meaning and Purpose, will continue to support and heal you as you work with these other approaches.

Don't be restricted by either/or. It can be both/and.

Before I provide guidance for choosing a therapist and describe these other therapies, I want to briefly discuss the value and place of a medical consultation.

If everything you've been doing, including faithfully using the program in *The Transformation*, isn't giving you all the benefit you hope for—and especially if you're experiencing physical as well as emotional symptoms—you should consult a physician, preferably one who practices "integrative" or "functional" medicine. She can do laboratory testing to explore, and nutritional prescribing to address, genetic variations, infections, biochemical disturbances, or gut abnormalities and other physical disorders and imbalances that may not have been resolved by the Trauma-Healing Diet. She can, if necessary, explore the possible usefulness of medication and herbal alternatives and/or refer you to a nutritionist.

I WANT NOW to share with you a few words that will help you choose among the people who may be offering any of these therapeutic approaches. Please keep in mind that who the therapist or physician is, and how you feel about her or him, is as important as the therapeutic modality you choose.

In an earlier book of mine—*Unstuck: Your Guide to the Seven-Stage Journey Out of Depression*—I discussed at length all the elements that go into selecting a therapist who's just right for you. Here, I want to summarize some of the most important points and add a few more.

Sixty years ago, the pioneering American psychologist Carl Rogers described the ideal relationship between doctor and patient or therapist and client (Rogers's use of *client* rather than *patient* reflected his challenge to a medical model he believed to be inappropriate and disempowering). The phrase he used for this relationship was "unconditional positive regard." *Regard* means not only "respect" but also "look at." The phrase is at once intimate and biological, philosophical and interpersonal. Over the years, it has been widely appreciated and embraced by clinicians of all kinds.

Unconditional positive regard is what I hope you've felt in this book. It's what I want to offer anyone who comes to see me. It's also what I believe every one of you should look for and expect from any therapist you might see, no matter her therapeutic perspective or what technique she is using.

This way of being with you and the connection it brings can itself help repair psychological damage produced by loss and other forms of early and later trauma.

What follows are questions to consider and steps to take as you look for a therapist who will treat you with unconditional positive regard:

- Ask someone who knows you well and cares about you—a physician, friend, or family member whom you respect—for a referral. And when he gives you one, ask why he thought this person (and the modality she uses) would be right for you.

- Check out the therapist's qualifications. You'll generally want someone who's licensed as a physician or nurse, psychologist, social worker, counselor, or pastoral counselor. This ensures a certain level of professional education, as well as recognition by a state government.

- Others who are certified as expert in a particular technique but not licensed can also provide important help. The most popular and effective trauma therapies are offered by licensed professionals who've also been certified as expert in a modality. Sometimes, however, certification without licensure can ensure excellence. This was the case for the rural high school teachers in Kosovo who provided extraordinarily effective Mind-Body Skills Groups for thousands of students and their families, and for Azhaar's group leader in Gaza, as well as others we're now training and certifying in the US: health coaches in the Veterans Administration system, and teachers, parents, clergy, and first responders in communities devastated by school shootings and climate change catastrophes.

- Arrange and be willing to pay for an interview with the person you're considering. During the interview, ask yourself if this is someone with whom you can be honest and vulnerable. Is she likely to be courageous enough to sit comfortably with you as you wail with pain and rage, and wise and generous enough to experience and value your strengths and help you call on them? Bob Coles did this for and with me. So did Shyam.

- Ask whatever questions seem important to you about her qualifications and methods. Why does she use the approach she does? What's the evidence for its effectiveness? In what ways have other patients/clients improved? Has she experienced benefits from this approach herself? How long does she expect the therapy to last? What are her attitudes toward possibly controversial personal challenges and issues that you're facing—for example, divorce or abortion; sexual harassment and racial or gender discrimination; the need for medication; or the importance of group support.

- It's a good idea to write down your questions before the meeting. Others will come to you during it. Afterward, write down your impressions of the therapist, alongside the answers you received. The answers to the questions and the way they were answered will help you make your decision. This is a person you want and need to trust. You may be particularly drawn to one of the therapeutic approaches I'll describe, but that doesn't mean the person you're meeting with will work well with you. Please take your time. Find someone who feels right for you.

- Ask to speak with someone who has worked with this therapist. The experience of this client/patient and the way she talks about it can often help you discern whether this is the right therapist and the right approach for you.

- Use the imaginative techniques you've learned—for example, Wise Guide or Dialogue with a Symptom, Problem, or Issue—to check out your impressions and help you make your decision about a prospective therapist. Perhaps talk over what you've learned with the person who referred you or another friend you trust.

NOW FOR THE therapies themselves. As you'll see, they share—with the exception of medication—certain commonalities: a greater or lesser attention to traumatic events; a method for desensitizing you to the memories and residue of the event; and the evocation of attitudes, perceptions, and experiences that are antidotes to trauma's destructive consequences. However, each therapy has its particular personality and appeal, as well as characteristics that may make it inappropriate for or unattractive to you.

A couple of other thoughts as you read these brief descriptions:

You may want to check out the research on an approach that's of interest to you. I did before I recommended them, but I encourage you to take a look for yourself. I cite a few key references in the Notes. You may want to read these papers or look for others, including ones published since my book went to press. You don't need to have an advanced degree to get the gist of the research. You may not understand the statistics, but the abstract, introduction, results, discussion, and conclusion sections should all be pretty comprehensible. The quantity of the research will give you more confidence in the approach. The kinds of people for whom it's been effective—for example, veterans, survivors of sexual abuse, or people dealing with chronic illness or loss of a spouse—may also help you decide whether it's appropriate for you.

If you do decide to use one of these approaches, give it a fair trial—at least two or three sessions. Remember that whenever concerns about the approach arise, you should bring them to the therapist's attention. Her answers should be direct and satisfying to you.

If, after a while, an approach that was beneficial is losing its effectiveness or appeal, talk it over with your therapist. You may need to recalibrate the way you're using it, or you may need to stop. Once again, use the intuitive techniques you've learned in *The Transformation* to help you evaluate your progress and make decisions. You're always changing. What worked at one time might be unappealing and ineffective at another.

And always remember that you're in charge. You're in therapy to help yourself, not to please your therapist.

HERE, NOW, are some of the therapies:

Cognitive-Behavioral Therapy (CBT) is currently the most widely taught and used therapy for depression and anxiety, as well as post-traumatic stress disorder and a host of other conditions. Developed by University of Pennsylvania psychiatrist Aaron Beck in the 1960s, CBT teaches you to challenge and change negative beliefs about yourself. It is, basically, a series of techniques for helping you see that the glass of water that represents your life is half full rather than half empty.

Beck and other CBT practitioners understand the intimate connections among cognitive beliefs, emotions, physiological functioning, and behavior. Their focus is on challenging and changing belief and behavior; they believe that these changes will affect all aspects of our lives.

CBT usually begins with a stabilization phase, which includes a discussion of trauma and its effects; instruction in relaxation skills; an overview of techniques for problem solving; development of a focus on present events; and replacing unjustified negative thoughts with more realistic, positive ones. So, for example, you learn that your belief that "I do everything wrong" is inaccurate. In fact, like everyone else, you do some things wrong and some things right.

The therapy continues with an assessment of the trauma narrative. This is designed to reveal the most disturbing parts of your traumas. It also helps you overcome the avoidance that compounds trauma's destructive effects.

The third phase, integration, focuses on ways to use thoughts and behavior to deal with your triggers, the real-life situations that reawaken traumatic experience.

There is a significant body of research on CBT's effectiveness for relieving symptoms of trauma, particularly with veterans and women who've been sexually abused, but also for others who've been traumatized by loss.

CBT usually consists of twelve to sixteen hour-long individual or group sessions. If you like problem solving, CBT can be quite appealing and absorbing. Many people find great benefit in integrating the perspective and techniques of CBT into the more comprehensive approach you've learned in *The Transformation*. Some, including a number of veterans I've met, feel CBT is superficial and too slow moving.

Trauma-Focused Cognitive Behavioral Therapy (TF-CBT) combines elements from CBT with aspects of family therapy and education about childhood trauma and PTSD, and skills to regulate emotions.

Therapists have effectively used TF-CBT with children, adolescents, and young adults who have been traumatized by their family, as well as with parents and other caregivers.

Dialectical Behavioral Therapy (DBT) was developed by the psychologist Marsha Linehan in the 1980s for disorganized, self-destructive, sometimes suicidal people, like Diana, who were diagnosed with borderline personality disorder. More recently, DBT has been used to address other conditions, like depression and eating disorders, in which trauma may have played an important role, as well as PTSD. DBT combines CBT with an emphasis on meditative awareness as a path to recognizing, dealing with, and accepting emotions. It is an intensive process and usually requires a dedicated commitment of months or years.

Cognitive Processing Therapy (CPT) combines CBT with detailed written accounts of traumatic experiences and a significant focus on trust, self-esteem, and intimacy. It has been used effectively to address triggers and to enhance the coping skills of military, first responders, and others who anticipate danger in their daily lives.

Acceptance and Commitment Therapy emphasizes openness to experiencing, but not being overwhelmed by or reacting automatically to, unpleasant feelings. It is a more meditative version of CBT.

Prolonged Exposure (PE) was developed by Edna Foa, the psychologist who directs the Center for the Treatment and Study of Anxiety at the University of Pennsylvania. It's designed to help people who've been traumatized to see that their current fears are not intrinsically dangerous. PE uses a deconditioning process in which repeated exposure to your fears—paired with relaxation and therapeutic guidance—reduces your vulnerability to those fears.

After initially explaining the therapy and teaching a breathing technique to reduce stress, PE focuses on talking about and using all of one's senses to evoke intense emotions and memories of trauma. Often these sessions are recorded so that you can listen to them between meetings with your therapist. As you reexperience the trauma, your therapist helps you stay grounded in the present. Over time, you learn to experience and understand the difference between what happened then and what's going on right now.

These sessions can be extremely anxiety provoking, so the relationship with and trust in your therapist is crucial. In addition, you're assigned homework in which you confront situations that would ordinarily trigger you—a dark alley that resembles the one where you were assaulted perhaps, or a war movie if you've been traumatized by combat.

PE is generally offered in weekly individual sessions of 60–120 minutes over a period of about three months. The research on people who participate in PE shows significant reduction in trauma symptoms for those who complete a course of therapy. However, many people are put off by the confrontative nature of the modality, and dropout rates are high.

Narrative Exposure Therapy (**NET**) combines principles of CBT with testimony therapy, a technique originally developed to enable political prisoners and refugees to tell the story of what happened to them.

Your NET therapist guides you in creating a chronological narrative that concentrates on your traumatic experiences but also places them in the larger context of your life. The therapist asks you to describe the emotions, thoughts, feelings, and physiological responses to traumatic events, while helping you stay connected to the present moment and to her.

By the end of this therapy, which usually requires four to ten individual or group sessions, you've created an identity-affirming autobiography in which traumatic events are recognized but ultimately seen as a part, but not the whole, of your life.

Published studies of NET with refugee populations are promising, but the research is not nearly as strong as for CBT and PE.

Mindfulness-Based Stress Reduction (**MBSR**) was developed by Jon Kabat-Zinn at the University of Massachusetts Medical School in the late 1970s. It includes eight weeks of two- to two-and-a-half-hour weekly group sessions and a full-day silent meditation retreat, usually around the sixth week, and is grounded in the moment-to-moment awareness of Buddhist Vipassana (mindfulness) meditation. MBSR combines extensive practice of sitting meditation with mindful walking and eating. It also includes the postures of hatha yoga and body scans.

Mindfulness practice has been shown in many studies (I've cited several of them in *The Transformation*) to enhance brain functioning and promote the growth of new brain cells, as well as to decrease stress and pain, improve immunity, and encourage compassion and loving kindness.

MBSR encourages people who have been traumatized to focus on moment-to-moment present experience rather than trauma symptoms and acceptance rather than avoidance of painful thoughts.

In recent years, MBSR and a hybrid of MBSR and cognitive therapy called Mindfulness-Based Cognitive Therapy (MBCT) have been used to treat post-traumatic stress disorder. Studies on the use of MBSR and MBCT to heal PTSD show promising results.

MBSR's approach to dealing with trauma is quite congruent with the one you've been practicing in *The Transformation*, and the two approaches share several techniques.

Transcendental Meditation (TM) was created by Maharishi Mahesh Yogi (the Beatles's guru) and introduced in India in the 1950s as a form of silent mantra (sound) meditation. The TM organization estimates that it's been taught to four million people worldwide. Practitioners sit on their own for twenty minutes twice a day, breathing normally and focusing on repeating the mantra they have been assigned by their certified TM instructor.

More than forty years of research has repeatedly demonstrated that regular practice of TM can decrease anxiety as well as relieve symptoms of cardiovascular disease and other chronic conditions. More recently, researchers have studied the effect of TM on PTSD. In one randomized controlled trial, they demonstrated that twelve weekly group sessions along with daily practice significantly reduced trauma symptoms.

Many people have successfully combined their TM practice with the approach you have been learning in *The Transformation*.

Eye Movement Desensitization and Reprocessing (EMDR) was discovered by the California psychologist Francine Shapiro in 1987, while Shapiro, who was troubled by disturbing thoughts, was taking a long walk in the woods. After looking for some time at the scenery around her, she noticed that the disturbing thoughts had dissipated. It occurred to her that the movement of her eyes as she scanned the scene around her had somehow dissolved the anxiety that went with the thoughts. The therapy she developed concentrates on memories to be desensitized and uses eye movements to accomplish the task.

After the initial phases of history taking and the discussion of imagery techniques, your EMDR therapist asks you to identify a visual image related to a traumatic memory, a negative belief about yourself that goes with it—for example, "I'm helpless"—and a positive belief that contradicts the negative one ("I'm capable").

The therapist then begins to move her fingers back and forth in front of your eyes, instructing you to follow them from side to side as you recall the disturbing image and the belief that goes with it. As the emotional charge connected to the thoughts dissipates, you begin to "install" the positive beliefs. An EMDR session is regarded as successful and complete when you can bring the original memory to mind without feeling anxious or tense.

EMDR appears to increase parasympathetic nervous system activity while decreasing limbic system hyperactivity and enhancing function in the prefrontal cortex. It has been successfully used with phobias, single fears, and also more complex traumatic experiences. However, the critical role of eye movement has been challenged by other studies, which obtained similar results when the person's eyes were fixed rather than moving.

Interpersonal Therapy (IPT) is a twelve-week structured psychotherapy developed in the 1980s by psychiatrists Gerald Klerman and Myrna Weissman. Originally used for depression, IPT has more recently been successful for people who've been traumatized.

Rather than focusing on traumatic events, IPT deals with the interpersonal origins of the trauma—from loss or conflict—and its impact. The emphasis is on recalling and recreating recent, emotionally charged life circumstances, and using the alliance with your therapist and her suggestions to help you deal with these problematic situations.

You're encouraged to mourn your losses, explore current relationships, and develop more successful options for dealing with these relationships. In the latter phases, there's an emphasis on helping you to become more independent and to anticipate and develop strategies for meeting future life challenges.

IPT dropout rates are generally low, but studies indicate that it is not as effective for severe trauma as PE and CBT.

Somatic Experiencing (SE) was developed by psychologist Peter Levine and is, as its name suggests, a body-oriented therapy. Levine had observed that animals who had been attacked or threatened shook or trembled afterward. He hypothesized that human symptoms of post-traumatic stress—including the anxiety and agitation of fight or flight and the rigidity and withdrawal of freezing—could be relieved by evoking a similar physical discharge.

SE begins with the therapist gently encouraging you to speak of your trauma and become aware of the physical responses connected to it. As the therapy unfolds, you learn to "pendulate," to go back and forth between thinking about traumatic events and discharging the emotions associated with them by physical movement, then returning to a quiet, relaxed, "grounded" state. This alternation between physically and emotionally experiencing helplessness and safety is designed to dissipate the effects of past trauma, reestablish physiological balance, and let you grow comfortable with trauma memories that may remain.

Levine and other SE practitioners emphasize that your emotional and physical reactions are normal responses to trauma. As you come into a state of balance, your therapist helps you experience inner feelings of safety, strength, comfort, and optimism.

The research on SE, still in its early stages, is promising. The approach is particularly attractive for those who wish to address their trauma physically rather than cognitively. There are, of course, significant similarities between PE and the way you've learned to use expressive meditations.

"Tapping" therapies, including Emotional Freedom Technique (EFT) and Thought Field Therapy (TFT), ask you to focus on disturbing thoughts or memories while tapping on acupuncture points. As you tap five to seven times each on fifteen acupuncture points on your face, chest, and hands, you speak aloud of a symptom and accept it and yourself. For example, each time you tap you might say, "Even though I feel this anxiety, I deeply and completely accept myself." Practitioners believe that these acupuncture points decrease activity in the amygdala and create a state of relaxation that promotes desensitization, relieves symptoms, and enhances positive attitudes and emotions.

TFT was originally developed by psychologist Roger Callahan. EFT is a simplified form created by Gary Craig. Both forms of tapping therapy hypothesize that "the cause of all negative emotions is a disruption in the body's energy system."

These self-care techniques are often taught by certified but unlicensed therapists and have been highly controversial. However, recent research on TFT and EFT, including studies by Audun Irgens and Dawson Church, show benefits for traumatized veterans and others.

Medication for trauma. Antidepressant drugs like the selective serotonin reuptake inhibitors (SSRIs) Prozac and Paxil have shown some effectiveness in relieving depressive symptoms associated with PTSD. There's little evidence, however, that they are of any help with the vast majority of trauma-related symptoms: agitation and fearfulness, flashbacks and nightmares, disturbed sleep and concentration, emotional numbing, and withdrawal. And these drugs have very significant side effects, including headaches, weight gain, GI disturbances, and suicidality. Regard them as a last resort, not a treatment of choice.

If medication seems appealing, you might also want to consult with your physician, nutritionist, or dietician about using S-adenosyl-L-methionine (SAM-e) or Saint-John's-wort as less side-effect burdened alternatives.

SAM-e plays a vital role in a variety of metabolic pathways, including the process of methylation (the adding of CH_3 or methyl groups), which is integral to the synthesis of dopamine, serotonin, and norepinephrine, the neurotransmitters that antidepressants also aim to increase. Although the studies are not definitive, there is considerable evidence that SAM-e is as effective in treating depression as antidepressant drugs. SAM-e has a small fraction of their negative side effects but occasionally can cause agitation and may, rarely, precipitate manic excitement in people with bipolar disorder. You can begin with 500–1,000 mg of SAM-e in the morning and early afternoon.

Saint-John's-wort, otherwise known by its Latin name, *Hypericum,* is a plant that has been used by European healers for hundreds of years. Modern research shows that, like SAM-e, it enhances the activity of dopamine, serotonin, and norepinephrine—with similar clinical results in relieving depression and few side effects. You can start with 300 mg twice a day and increase to 600 mg twice a day. The brand you use should be standardized to contain 0.3 percent of the most important active ingredient, hypericin.

There have been no clinical trials on SAM-e or Saint-John's-wort for traumatic stress, but results are likely to be similar to those for antidepressant drugs. Don't, however, take SAM-e or Saint-John's-wort along with antidepressants; the interactions may be harmful.

Notes

INTRODUCTION

1 "Studies of adverse childhood experiences": V. J. Felitti, R. F. Anda, D. Nordenberg, D. F. Williamson, A. M. Spitz, V. Edwards, M. Koss, and J. S. Marks, "Relationship of childhood abuse and household dysfunction to many of the leading causes of death in adults: The Adverse Childhood Experiences (ACE) Study," *American Journal of Preventive Medicine* 14, no. 4 (May 1998): 245–58.

2 "Having a life-threatening illness": F. Stoddard and G. Saxe, "Ten-year research review of physical injuries," *Journal of the American Academy of Child & Adolescent Psychiatry* 40, no. 10 (October 2001): 1128–45.

2 "So is caring for someone": S. Isobel, M. Goodyear, and K. Foster, "Psychological trauma in the context of familial relationships: A concept analysis," *Trauma, Violence, & Abuse* (August 2017): 1–11, doi: 10.1177/1524838017726424.

2 "Poverty is traumatizing": J. A. Parto, M. K. Evans, and A. B. Zonderman, "Symptoms of posttraumatic stress disorder among urban residents," *Journal of Nervous and Mental Disease* 199, no. 7 (July 2011): 436–39.

2 "racism": R. T. Carter, "Racism and psychological and emotional injury: Recognizing and assessing race-based traumatic stress," *Counseling Psychologist* 35, no. 1 (January 2007): 105.

2 "gender discrimination": J. Kucharska, "Cumulative trauma, gender discrimination and mental health in women: mediating role of self-esteem," *Journal of Mental Health* 27, no. 5 (October 2018): 416–23.

2 "Loss of a loving relationship": K. M. Keyes, C. Pratt, S. Galea, K. A. McLaughlin, K. C. Koenen, and M. K. Shear, "The burden of loss: Unexpected death of a loved one and psychiatric disorders across the life course in a national study," *American Journal of Psychiatry* 171, no. 8 (2014): 864–71.

2 "So is the loss of a job": J. Brand, "The far-reaching impact of job loss and unemployment," *Annual Review of Sociology* 41 (August 2015): 359–75.

2 "And all of us": L. K. Lapp, C. Agbokou, and F. Ferreri, "PTSD in the elderly: The inter-

action between trauma and aging," *International Psychogeriatrics* 23, no. 6 (August 2011): 858–68.

3 "Early on": V. Frankl, *Man's Search for Meaning* (Boston: Beacon Press, 2006).

6 "Many psychiatrists": H. Praag, "The position of biological psychiatry among the psychiatric disciplines," *Comprehensive Psychiatry* 12, no. 1 (January 1971): 1–7, doi: 10.1016/0010–440X(71)90050–2.

6 "Studies were even then": J. T. Hartford, "How to minimize side effects of psychotropic drugs," *Geriatrics* 34, no. 6 (June 1979): 83–93.

7 "The research was telling us": R. K. Wallace, "Physiological Effects of Transcendental Meditation," *Science* 167, no. 3926 (1970): 1751–54; H. Benson, J. F. Beary, and M. P. Carol, "The relaxation response," *Psychiatry* 37, no. 1 (February 1974): 37–46.

7 "But concerns about": Committee on Psychiatry and Religion, *The Psychic Function of Religion in Mental Illness and Health* (Dallas: Group for the Advancement of Psychiatry, 1968).

8 "I coedited two books": J. S. Gordon, D. T. Jaffe, and D. E. Bresler, *Mind, Body and Health: Toward an Integral Medicine* (New York: Human Sciences Press, 1984); A. C. Hastings, J. Fadiman, and J. S. Gordon, *Health for the Whole Person: The Complete Guide to Holistic Medicine* (Boulder, CO: Westview Press, 1980).

12 "We published a pilot study": J. S. Gordon, J. K. Staples, A. Blyta, and M. Bytyqi, "Treatment of posttraumatic stress disorder in postwar Kosovo high school students using mind-body skills groups: A pilot study." *Journal of Traumatic Stress* 17, no. 2 (April 2004): 143–47.

12 "The RCT compared": J. Gordon, J. Staples, A. Blyta, M. Bytyqi, and A. Wilson, "Treatment of posttraumatic stress disorder in postwar Kosovar adolescents using mind-body skills groups," *Journal of Clinical Psychiatry* 69, no. 9 (September 2008): 1469–76.

14 "Published in medical": J. K. Staples and J. S. Gordon, "Effectiveness of a mind-body skills training program for healthcare professionals," *Alternative Therapies in Health and Medicine* 11, no. 4 (July–August 2005): 36–41; P. A. Saunders, R. E. Tractenberg, R. Chaterji, H. Amri, N. Harazduk, J. S. Gordon, M. Lumpkin, and A. Haramati, "Promoting self-awareness and reflection through an experiential mind-body skills course for first year medical students," *Medical Teacher* 29, no. 8 (October 2007): 778–84; J. S. Gordon, "Mind-body skills groups for medical students: Reducing stress, enhancing commitment, and promoting patient-centered care," *BMC Medical Education* 14, no. 1 (2014): 198; C. Finkelstein, A. Brownstein, C. Scott, and Y. L. Lan, "Anxiety and stress reduction in medical education: An intervention," *Medical Education* 41, no. 3 (March 2007): 258–64; J. M. Greeson, M. J. Toohey, and M. J. Pearce, "An adapted, four-week mind-body skills group for medical students: Reducing stress, increasing mindfulness, and enhancing self-care," *Explore: The Journal of Science and Healing* 11, no. 3 (May–June 2015): 186–92; J. K. Staples, A. Atti, J. Ahmed, and J. S. Gordon, "Mind-body skills groups for posttraumatic stress disorder and depression symptoms in Palestinian children and adolescents in Gaza," *International Journal of Stress Management* 18, no. 3 (2011): 246–62; J. S. Gordon, J. K. Staples, D. Y. He, and J. A. A. Atti, "Mind-body skills groups for posttraumatic stress disorder in Palestinian adults in Gaza," *Traumatology* 22, no. 3 (2016): 155–64.

CHAPTER 1

17 "When she sits": Center for Mind-Body Medicine, "The Center's Work Featured on CBS 60 Minutes," *Center Blog*, May 31, 2015, https://cmbm.org/blog/gaza/60-minutes/.

CHAPTER 2

27 "This response": S. W. Porges, "Orienting in a defensive world: Mammalian modifications of our evolutionary heritage; A Polyvagal Theory," *Psychophysiology* 32, no. 4 (July 1995): 301–18.

27 "Fight or flight": W. Cannon, *Bodily Changes in Pain, Hunger, Fear and Rage: An Account of Recent Researches into the Function of Emotional Excitement* (New York: Appleton, 1922), http://hdl.handle.net/2027/hvd.32044031655350.

28 "Hans Selye": H. Selye, *The Stress of Life* (New York: McGraw-Hill, 1978).

29 "Freezing is mediated": K. Kozlowska, P. Walker, L. McLean, and P. Carrive, "Fear and the defense cascade: Clinical implications and management," *Harvard Review of Psychiatry* 23, no. 4 (July–August 2015): 263–87.

29 "These memories can affect us": Duke University, "Emotional memories function in self-reinforcing loop," *Science Daily*, March 24, 2005, www.sciencedaily.com /releases/2005/03/050323130625.htm.

30 "High levels of cortisol that persist": K. Szabo and M. G. Hennerici, eds., *The Hippocampus in Clinical Neuroscience* (Basel: Karger Medical and Scientific Publishers, 2014).

30 "They can also diminish": A. Lim, "Stress, cortisol, and the immune system: What makes us get sick?," *Science Creative Quarterly*, December 2007.

30 "and to autoimmune disorders": A. W. Evers, E. W. Verhoeven, H. van Middendorp, F. C. Sweep, F. W. Kraaimaat, A. R. Donders, A. E. Eijsbouts, et al., "Does stress affect the joints? Daily stressors, stress vulnerability, immune and HPA axis activity, and short-term disease and symptom fluctuations in rheumatoid arthritis," *Annals of the Rheumatic Diseases* 73, no. 9 (September 2014): 1683–88.

30 "Over time": J. L. Wilson, "Clinical perspective on stress, cortisol and adrenal fatigue," *Advances in Integrative Medicine* 1, no. 2 (May 2014): 93–96, doi: 10.1016/j .aimed.2014.05.002.

30 "The level of the energizing": J. E. Sherin and C. B. Nemeroff, "Post-traumatic stress disorder: The neurobiological impact of psychological trauma," *Dialogues in Clinical Neuroscience* 13, no. 3 (September 2011): 263–78.

30 "Many people": E. J. Dansie, P. Heppner, H. Furberg, J. Goldberg, D. Buchwald, and N. Afari, "The comorbidity of self-reported chronic fatigue syndrome, post-traumatic stress disorder, and traumatic symptoms," *Psychosomatics* 53, no. 3 (May 2012): 250–57.

30 "Trauma diminishes functioning": J. Douglas Bremner, "Traumatic stress: Effects on the brain," *Dialogues in Clinical Neuroscience* 8, no. 4 (December 2006): 445–61.

30 "Sometimes communication between the two hemispheres": R. A. Lanius, P. A. Frewen, M. Tursich, R. Jetly, and M. C. McKinnon, "Restoring large-scale brain networks in PTSD and related disorders: A proposal for neuroscientifically-informed treatment interventions," *European Journal of Psychotraumatology* 6, no. 1 (2015): 27313.

30 "We cannot concentrate or relax": K. S. Gilbert, S. M. Kark, P. Gehrman, and Y. Bog-danova, "Sleep disturbances, TBI and PTSD: Implications for treatment and recovery," *Clinical Psychology Review* 40 (August 2015): 195–212.

31 "When trauma causes prolonged freezing": L. Margolies, "Understanding the effects of trauma: Post-traumatic stress disorder (PTSD)," *Psych Central*, October 2018, https://psychcentral.com/lib/understanding-the-effects-of-trauma-post-traumatic-stress-disorder-ptsd/.

31 "Suicide may seem": S. M. Rojas, S. Bujarski, K. A. Babson, C. E. Dutton, and M. T. Feld-ner, "Understanding PTSD comorbidity and suicidal behavior: Associations among histories of alcohol dependence, major depressive disorder, and suicidal ideation and attempts," *Journal of Anxiety Disorders* 28, no. 3 (April 2014): 318–25, doi: 10.1016/j.janxdis .2014.02.004.

31 "Twenty US veterans": U.S. Department of Veterans Affairs, "VA Releases Veteran Suicide Statistics by State," *News release* 8 (2017), https://www.va.gov/opa/pressrel /pressrelease.cfm?id=2951.

31 "Very large numbers of American children": V. J. Felitti and R. F. Anda, "The relation-ship of adverse childhood experiences to adult medical disease, psychiatric disorders, and sexual behavior: Implications for healthcare," in *The Impact of Early Life Trauma on Health and Disease: The Hidden Epidemic*, R. A. Lanius, E. Vermetten, and C. Pain, eds. (Cambridge: Cambridge Univ. Press, 2010), 77–87.

31 "As adults, 66 percent": Felitti et al., "Relationship of childhood abuse and household dysfunction."

32 "This, in turn, makes us more vulnerable": Felitti and Anda, "The relationship of adverse childhood experiences."

32 "Trauma can cause epigenetic": C. Rampp, E. B. Binder, and N. Provençal, "Epigenetics in posttraumatic stress disorder," *Progress in Molecular Biology and Translational Science* 128 (2014): 29–50.

32 "the shortening of telomeres": A. O'Donovan, E. Epel, J. Lin, O. Wolkowitz, B. Cohen, S. Maguen, T. Metzler, M. Lenoci, E. Blackburn, and T. C. Neylan, "Childhood trauma associated with short leukocyte telomere length in posttraumatic stress disorder," *Bio-logical Psychiatry* 70, no. 5 (September 2011): 465–71.

33 "Trauma disrupts our digestion": D. A. Drossman, "Abuse, trauma, and GI illness: Is there a link?," *American Journal of Gastroenterology* 106, no. 1 (January 2011): 14–25, doi: 10.1038/ajg.2010.453.

34 "When we're stressed": J. V. Esplugues, M. D. Barrachina, S. Beltran, S. Calatayud, B. J. R. Whittle, and S. Moncada, "Inhibition of gastric acid secretion by stress: A pro-tective reflex mediated by cerebral nitric oxide," *Proceedings of the National Academy of Sciences* 93, no. 25 (December 1996): 14839–44.

34 "If we take proton pump inhibitors": M. Sanaka, T. Yamamoto, and Y. Kuyama, "Effects of proton pump inhibitors on gastric emptying: A systematic review," *Digestive Diseases and Sciences* 55, no. 9 (September 2010): 2431–40.

35 "stress can produce ulcers": M. P. Plummer, A. R. Blaser, and A. M. Deane, "Stress ulceration: Prevalence, pathology and association with adverse outcomes," *Critical Care* 18, no. 2 (March 2014): 213.

35 "It can damage the villi": G. Davidson, S. Kritas, and R. Butler, "Stressed mucosa," in *Nutrition Support for Infants and Children at Risk*, ed. R. J. Cooke, Y. Vandenplas, and U. Wahn (Basel: Karger Medical and Scientific Publishers, 2007), 133–46.

35 "loosen the tight junctions": Davidson, Kritas, and Butler, "Stressed mucosa."

35 "These molecules, among them": M. Hadjivassiliou, D. S. Sanders, R. A. Grünewald, N. Woodroofe, S. Boscolo, and D. Aeschlimann, "Gluten sensitivity: From gut to brain." *Lancet Neurology* 9, no. 3 (March 2010): 318–30.

35 "a powerful effect on the microbiome": J. A. Foster, L. Rinaman, and C. F. Cryan, "Stress & the gut-brain axis: Regulation by the microbiome," *Neurobiology of Stress* 7 (March 2017): 124–36.

36 "the population of good bacteria decreases": Foster, Rinaman, and Cryan, "Stress & the gut-brain axis."

36 "Under stress, bacteria that belong": A. C. Bested, A. C. Logan, and E. M. Selhub, "Intestinal microbiota, probiotics and mental health: From Metchnikoff to modern advances; Part II—Contemporary contextual research," *Gut Pathogens* 5, no. 1 (March 2013): 3.

37 "That's when we reach": M. F. Dallman, N. Pecoraro, S. F. Akana, S. E. La Fleur, F. Gomez, H. Houshyar, M. E. Bell, S. Bhatnagar, K. D. Laugero, and S. Manalo, "Chronic stress and obesity: A new view of 'comfort food,'" *Proceedings of the National Academy of Sciences* 100, no. 20 (September 2003): 11696–701.

37 "And when we eat sugar": B. Spring, J. Chiodo, and D. J. Bowen, "Carbohydrates, tryptophan, and behavior: A methodological review," *Psychological Bulletin* 102, no. 2 (September 1987): 234–56.

38 "Dishes high in fats": Z. A. Cordner and K. L. Tamashiro, "Effects of high-fat diet exposure on learning & memory," *Physiology & Behavior* 152, pt. B (December 2015): 363–71, doi: 10.1016/j.physbeh.2015.06.008.

38 "And sweet-tasting foods": C. Colantuoni, P. Rada, J. McCarthy, C. Patten, N. M. Avena, A. Chadeayne, and Bartley G. Hoebel, "Evidence that intermittent, excessive sugar intake causes endogenous opioid dependence," *Obesity Research* 10, no. 6 (June 2002): 478–88.

38 "high-sugar, high-fat diets": Colantuoni et al., "Intermittent, excessive sugar intake."

38 "Brain-derived neurotrophic factor (BDNF)": J. R. Pfeiffer, L. Mutesa, and M. Uddin, "Traumatic stress epigenetics," *Current Behavioral Neuroscience Reports* 5, no. 1 (March 2018): 81–93, doi: 10.1007/s40473-018-0143-z.

38 "Over time, inflammation": A. Manzel, D. N. Muller, D. A. Hafler, S. E. Erdman, R. A. Linker, and M. Kleinewietfeld, "Role of 'Western diet' in inflammatory autoimmune diseases," *Current Allergy and Asthma Reports* 14, no. 1 (January 2014): 404, doi: 10.1007/s11882-013-0404-6.

38 "The dangerous combination": V. Drapeau, F. Therrien, D. Richard, and A. Tremblay, "Is visceral obesity a physiological adaptation to stress?," *Panminerva Medica* 45, no. 3 (September 2003): 189–95.

39 "In time it may increase": A. Shuster, M. Patlas, J. H. Pinthus, and M. Mourtzakis, "The clinical importance of visceral adiposity: A critical review of methods for visceral adipose tissue analysis," *British Journal of Radiology* 85, no. 1009 (January 2012): 1–10.

39 "Accumulated visceral fat": C. Finelli, L. Sommella, S. Gioia, N. La Sala, and G. Tarantino, "Should visceral fat be reduced to increase longevity?," *Ageing Research Reviews* 12, no. 4 (September 2013): 996–1004, doi: 10.1016/j.arr.2013.05.007.

CHAPTER 3

40 "And trauma may override": Sherin and Nemeroff, "Post-traumatic stress disorder."

41 "It quiets the amygdala's frenzy": A. A. Taren, P. J. Gianaros, C. M. Greco, E. K. Lindsay, A. Fairgrieve, K. W. Brown, R. K. Rosen, et al., "Mindfulness meditation training alters stress-related amygdala resting state functional connectivity: A randomized controlled trial," *Social Cognitive and Affective Neuroscience* 10, no. 12 (December 2015): 1758–68.

41 "if you meditate regularly": S. Breit, A. Kupferberg, G. Rogler, and G. Hasler, "Vagus nerve as modulator of the brain-gut axis in psychiatric and inflammatory disorders," *Frontiers in Psychiatry* 9 (March 2018): 44.

41 "Meditation enhances functioning": E. Luders, P. M. Thompson, and F. Kurth, "Larger hippocampal dimensions in meditation practitioners: Differential effects in women and men," *Frontiers in Psychology* 6 (March 2015): 186, doi: 10.3389/fpsyg.2015.00186.

41 "promotes the growth of new brain tissue": S. W. Lazar, C. E. Kerr, R. H. Wasserman, J. R. Gray, D. N. Greve, M. T. Treadway, M. McGarvey, et al., "Meditation experience is associated with increased cortical thickness," *Neuroreport* 16, no. 17 (November 2005): 1893–97; B. K. Hölzel, J. Carmody, M. Vangel, C. Congleton, S. M. Yerramsetti, T. Gard, and Sara. W. Lazar, "Mindfulness practice leads to increases in regional brain gray matter density," *Psychiatry Research* 191, no. 1 (January 2011): 36–43, doi: 10.1016/j.pscychresns.2010.08.006.

41 "Meditation reliably reduces high blood pressure": C. M. Goldstein, R. Josephson, S. Xie, and J. W. Hughes, "Current perspectives on the use of meditation to reduce blood pressure," *International Journal of Hypertension* 2012 (2012): 578397.

41 "and decreases the inflammation": I. Buric, M. Farias, J. Jong, C. Mee, and I. A. Brazil, "What is the molecular signature of mind–body interventions? A systematic review of gene expression changes induced by meditation and related practices," *Frontiers in Immunology* 8 (June 2017): 670.

42 "helps preserve the length of the telomeres": E. Epel, J. Daubenmier, J. T. Moskowitz, S. Folkman, and E. Blackburn, "Can meditation slow rate of cellular aging? Cognitive stress, mindfulness, and telomeres," *Annals of the New York Academy of Sciences* 1172, no. 1 (August 2009): 34–53.

42 "reverse the epigenetic damage": Epel et al., "Can meditation slow rate of cellular aging?"

42 "In one of Lazar's studies": Hölzel et al., "Mindfulness practice leads to increases."

42 "And in another study by Fennell": A. B. Fennell, E. M. Benau, and R. A. Atchley, "A single session of meditation reduces of [sic] physiological indices of anger in both experienced and novice meditators," *Consciousness and Cognition* 40 (February 2016): 54–66.

43 "One ancient Indian tantric text": S. S. Saraswati, *Asana Pranayama Mudra Bandha*, 4th ed. (Munger, Bihar, India: Yoga Publications Trust, 2008).

43 "Though there are many forms": C. Naranjo and R. E. Ornstein, *On the Psychology of Meditation* (New York: Penguin Books, 1976).

44 "I learned Soft Belly": Stephen Levine, *Unattended Sorrow: Recovering from Loss and Reviving the Heart* (Emmaus, PA: Rodale, 2005).

50 "Research by the University of Wisconsin's Richard Davidson": T. R. A. Kral, B. S. Schuyler, J. A. Mumford, M. A. Rosenkranz, A. Lutz, and R. J. Davidson, "Impact of short- and long-term mindfulness meditation training on amygdala reactivity to emotional stimuli," *NeuroImage* 181 (November 2018): 301–13.

50 "If you practice Soft Belly regularly": V. Perciavalle, M. Blandini, P. Fecarotta, A. Buscemi, D. Di Corrado, L. Bertolo, F. Fichera, and M. Coco, "The role of deep breathing on stress," *Neurological Sciences* 38, no. 3 (March 2017): 451–58; M. A. Russo, D. M. Santarelli, and D. O'Rourke, "The physiological effects of slow breathing in the healthy human," *Breathe* 13, no. 4 (December 2017): 298–309.

CHAPTER 4

55 "Over the last sixty years": D. D. Price, D. G. Finniss, and F. Benedetti, "A comprehensive review of the placebo effect: Recent advances and current thought," *Annual Review of Psychology* 59 (2008): 565–90; H. Benson and M. D. Epstein, "The placebo effect: A neglected asset in the care of patients," in *Health for the Whole Person: The Complete Guide to Holistic Medicine* , ed. A. C. Hastings, J. E. Gordon, and J. Fadiman (Boulder, CO: Westview Press, 1975), 179–85; A. H. Roberts, D. G. Kewman, L. Mercier, and M. Hovell, "The power of nonspecific effects in healing: Implications for psychosocial and biological treatments," *Clinical Psychology Review* 13, no. 5 (December 1993): 375–91.

56 "Placebos can calm the anxiety": Harvard Men's Health Watch, "The power of the placebo effect: Treating yourself with your mind is possible, but there is more to it than positive thinking," *Harvard Health Publishing*, May 2017, https://www.health.harvard .edu/mental-health/the-power-of-the-placebo-effect.

56 "Studies have shown": F. Benedetti, E. Carlino, and A. Pollo, "How placebos change the patient's brain," *Neuropsychopharmacology* 36, no. 1 (January 2011): 339–54, doi: 10.1038 /npp.2010.81.

56 "Hope significantly improves": J. E. Brody, "Nourishing hope when illness seems hopeless," *New York Times*, September 6, 2005, https://www.nytimes.com/2005/09/06 /health/psychology/nourishing-hope-when-illness-seems-hopeless.html.

56 "Children and young people who are hopeful": C. R. Snyder, H. S. Shorey, J. Cheavens, K. M. Pulvers, V. H. Adams III, and C. Wiklund, "Hope and academic success in college," *Journal of Educational Psychology* 94, no. 4 (December 2002): 820–26, doi: 10.1037/0022–0663.94.4.820.

56 "In one study, 'high hope'": C. Zuber and A. Conzelmann, "The impact of the achievement motive on athletic performance in adolescent football players," *European Journal of Sport Science* 14, no. 5 (2014): 475–83, doi: 10.1080/17461391.2013.837513.

56 "Hopeful adults are more flexible": S. J. Lopez, "Want more productive workers—give them hope," *CNBC*, March 8, 2013, https://www.cnbc.com/id/100537689.

CHAPTER 5

72 "'Archaic techniques of ecstasy'": M. Eliade, *Shamanism: Archaic Techniques of Ecstasy* (Princeton, NJ: Princeton Univ. Press, 2004).

72 "Peter Levine, a researcher": P. A. Levine, *Waking the Tiger: Healing Trauma* (Berkeley: North Atlantic Books, 1997).

73 "Nobel Prize winner Ilya Prigogine's work": I. Prigogine and R. Lefever, "Theory of dissipative structures," in *Synergetics: Cooperative Phenomena in Multi-Component Systems*, ed. H. Haken (Wiesbaden: Vieweg+Teubner Verlag, 1973), 124–35.

77 "'Kundalini' CD listed": Osho Deuter, Osho Kundalini Meditation, New Earth Records, 1990.

CHAPTER 6

80 "Enough recalled childhood sexual abuse": U.S. Department of Health & Human Services, Administration for Children and Families, Children's Bureau, *Child Maltreatment 2016* (February 1, 2018), https://www.acf.hhs.gov/cb/resource/child-maltreatment-2016.

84 "In the early 1970s, cardiologists Ray Rosenman and Meyer Friedman": R. H. Rosenman, R. J. Brand, R. I. Sholtz, and M. Friedman, "Multivariate prediction of coronary heart disease during 8.5 year follow-up in the Western Collaborative Group Study," *American Journal of Cardiology* 37, no. 6 (May 1976): 903–10, doi: 10.1016/0002–9149(76)90117-x.

84 "More recently, Redford Williams": R. B. Williams, *The Trusting Heart: Great News About Type A Behavior* (New York: Times Books, 1989).

84 "Trauma often provokes anger": U.S. Department of Veterans Affairs, PTSD: National Center for PTSD, "Anger and Trauma," https://www.ptsd.va.gov/understand/related/anger.asp.

85 "as Freud observed a century ago": S. Freud, "Mourning and melancholia," in *The Standard Edition of the Complete Psychological Works of Sigmund Freud, Volume XIV (1914-1916): On the History of the Psycho-Analytic Movement, Papers on Metapsychology and Other Works* (London: The Hogarth Press and The Institute of Psycho-Analysis, 1957), 237–58.

85 "affects close to twenty million Americans": National Institute of Mental Health, "Depression," https://www.nimh.nih.gov/health/topics/depression/index.shtml.

87 "It enhances activity in the hippocampus": E. Luders, P. M. Thompson, and F. Kurth, "Larger hippocampal dimensions in meditation practitioners: Differential effects in women and men," *Frontiers in Psychology* 6 (March 2015): 186.

88 "Freud famously wrote": J. Vives, "Catharsis: Psychoanalysis and the theatre," *International Journal of Psychoanalysis* 92, no. 4 (August 2011): 1009–27.

89 "As we express what's been inside": B. K. Hölzel, J. Carmody, K. C. Evans, E. A. Hoge, J. A. Dusek, L. Morgan, R. K. Pitman, and S. W. Lazar, "Stress reduction correlates with structural changes in the amygdala," *Social Cognitive and Affective Neuroscience* 5, no. 1 (March 2010): 11–17.

89 "Putting into words": UCSF Memory and Aging Center, "Speech & Language," https://memory.ucsf.edu/speech-language.

91 "University of Texas psychologist James Pennebaker": J. W. Pennebaker and J. D. Seagal, "Forming a story: The health benefits of narrative." *Journal of Clinical Psychology* 55, no. 10 (October 1999): 1243–54.

CHAPTER 7

97 "It's built into our biology": G. Cook, "Why we are wired to connect," *Scientific American*, October 27, 2013, https://www.scientificamerican.com/article/why-we-are-wired-to-connect/.

97 "In fact, researchers, beginning with René Spitz": R. A. Spitz, "Hospitalism: An inquiry into the genesis of psychiatric conditions in early childhood," *Psychoanalytic Study of the Child* 1, no. 1 (1945): 53–74.

98 "The medical literature tells us that social support": R. A. Bryant, "Social attachments and traumatic stress," *European Journal of Psychotraumatology* 7, no.1 (2016): 29065.

98 "Highly sociable children": M. Reblin and B. N. Uchino, "Social and emotional support and its implication for health," *Current Opinion in Psychiatry* 21, no. 2 (March 2008): 201–5, doi: 10.1097/YCO.0b013e3282f3ad89.

98 "Lack of these social connections": J. Holt-Lunstad, T. B. Smith, and J. B. Layton, "Social relationships and mortality risk: A meta-analytic review," *PLoS Medicine* 7, no. 7 (July 2010): e1000316, doi: 10.1371/journal.pmed.1000316.

98 "Trauma numbs and isolates": Margolies, "Understanding the effects of trauma."

98 "Even when we know intellectually": J. McAloon, "Complex trauma: How abuse and neglect can have life-long effects," *The Conversation*, October 27, 2014, http://theconversation.com/complex-trauma-how-abuse-and-neglect-can-have-life-long-effects-32329.

98 "This sense of isolation": S. B. Baek, "Psychopathology of social isolation," *Journal of Exercise Rehabilitation* 10, no. 3 (June 2014): 143–47, doi: 10.12965/jer.140132.

98 "When we are finally able to connect": Bryant, "Social attachments and traumatic stress."

99 "As we share with others": R. Kearney, "Narrating pain: The power of catharsis," *Paragraph* 30, no. 1 (March 2007): 51–66, doi: 10.3366/prg.2007.0013.

99 "In sharing ourselves and our story": S. E. Taylor, "Social Support: A Review," in *The Oxford Handbook of Health Psychology*, ed. H. S. Friedman (Oxford: Oxford Univ. Press, 2011), 189–214.

CHAPTER 8

106 "Imagery is the language"; B. Brogaard and D. E. Gatzia, "Unconscious imagination and the mental imagery debate," *Frontiers in Psychology* 8 (2017): 799, doi: 10.3389/fpsyg.2017.00799.

106 "Imagery also reawakens right-brain activity": E. Virshup and B. Virshup, "Visual imagery: The language of the right brain," in *Imagery*, ed. J. E. Shorr, G. E. Sobel, P. Robin, and J. A. Connella (Boston: Springer, 1980), 107–12.

106 "The brain centers where images are formed": J. N. Lundstrom, S. Boesveldt, and J. Albrecht, "Central processing of the chemical senses: An overview," *Chemical Neuroscience* 2, no. 1 (January 2011): 5–16.

107 "Forty years of published research": J. H. Gruzelier, "A review of the impact of hypnosis, relaxation, guided imagery and individual differences on aspects of immunity and health," *Stress* 5, no. 2 (June 2002): 147–63, doi: 10.1080/10253890290027877; J. L. Apóstolo and K. Kolcaba, "The effects of guided imagery on comfort, depression, anxiety, and stress of psychiatric inpatients with depressive disorders," *Archives of Psychiatric Nursing* 23, no. 6 (December 2009): 403–11, doi: 10.1016/j.apnu.2008.12.003.

107 "Imagery, we now know, reduces the biological and psychological symptoms": C. H. McKinney, M. H. Antoni, M. Kumar, F. C. Tims, and P. M. McCabe, "Effects of guided imagery and music (GIM) therapy on mood and cortisol in healthy adults," *Health Psychology* 16, no. 4 (July 1997): 390–400, doi: 10.1037/0278–6133.16.4.390.

107 "It decreases the intensity of traumatic events": D. J. A. Edwards, "Cognitive therapy and the restructuring of early memories through guided imagery," *Journal of Cognitive Psychotherapy* 4, no. 1 (November 1990): 33–50.

109 "It's called Autogenics and Biofeedback Therapy (ABT)": P. Norris, S. Fahrion, and L. Oikawa, "Autogenic biofeedback training in psychophysiological therapy and stress management." In *Principles and Practice of Stress Management*, 3rd ed., ed. P. M. Lehrer, R. L. Woolfolk, and W. E. Sime (New York: Guilford Press, 2007), 175–206; M. L. Esty, "The development of mind-body self-regulation groups," *Biofeedback* 33, no. 4 (Winter 2005): 161–62.

110 "Autogenic training was developed"; J. H. Schultz and W. Luthe, *Autogenic Training: A Psychophysiologic Approach to Psychotherapy* (New York: Grune & Stratton, 1959).

110 "thousands of papers have been published": Y. Watanabe, G. Cornélissen, F. Halberg, Y. Saito, K. Fukuda, K. Otsuka, and T. Kikuchi, "Chronobiometric assessment of autogenic training effects upon blood pressure and heart rate," *Perceptual and Motor Skills* 83, no. 3, pt. 2 (December 1996): 1395–1410, doi: 10.2466/pms.1996.83.3f.1395; "The benefits of autogenic relaxation," https://www.anxiety.org/autogenic-relaxation; G. Marafante, L. Bidin, P. Seghini, and L. Cavanna, "Mood and distress in cancer patients after Autogenic Training (AT): A pilot study in an Italian oncologic unit," *Annals of Oncology* 27, suppl. 4 (September 2016): 93–94; F. J. Keefe, R. S. Surwit, and R. N. Pilon, "Biofeedback, autogenic training, and progressive relaxation in the treatment of Raynaud's disease: A comparative study," *Journal of Applied Behavior Analysis* 13, no. 1 (Spring 1980): 3–11, doi: 10.1901/jaba.1980.13–3.

111 "In his laboratory at Yale": N. E. Miller and L. Dicara, "Instrumental learning of heart rate changes in curarized rats: Shaping, and specificity to discriminative stimulus," *Journal of Comparative and Physiological Psychology* 63, no. 1 (February 1967): 12–19; N. E. Miller, "Biofeedback and visceral learning," *Annual Review of Psychology* 29 (1978): 373–404.

111 "At about the same time, Elmer Green": E. Green and A. Green, *Beyond Biofeedback* (Boca Raton, FL: Knoll, 1983).

112 "You're going to have to order the temperature-sensitive Biodots": "Stress Squares–1 SHEET Stress Squares, 972 per sheet." Amazon.com. https://www.amazon.com/Stress-Squares-SHEET-972-sheet/dp/B002IGFZ7W.

114 "When you successfully go to your Safe Place": J. L. Strauss, P. S. Calhoun, and C. E. Marx, "Guided imagery as a therapeutic tool in post-traumatic stress disorder," in *Post-*

Traumatic Stress Disorder: Basic Science and Clinical Practice, ed. P. J. Shiromani, T. M. Keane, and J. E. LeDoux (New York: Humana Press, 2009), 363–73.

117 "Carl Jung brought the practice": S. Mehrtens, "Senex play and puer play: A Jungian interpretation of the varieties of recreation," *Jungian Center for the Spiritual Sciences*, http://jungiancenter.org/wp/senex-play-and-puer-play-a-jungian-interpretation-of -the-varieties-of-recreation/.

117 "I first learned Wise Guide imagery": R. C. Stapleton, *The Gift of Inner Healing* (London: Hodder and Stoughton, 1979).

117 "For aboriginal healers, the Guide's words": "Psychic and mystical experiences of the Aborigines," Australian Institute of Parapsychological Research, https://www.aiprinc .org/aboriginal/.

117 "For Jung, the Wise Guide": J. A. Graham, "Reimagining the self: The sage, the wise old one, and the elder," Jung Society of Atlanta, www.jungatlanta.com/articles /summer13-the-sage.pdf.

117 "Most scientific researchers believe the Wise Guide": J. Achterberg, *Imagery in Healing: Shamanism and Modern Medicine* (Boston: Shambhala, 2002).

CHAPTER 9

125 "Long after the threats are over": Bremner, "Traumatic stress"; U.S. Department of Veterans Affairs, "Chronic pain and PTSD: A guide for patients," https://www.ptsd .va.gov/understand/related/chronic_pain.asp.

125 "Many people who've been raped": A. Möller, H. P. Söndergaard, and L. Helström, "Tonic immobility during sexual assault—a common reaction predicting post-traumatic stress disorder and severe depression," *Acta Obstetricia et Gynecologica Scandinavica* 96, no. 8 (August 2017): 932–38, doi: 10.1111/aogs.13174.

125 "And sometimes those of us": E. F. Loftus, "The reality of repressed memories," *American Psychologist* 48, no. 5 (1993): 518–37, doi: 10.1037/0003–066X.48.5.518.

126 "The chronic stress that is trauma's": R. Yehuda, "Biology of posttraumatic stress disorder," *Journal of Clinical Psychiatry* 62, suppl. 17 (2001): 41–46.

126 "It can push our blood pressure": Sherin and Nemeroff, "Post-traumatic stress disorder."

126 "open gaps in our small intestine": Davidson, Kritas, and Butler, "Stressed mucosa."

126 "Chronic stress can contribute to insulin resistance": M. Solas, B. Aisa, R. M. Tordera, M. C. Mugueta, and M. J. Ramírez, "Stress contributes to the development of central insulin resistance during aging: Implications for Alzheimer's disease," *Biochimica et Biophysica Acta (BBA)—Molecular Basis of Disease* 1832, no. 12 (2013): 2332–39.

126 "and fell us with migraine headaches": K. M. Sauro and W. J. Becker, "The stress and migraine interaction," *Headache: The Journal of Head and Face Pain* 49, no. 9 (October 2009): 1378–86, doi: 10.1111/j.1526–4610.2009.01486.x.

126 "Sometimes the symptoms and illnesses": UCSF Urology, "PTSD Increases Risk for Sexual and Urinary Problems," *UCSF Department of Urology*, May 14, 2014, https://urology .ucsf.edu/news/all/201405/ptsd-increases-risk-sexual-and-urinary-problems# .W20ICNJKg2w.

126 "Some of us who felt neglected": Robert L. Marrone, *Body of Knowledge: An Introduction to Body/Mind Psychology* (Albany: SUNY Press, 1990).

127 "Water is a time- and tradition-honored way": Cynthia Kosso and Anne Scott, eds., *The Nature and Function of Water, Baths, Bathing, and Hygiene from Antiquity Through the Renaissance*, vol. 11 (Leiden: E. J. Brill, 2009), doi: 10.1163/ej.9789004173576.i-538.

127 "When we're under stress": S. M. J. Hemmings, S. Malan-Müller, L. L. van den Heuvel, B. A. Demmitt, M. A. Stanislawski, D. G. Smith, A. D. Bohr, et al., "The microbiome in posttraumatic stress disorder and trauma-exposed controls: An exploratory study," *Psychosomatic Medicine* 79, no. 8 (October 2017): 936–46.

128 "Some researchers have been impressed": M. Kawahara and M. Kato-Negishi, "Link between aluminum and the pathogenesis of Alzheimer's disease: The integration of the aluminum and amyloid cascade hypotheses," *International Journal of Alzheimer's Disease* 2011 (March 2011), https://www.hindawi.com/journals/ijad/2011/276393/abs/.

128 "Bisphenol A (BPA), which is present in plastic": M. Murata and J. H. Kang, "Bisphenol A (BPA) and cell signaling pathways," *Biotechnology Advances* 36, no. 1 (January–February 2018): 311–27, doi: 10.1016/j.biotechadv.2017.12.002.

128 "GMOs were invented because": T. Phillips, "Genetically modified organisms (GMOs): Transgenic crops and recombinant DNA technology," *Scitable*, https://www.nature.com/scitable/topicpage/genetically-modified-organisms-gmos-transgenic-crops-and-732.

128 "Glyphosate, which was patented by Monsanto": G. Chaufan, I. Coalova, and M. del Carmen Ríos de Molina, "Glyphosate commercial formulation causes cytotoxicity, oxidative effects, and apoptosis on human cells: Differences with its active ingredient," *International Journal of Toxicology* 33, no. 1 (January–February 2014): 29–38.

128 "There may be other reasons to avoid GMOs": G. A. Kleter, A. A. Peijnenburg, and H. J. Aarts, "Health considerations regarding horizontal transfer of microbial transgenes present in genetically modified crops," *Journal of Biomedicine and Biomedical Technology* 2005, no. 4 (2005): 326–52.

129 "Drink plenty of water": Y. Elkaim, "The truth about how much water you should really drink," *U.S. News and World Report*, September 13, 2013, https://health.usnews.com/health-news/blogs/eat-run/2013/09/13/the-truth-about-how-much-water-you-should-really-drink.

129 "Add a filter to your faucet": J. Gibbons and S. Laha, "Water purification systems: A comparative analysis based on the occurrence of disinfection by-products," *Environmental Pollution* 106, no. 3 (September 1999): 425–28.

130 "If you need some encouragement": S. Nair, M. Sagar, J. Sollers III, N. Consedine, and E. Broadbent, "Do slumped and upright postures affect stress responses? A randomized trial," *Health Psychology* 34, no. 6 (June 2015): 632–41.

130 "The scientific literature on the benefits of massage": T. Field, "Massage therapy research review," *Complementary Therapies in Clinical Practice* 24 (August 2016): 19–31, doi: 10.1016/j.ctcp.2014.07.002.

130 "And movement": S. Pillay, "How simply moving benefits your mental health," *Harvard Health Publishing*, March 28, 2016, www.health.harvard.edu/blog/how-simply-moving-benefits-your-mental-health-201603289350.

131 *"Aerobic exercise"*: S. Heijnen, B. Hommel, A. Kibele, and L. S. Colzato, "Neuromodulation of aerobic exercise—a review," *Frontiers in Psychology* 6 (January 2016): 1890, doi: 10.3389/fpsyg.2015.01890.

131 "Very good clinical research": M. T. Schmolesky, D. L. Webb, and R. A. Hansen, "The effects of aerobic exercise intensity and duration on levels of brain-derived neurotrophic factor in healthy men," *Journal of Sports Science & Medicine* 12, no. 3 (September 2013): 502–11.

131 "Clinical trials have also shown": P. J. Smith, J. A. Blumenthal, B. M. Hoffman, H. Cooper, T. A. Strauman, K. Welsh-Bohmer, J. N. Browndyke, and A. Sherwood, "Aerobic exercise and neurocognitive performance: A meta-analytic review of randomized controlled trials," *Psychosomatic Medicine* 72, no. 3 (2010): 239, doi: 10.1097/PSY.0b013e3181d14633; S. Rosenbaum, C. Sherrington, and A. Tiedemann, "Exercise augmentation compared with usual care for post-traumatic stress disorder: A randomized controlled trial," *Acta Psychiatrica Scandinavica* 131, no. 5 (May 2015): 350–59, doi: 10.1111/acps.12371.

131 "One fascinating study": G. Shivakumar, E. H. Anderson, A. M. Surís, and C. S. North, "Exercise for PTSD in women veterans: A proof-of-concept study," *Military Medicine* 182, no. 11 (November 2017): e1809–14, doi: 10.7205/milmed-d-16–00440.

132 "Recent scientific studies": J. West, B. Liang, and J. Spinazzola, "Trauma sensitive yoga as a complementary treatment for posttraumatic stress disorder: A qualitative descriptive analysis," *International Journal of Stress Management* 24, no. 2 (May 2017): 173–95, doi: 10.1037/str0000040.

132 "the postures of hatha yoga and the yogic breathing techniques": H. Cramer, D. Anheyer, F. J. Saha, and G. Dobos, "Yoga for posttraumatic stress disorder—a systematic review and meta-analysis," *BMC Psychiatry* 18, no. 1 (March 2018): 72, doi: 10.1186/s12888–018–1650-x; B. A. van der Kolk, L. Stone, J. West, A. Rhodes, D. Emerson, M. Suvak, and J. Spinazzola, "Yoga as an adjunctive treatment for posttraumatic stress disorder: A randomized controlled trial," *Journal of Clinical Psychiatry* 75, no. 6 (June 2014): e559–65.

132 "The Chinese moving meditations": B. L. Niles, D. L. Mori, C. P. Polizzi, A. Pless Kaiser, A. M. Ledoux, and C. Wang, "Feasibility, qualitative findings and satisfaction of a brief Tai Chi mind-body programme for veterans with post-traumatic stress symptoms," *BMJ Open* 6, no. 11 (November 2016): e012464, doi: 10.1136/bmjopen-2016–012464.

132 "And exercise, as we continue to discover": S. K. Agarwal, "Cardiovascular benefits of exercise," *International Journal of General Medicine* 5 (2012): 541–45, doi: 10.2147/IJGM .S30113; K. A. Ashcraft, R. M. Peace, A. S. Betof, M. W. Dewhirst, and L. W. Jones, "Efficacy and mechanisms of aerobic exercise on cancer initiation, progression, and metastasis: A critical systematic review of *in vivo* preclinical data," *Cancer Research* 76, no. 14 (July 2016): 4032–50, doi: 10.1158/0008–5472.CAN-16–0887; K. R. Ambrose and Y. M. Golightly, "Physical exercise as non-pharmacological treatment of chronic pain: Why and when," *Best Practice & Research Clinical Rheumatology* 29, no. 1 (February 2015): 120–30, doi: 10.1016/j.berh.2015.04.022.

132 "Mindful walking": M. Teut, E. J. Roesner, M. Ortiz, F. Reese, S. Binting, S. Roll, H. F. Fischer, A. Michalsen, S. N. Willich, and B. Brinkhaus, "Mindful walking in psycho-

logically distressed individuals: A randomized controlled trial," *Evidence-Based Complementary and Alternative Medicine* 2013, no. 3171 (July 2013), doi: 10.1155/2013/489856.

133 "The genes we carry": L. Kravitz, "The age antidote," *IDEA Today* 14 (1996): 28–35.

135 "Trauma of all kinds twists and tortures our relationship to food": J. Y. Breland, R. Donalson, J. V. Dinh, and S. Maguen, "Trauma exposure and disordered eating: A qualitative study," *Women & Health* 58, no. 2 (February 2018): 160–74.

CHAPTER 10

141 "Eating in a trauma-healing way": M. A. Ricker and W. C. Haas, "Anti-inflammatory diet in clinical practice: A review," *Nutrition in Clinical Practice* 32, no. 3 (June 2017): 318–25, doi: 10.1177/0884533617700353.

141 "It will ease you away": Y. H. C. Yau and M. N. Potenza, "Stress and eating behaviors," *Minerva Endocrinologica* 38, no. 3 (September 2013): 255–67.

141 "It will improve your mood": A. O'Neil, S. E. Quirk, S. Housden, S. L. Brennan, L. J. Williams, J. A. Pasco, M. Berk, and F. N. Jacka, "Relationship between diet and mental health in children and adolescents: A systematic review," *American Journal of Public Health* 104, no. 10 (October 2014): e31–42, doi: 10.2105/AJPH.2014.302110.

141 "And keeping to a Trauma-Healing Diet": J. K. Kiecolt-Glaser, "Stress, food, and inflammation: Psychoneuroimmunology and nutrition at the cutting edge," *Psychosomatic Medicine* 72, no. 4 (May 2010): 365–69, doi: 10.1097/PSY.0b013e3181dbf489.

141 "The withdrawal may": S. L. Parylak, G. F. Koob, and E. P. Zorrilla, "The dark side of food addiction," *Physiology & Behavior* 104, no. 1 (July 2011): 149–56, doi: 10.1016/j.physbeh.2011.04.063.

142 "When food is processed": E. M. Steele, B. M. Popkin, B. Swinburn, and C. A. Monteiro, "The share of ultra-processed foods and the overall nutritional quality of diets in the US: Evidence from a nationally representative cross-sectional study," *Population Health Metrics* 15, no. 1 (February 2017): 6, doi: 10.1186/s12963–017–0119–3.

142 "For example, grinding and bleaching flour": J. L. Slavin, "Whole grains, refined grains and fortified refined grains: What's the difference?," *Asia Pacific Journal of Clinical Nutrition* 9, suppl. 1 (September 2000): S23–27.

142 "Refined flour may also interfere with leptin": J. P. Karl and E. Saltzman, "The role of whole grains in body weight regulation," *Advances in Nutrition* 3, no. 5 (September 2012): 697–707, doi: 10.3945/an.112.002782.

142 "Study after study has shown": Kiecolt-Glaser, "Stress, food, and inflammation."

143 "All contain antioxidants": V. Lobo, A. Patil, A. Phatak, and N. Chandra, "Free radicals, antioxidants and functional foods: Impact on human health," *Pharmacognosy Reviews* 4, no. 8 (July 2010): 118–26, doi: 10.4103/0973–7847.70902; H. D. Holscher, "Dietary fiber and prebiotics and the gastrointestinal microbiota," *Gut Microbes* 8, no. 2 (March 2017): 172–84, doi: 10.1080/19490976.2017.1290756.

143 "They all have a low glycemic index": G. Radulian, E. Rusu, A. Dragomir, and M. Posea, "Metabolic effects of low glycaemic index diets," *Nutrition Journal* 8 (January 2009): 5, doi: 10.1186/1475–2891–8–5.

143 "Each veggie also has": M. M. Murphy, L. M. Barraj, J. H. Spungen, D. R. Herman, and

R. K. Randolph, "Global assessment of select phytonutrient intakes by level of fruit and vegetable consumption," *British Journal of Nutrition* 112, no. 6 (September 2014): 1004–18, doi: 10.1017/S0007114514001937.

143 "For example, many mushrooms": A. G. Guggenheim, K. M. Wright, and H. L. Zwickey, "Immune modulation from five major mushrooms: Application to integrative oncology," *Integrative Medicine: A Clinician's Journal* 13, no. 1 (February 2014): 32.

143 "Okinawans, who use purple sweet potatoes": D. C. Willcox, G. Scapagnini, and B. J. Willcox, "Healthy aging diets other than the Mediterranean: A focus on the Okinawan diet," *Mechanisms of Ageing and Development* 136–37 (March–April 2014): 148–62.

144 "Corn and peas": Y. Ai and J. Jane, "Macronutrients in corn and human nutrition," *Comprehensive Reviews in Food Science and Food Safety* 15, no. 3 (February 2016): 581–98, doi: 10.1111/1541–4337.12192; W. J. Dahl, L. M. Foster, and R. T. Tyler, "Review of the health benefits of peas (Pisum sativum L.)," *British Journal of Nutrition* 108, suppl. 1 (August 2012): S3–10, doi: 10.1017/s0007114512000852.

144 "So, too, are white potatoes": J. C. King and J. L. Slavin, "White potatoes, human health, and dietary guidance," *Advances in Nutrition* 4, no. 3 (May 2013): 393S–401S, doi: 10.3945/an.112.003525.

144 "Fried potatoes and chips": SELFNutritionData, "Foods highest in total omega-6 fatty acids," https://nutritiondata.self.com/foods-011141000000000000000-1w.html.

144 "Frying also brings out": R. J. Foot, N. U. Haase, K. Grob, and P. Gondé, "Acrylamide in fried and roasted potato products: A review on progress in mitigation," *Food Additives and Contaminants* 24, suppl. 1 (2007): 37–46, doi: 10.1080/02652030701439543.

144 "Fruits contain a wide variety of phytonutrients": A. Rodriguez-Casado, "The health potential of fruits and vegetables phytochemicals: Notable examples," *Critical Reviews in Food Science and Nutrition* 56, no. 7 (May 2016): 1097–1107.

144 "and, in particular, blueberries": S. Lee, K. I. Keirsey, R. Kirkland, Z. I. Grunewald, J. G. Fischer, and C. B. de La Serre, "Blueberry supplementation influences the gut microbiota, inflammation, and insulin resistance in high-fat-diet–fed rats." *Journal of Nutrition* 148, no. 2 (February 2018): 209–19, doi: 10.1093/jn/nxx027.

145 "They can, however, be a problem": M. A. Daulatzai, "Non-celiac gluten sensitivity triggers gut dysbiosis, neuroinflammation, gut-brain axis dysfunction, and vulnerability for dementia," *CNS & Neurological Disorders Drug Targets* 14, no. 1 (2015): 110–31.

145 "People with celiac disease": N. Gujral, H. J. Freeman, and A. B. R. Thomson, "Celiac disease: Prevalence, diagnosis, pathogenesis and treatment," *World Journal of Gastroenterology* 18, no. 42 (November 2012): 6036–59, doi: 10.3748/wjg.v18.i42.6036.

145 "Perhaps 6 percent of us": S. O. Igbinedion, J. Ansari, A. Vasikaran, F. N. Gavins, P. Jordan, M. Boktor, and J. S. Alexander, "Non-celiac gluten sensitivity: All wheat attack is not celiac," *World Journal of Gastroenterology* 23, no. 40 (October 2017): 7201–10.

145 "They also damage the intestinal wall": J. R. Biesiekierski and J. Iven, "Non-coeliac gluten sensitivity: Piecing the puzzle together," *United European Gastroenterology Journal* 3, no. 2 (April 2015): 160–65, doi: 10.1177/2050640615578388.

146 "When we've been traumatized and eat gluten": Davidson, Kritas, and Butler, "Stressed mucosa."

146 "A number of studies have shown": A. Mie, H. R. Andersen, S. Gunnarsson, J. Kahl,

E. Kesse-Guyot, E. Rembiałkowska, G. Quaglio, and P. Grandjean, "Human health implications of organic food and organic agriculture: A comprehensive review," *Environmental Health* 16, no. 1 (October 2017): 111.

146 "And many of the pesticides and herbicides": J. Rothlein, D. Rohlman, M. Lasarev, J. Phillips, J. Muniz, and L. McCauley, "Organophosphate pesticide exposure and neurobehavioral performance in agricultural and non-agricultural Hispanic workers," *Environmental Health Perspectives* 114, no. 5 (May 2006): 691–96, doi: 10.1289 /ehp.8182.

147 "The EWG strongly recommends": Environmental Working Group, "Dirty dozen: EWG's 2018 shopper's guide to pesticides in produce," www.ewg.org/foodnews /dirty-dozen.php.

148 "Make beans and other legumes": T. P. Trinidad, A. C. Mallillin, A. S. Loyola, R. S. Sagum, and R. R. Encabo, "The potential health benefits of legumes as a good source of dietary fibre," *British Journal of Nutrition* 103, no. 4 (February 2010): 569–74.

148 "Walnuts, pecans, Brazil nuts, and almonds": E. Ros, "Health benefits of nut consumption," *Nutrients* 2, no. 7 (July 2010): 652–82, doi: 10.3390/nu2070652.

148 "Fish are rich": D. Swanson, R. Block, and S. A. Mousa, "Omega-3 fatty acids EPA and DHA: Health benefits throughout life," *Advances in Nutrition* 3, no. 1 (January 2012): 1–7, doi: 10.3945/an.111.000893.

148 "And one dramatic experiment": K. Matsumura, H. Noguchi, D. Nishi, K. Hamazaki, T. Hamazaki, and Y. J. Matsuoka, "Effects of omega-3 polyunsaturated fatty acids on psychophysiological symptoms of post-traumatic stress disorder in accident survivors: A randomized, double-blind, placebo-controlled trial," *Journal of Affective Disorders* 224 (December 2017): 27–31, doi: 10.1016/j.jad.2016.05.054.

148 "Small fish are far less likely": A. Abelsohn, L. D. Vanderlinden, F. Scott, J. A. Archbold, and T. L. Brown, "Healthy fish consumption and reduced mercury exposure: Counseling women in their reproductive years," *Canadian Family Physician* 57, no. 1 (January 2011): 26–30.

149 "Seafood, including shrimp, mussels": Ann L. Yaktine and Malden C. Nesheim, eds., *Seafood Choices: Balancing Benefits and Risks* (Washington: National Academies Press, 2007).

149 "Eggs have had a long and undeserved": Bruce A. Griffin, "Eggs: Good or bad?," *Proceedings of the Nutrition Society* 75, no. 3 (August 2016): 259–64.

149 "When they could, our hunter-gatherer ancestors ate meat": K. Milton, "Hunter-gatherer diets—a different perspective," *American Journal of Clinical Nutrition* 71, no. 3 (March 2000): 665–67, doi: 10.1093/ajcn/71.3.665.

149 "The fat composition of wild animal meat": A. P. Simopoulos, "An increase in the omega-6/omega-3 fatty acid ratio increases the risk for obesity," *Nutrients* 8, no. 3 (March 2016): 128, doi: 10.3390/nu8030128.

150 "Modern meat also contains saturated fats": T. A. O'Sullivan, K. Hafekost, F. Mitrou, and D. Lawrence, "Food sources of saturated fat and the association with mortality: A meta-analysis," *American Journal of Public Health* 103, no. 9 (September 2013): e31–42.

150 "It will be free of chemicals": T. F. Landers, B. Cohen, T. E. Wittum, and E. L. Larson,

"A review of antibiotic use in food animals: Perspective, policy, and potential," *Public Health Reports* 127, no. 1 (January–February 2012): 4–22.

150 "Also, if animals are free to roam": A. J. Yun, P. Y. Lee, and J. D. Doux, "Are we eating more than we think? Illegitimate signaling and xenohormesis as participants in the pathogenesis of obesity," *Medical Hypotheses* 67, no. 1 (2006): 36–40.

150 "the Mediterranean diet": R. Casas, E. Sacanella, and R. Estruch, "The immune protective effect of the Mediterranean diet against chronic low-grade inflammatory diseases," *Endocrine, Metabolic & Immune Disorders Drug Targets* 14, no. 4 (2014): 245–54, doi: 10.2174/1871530314666140922153350.

150 "Extra virgin olive oil": M. Gorzynik-Debicka, P. Przychodzen, F. Cappello, A. Kuban-Jankowska, A. Marino Gammazza, N. Knap, M. Wozniak, and M. Gorska-Ponikowska, "Potential health benefits of olive oil and plant polyphenols," *International Journal of Molecular Sciences* 19, no. 3 (February 2018): 686, doi: 10.3390/ijms19030686.

151 "coconut oil": S. Intahphuak, P. Khonsung, and A. Panthong, "Anti-inflammatory, analgesic, and antipyretic activities of virgin coconut oil," *Pharmaceutical Biology* 48, no. 2 (February 2010): 151–57, doi: 10.3109/13880200903062614.

151 "sesame oil": E. Hsu and S. Parthasarathy, "Anti-inflammatory and antioxidant effects of sesame oil on atherosclerosis: A descriptive literature review," *Cureus* 9, no. 7 (July 2017): e1438, doi: 10.7759/cureus.1438.

151 "In fact, they're high in the omega-6s": J. K. Innes and P. C. Calder, "Omega-6 fatty acids and inflammation." *Prostaglandins, Leukotrienes and Essential Fatty Acids* 132 (May 2018): 41–48.

151 "trans fats contribute": F. A. Kummerow, "The negative effects of hydrogenated trans fats and what to do about them," *Atherosclerosis* 205, no. 2 (August 2009): 458–65, doi: 10.1016/j.atherosclerosis.2009.03.009.

151 "often intolerant of lactose": S. Bhatnagar and R. Aggarwal, "Lactose intolerance," *BMJ* 334, no. 7608 (June 2007): 1331–32.

151 "the interaction between lactose and our microbiome": R. K. Singh, H. W. Chang, D. Yan, K. M. Lee, D. Ucmak, K. Wong, M. Abrouk, et al., "Influence of diet on the gut microbiome and implications for human health," *Journal of Translational Medicine* 15, no. 1 (April 2017): 73, doi: 10.1186/s12967-017-1175-y.

151 "When we're under stress and our gut is leaking": M. Clapp, N. Aurora, L. Herrera, M. Bhatia, E. Wilen, and S. Wakefield, "Gut microbiota's effect on mental health: The gut-brain axis," *Clinics and Practice* 7, no. 4 (September 2017), doi: 10.4081/cp.2017.987.

152 "yogurt, which is rich in the good bacteria": M. Kechagia, D. Basoulis, S. Konstantopoulou, D. Dimitriadi, K. Gyftopoulou, N. Skarmoutsou, and E. M. Fakiri, "Health benefits of probiotics: A review," *ISRN Nutrition* 2013 (January 2013), doi: 10.5402/2013/481651.

152 "Insoluble fiber includes": U.S. National Library of Medicine, "Soluble vs. insoluble fiber," *Medline Plus*, www.medlineplus.gov/ency/article/002136.htm.

152 "Foods that contain it are prebiotic": J. Slavin, "Fiber and prebiotics: Mechanisms and health benefits," *Nutrients* 5, no. 4 (April 2013): 1417–35, doi: 10.3390/nu5041417.

152 "Their diet of plants, seeds, and wild game": S. B. Eaton, S. B. Eaton III, M. J. Konner, and M. Shostak, "An evolutionary perspective enhances understanding of human nutritional requirements," *Journal of Nutrition* 126, no. 6 (June 1996): 1732–40, doi: 10.1093/jn/126.6.1732.

152 "When we've been traumatized, low fiber intake": D. A. Timm and J. L. Slavin, "Dietary fiber and the relationship to chronic diseases," *American Journal of Lifestyle Medicine* 2, no. 3 (March 2008): 233–40, doi: 10.1177/1559827608314149.

153 "Probiotics are the healthy bacteria": Holscher, "Dietary fiber and prebiotics."

153 "Probiotics send messages": H. Wang, I. S. Lee, C. Braun, and P. Enck, "Effect of probiotics on central nervous system functions in animals and humans: A systematic review," *Journal of Neurogastroenterology and Motility* 22, no. 4 (October 2016): 589–605, doi: 10.5056/jnm16018.

153 "They include sauerkraut": M. L. Marco, D. Heeney, S. Binda, C. J. Cifelli, P. D. Cotter, B. Foligné, M. Gänzle, et al., "Health benefits of fermented foods: Microbiota and beyond," *Current Opinion in Biotechnology* 44 (April 2017): 94–102, doi: 10.1016/j.copbio.2016.11.010.

153 "I use blueberries": S. Skrovankova, D. Sumczynski, J. Mlcek, T. Jurikova, and J. Sochor, "Bioactive compounds and antioxidant activity in different types of berries," *International Journal of Molecular Sciences* 16, no. 10 (October 2015): 24673–706, doi: 10.3390/ijms161024673.

154 "Sugar, as I've explained": Yau and Potenza, "Stress and eating behaviors."

154 "In some animal studies, sugar has proved": M. Lenoir, F. Serre, L. Cantin, and S. H. Ahmed, "Intense sweetness surpasses cocaine reward," *PLoS One* 2, no. 8 (2007): e698, doi: 10.1371/journal.pone.0000698.

154 "Sugar directly leads to weight gain": K. L. Stanhope, "Sugar consumption, metabolic disease and obesity: The state of the controversy," *Critical Reviews in Clinical Laboratory Sciences* 53, no. 1 (2016): 52–67.

154 "Sugar increases cholesterol and triglycerides": L. H. Glimcher and A. H. Lee, "From sugar to fat: How the transcription factor XBP1 regulates hepatic lipogenesis," *Annals of the New York Academy of Sciences* 1173, suppl. 1 (September 2009): E2–9.

154 "The excessive quantities of sugar": J. Rippe and T. Angelopoulos, "Relationship between added sugars consumption and chronic disease risk factors: Current understanding," *Nutrients* 8, no. 11 (November 2016): 697, doi: 10.3390/nu8110697.

154 "When sugar is contained in fruits and root vegetables": J. L. Slavin and B. Lloyd, "Health benefits of fruits and vegetables," *Advances in Nutrition* 3, no. 4 (July 2012): 506–16.

155 "When sugar is added at the table": E. Martínez, B. Popkin, B. Swinburn, and C. Monteiro, "The share of ultra-processed foods and the overall nutritional quality of diets in the US: Evidence from a nationally representative cross-sectional study," *Population Health Metrics* 15, no. 1 (February 2017): 6, doi: 10.1186/s12963–017–0119–3.

155 "High fructose corn syrup (HFCS)": J. M. Rippe and T. J. Angelopoulos, "Sucrose, high-fructose corn syrup, and fructose, their metabolism and potential health effects: What do we really know?," *Advances in Nutrition* 4, no. 2 (March 2013): 236–45.

155 "Artificial sweeteners": Q. Yang, "Gain weight by 'going diet'? Artificial sweeteners and the neurobiology of sugar cravings," *Yale Journal of Biology and Medicine* 83, no. 2 (June 2010): 101–8.

155 "Unfiltered, unheated honey": K. M. Phillips, M. H. Carlsen, and R. Blomhoff, "Total antioxidant content of alternatives to refined sugar," *Journal of the American Dietetic Association* 109, no. 1 (January 2009): 64–71, doi: 10.1016/j.jada.2008.10.014.

155 "Stevia is a sweetening leaf": A. A. Momtazi-Borojeni, S. A. Esmaeili, E. Abdollahi, and A. Sahebkar, "A review on the pharmacology and toxicology of steviol glycosides extracted from Stevia rebaudiana," *Current Pharmaceutical Design* 23, no. 11 (2017): 1616–22, doi: 10.2174/1381612822666161021142835.

156 "Every year, the evidence for their therapeutic importance": K. Singh, "Nutrient and stress management," *Journal of Nutrition and Food Sciences* 6, no. 4 (2016), doi: 10.4172/2155–9600.1000528.

156 "The need for B vitamins": D. O. Kennedy, "B vitamins and the brain: Mechanisms, dose and efficacy—a review," *Nutrients* 8, no. 2 (January 2016): 68, doi: 10.3390 /nu8020068.

156 "Recently, researchers from New Zealand": J. J. Rucklidge, R. Andridge, B. Gorman, N. Blampied, H. Gordon, and A. Boggis, "Shaken but unstirred? Effects of micronutrients on stress and trauma after an earthquake: RCT evidence comparing formulas and doses," *Human Psychopharmacology: Clinical and Experimental* 27, no. 5 (September 2012): 440–54, doi: 10.1002/hup.2246.

158 "As many as 50–60 percent of Americans": K. Y. Forrest and W. L. Stuhldreher, "Prevalence and correlates of vitamin D deficiency in US adults," *Nutrition Research* 31, no. 1 (January 2011): 48–54, doi: 10.1016/j.nutres.2010.12.001.

158 "Its deficiency has repeatedly been correlated": E. R. Bertone-Johnson, "Vitamin D and the occurrence of depression: Causal association or circumstantial evidence?," *Nutrition Reviews* 67, no. 8 (August 2009): 481–92, doi: 10.1111/j.1753–4887.2009.00220.x.

158 "If it's normal": S. T. Haines and S. K. Park, "Vitamin D supplementation: What's known, what to do, and what's needed," *Pharmacotherapy: The Journal of Human Pharmacology and Drug Therapy* 32, no. 4 (April 2012): 354–82, doi: 10.1002/phar.1037.

158 "Zinc, which is so important": C. Pifl, A. Wolf, P. Rebernik, H. Reither, and M. L. Berger, "Zinc regulates the dopamine transporter in a membrane potential and chloride dependent manner," *Neuropharmacology* 56, no. 2 (February 2009): 531–40, doi: 10.1016/j.neuropharm.2008.10.009.

158 "It also supports BDNF production": E. Ranjbar, M. S. Kasaei, M. Mohammad-Shirazi, J. Nasrollahzadeh, B. Rashidkhani, J. Shams, S. A. Mostafavi, and M. R. Mohammadi, "Effects of zinc supplementation in patients with major depression: A randomized clinical trial," *Iranian Journal of Psychiatry* 8, no. 2 (June 2013): 73–79.

158 "Selenium has been shown": V. V. Voĭtsekhovskis, I. G. Voĭtsekhovska, A. Shkesters, G. Antsane, A. Silova, T. Ivashchenko, I. Michans, and N. Vaĭvads, "Advances of selenium supplementation in posttraumatic stress disorder risk group patients" [in Russian], *Biomeditsinskaia Khimiia* 60, no. 1 (January–February 2014): 125–32, doi: 10.18097 /pbmc20146001125.

158 "It also reduces oxidative stress": J. E. Kim, S. I. Choi, H. R. Lee, I. S. Hwang, Y. J. Lee, B. S. An, S. H. Lee, H. J. Kim, B. C. Kang, and D. Y. Hwang, "Selenium significantly

inhibits adipocyte hypertrophy and abdominal fat accumulation in OLETF rats via induction of fatty acid β-oxidation," *Biological Trace Element Research* 150, nos. 1–3 (December 2012): 360–70, doi: 10.1007/s12011–012–9519–1.

159 "Omega-3 fatty acids, as I've said": Stephen C. Heinrichs, "Dietary ω-3 fatty acid supplementation for optimizing neuronal structure and function," *Molecular Nutrition & Food Research* 54, no. 4 (April 2010): 447–56, doi: 10.1002/mnfr.200900201.

159 "They have repeatedly demonstrated significant antidepressant effects": G. Grosso, F. Galvano, S. Marventano, M. Malaguarnera, C. Bucolo, F. Drago, and F. Caraci, "Omega-3 fatty acids and depression: Scientific evidence and biological mechanisms," *Oxidative Medicine and Cellular Longevity* 2014 (2014), doi: 10.1155/2014/313570.

159 "Some research suggests that higher EPA content": P. Bozzatello, E. Brignolo, E. De Grandi, and S. Bellino, "Supplementation with omega-3 fatty acids in psychiatric disorders: A review of literature data," *Journal of Clinical Medicine* 5, no. 8 (July 2016): 67, doi: 10.3390/jcm5080067.

159 "Turmeric, a yellow spice": M. S. Monsey, D. M. Gerhard, L. M. Boyle, M. A. Briones, M. Seligsohn, and G. E. Schafe, "A diet enriched with curcumin impairs newly acquired and reactivated fear memories," *Neuropsychopharmacology* 40, no. 5 (March 2015): 1278–88, doi: 10.1038/npp.2014.315.

159 "Add some black pepper": G. Shoba, D. Joy, T. Joseph, M. Majeed, R. Rajendran, and P. S. S. R. Srinivas, "Influence of piperine on the pharmacokinetics of curcumin in animals and human volunteers," *Planta Medica* 64, no. 4 (May 1998): 353–56, doi: 10.1055/s-2006–957450.

159 "Phosphatidylserine decreases the hyperactivity": J. Hellhammer, E. Fries, C. Buss, V. Engert, A. Tuch, D. Rutenberg, and D. Hellhammer, "Effects of soy lecithin phosphatidic acid and phosphatidylserine complex (PAS) on the endocrine and psychological responses to mental stress," *Stress* 7, no. 2 (June 2004): 119–26.

160 "It regulates our circadian (daily waking and sleeping) cycle": V. Cassone, W. Warren, D. Brooks, and J. Lu, "Melatonin, the pineal gland, and circadian rhythms," *Journal of Biological Rhythms* 8, suppl. (February 1993): S73–81, http://handle.dtic.mil/100.2/ADA268200.

160 "Passion flower extract": S. E. Lakhan and K. F. Vieira, "Nutritional and herbal supplements for anxiety and anxiety-related disorders: systematic review," *Nutrition Journal* 9 (October 2010): 42, doi: 10.1186/1475–2891–9–42.

160 "Recently, researchers have demonstrated its benefits": J. J. Mao, S. X. Xie, J. Zee, I. Soeller, Q. S. Li, K. Rockwell, and J. D. Amsterdam, "Rhodiola rosea versus sertraline for major depressive disorder: A randomized placebo-controlled trial," *Phytomedicine* 22, no. 3 (March 2015): 394–99, doi: 10.1016/j.phymed.2015.01.010.

161 "Black and green tea both contain caffeine": S. M. Chacko, P. T. Thambi, R. Kuttan, and I. Nishigaki, "Beneficial effects of green tea: A literature review," *Chinese Medicine* 5 (April 2010): 13.

161 "Both, and green tea in particular": A. C. Nobre, A. Rao, and G. N. Owen, "L-theanine, a natural constituent in tea, and its effect on mental state," *Asia Pacific Journal of Clinical Nutrition* 17, suppl. 1 (2008): 167–68.

161 "For years coffee was demonized": P. Broderick and A. B. Benjamín, "Caffeine and psychiatric symptoms: A review," *Journal of the Oklahoma State Medical Association* 97, no. 12

(December 2004): 538–42; M. Ding, S. N. Bhupathiraju, A. Satija, R. M. van Dam, and F. B. Hu, "Long-term coffee consumption and risk of cardiovascular disease: A systematic review and a dose-response meta-analysis of prospective cohort studies," *Circulation* 129, no. 6 (February 2013): 643–59.

161 "For many of us": K. Nieber, "The impact of coffee on health," *Planta Medica* 83, no. 16 (November 2017): 1256–63.

161 "In recent years, research on the rate": P. Palatini, G. Ceolotto, F. Ragazzo, F. Dorigatti, F. Saladini, I. Papparella, L. Mos, G. Zanata, and M. Santonastaso, "CYP1A2 genotype modifies the association between coffee intake and the risk of hypertension," *Journal of Hypertension* 27, no. 8 (August 2009): 1594–1601.

161 "Alcohol, like comfort foods": J. A. Bisby, C. R. Brewin, J. R. Leitz, and H. Valerie Curran, "Acute effects of alcohol on the development of intrusive memories," *Psychopharmacology* 204, no. 4 (July 2009): 655–66.

162 "alcohol also inhibits areas": Y. Tu, S. Kroener, K. Abernathy, C. Lapish, J. Seamans, L. J. Chandler, and J. J. Woodward, "Ethanol inhibits persistent activity in prefrontal cortical neurons," *Journal of Neuroscience* 27, no. 17 (April 2007): 4765–75, doi: 10.1523 /JNEUROSCI.5378–06.2007.

162 "Chronic high consumption of alcohol": P. Hartmann, C. T. Seebauer, and B. Schnabl, "Alcoholic liver disease: The gut microbiome and liver cross talk," *Alcoholism: Clinical and Experimental Research* 39, no. 5 (May 2015): 763–75, doi: 10.1111/acer.12704.

162 "And of course, with its empty calories": G. Traversy and J. P. Chaput, "Alcohol consumption and obesity: An update," *Current Obesity Reports* 4, no. 1 (March 2015): 122–30, doi: 10.1007/s13679–014–0129–4.

163 "acupuncture is a safe, side-effect-free way": X. Liu, Z. Qin, X. Zhu, Q. Yao, and Z. Liu, "Systematic review of acupuncture for the treatment of alcohol withdrawal syndrome," *Acupuncture in Medicine* 36, no. 5 (October 2018): 275–83, doi: 10.1136 /acupmed-2016–011283.

163 "The smoking rates among those who've been traumatized": M. T. Feldner, K. A. Babson, and M. J. Zvolensky, "Smoking, traumatic event exposure, and post-traumatic stress: A critical review of the empirical literature," *Clinical Psychology Review* 27, no. 1 (January 2007): 14–45, doi: 10.1016/j.cpr.2006.08.004.

163 "Nicotine and tobacco can": T. M. Powledge, "Nicotine as therapy," *PLoS Biology* 2, no. 11 (November 2004): e404.

163 "The problem is long-term use": A. Mishr, P. Chaturvedi, S. Datta, S. Sinukumar, P. Joshi, and A. Garg, "Harmful effects of nicotine," *Indian Journal of Medical and Paediatric Oncology* 36, no. 1 (January–March 2015): 24–31, doi: 10.4103/0971–5851.151771.

163 "Acupuncture has repeatedly been shown": D. He, J. I. Medbø, and A. T. Høstmark, "Effect of acupuncture on smoking cessation or reduction: An 8-month and 5-year follow-up study," *Preventive Medicine* 33, no. 5 (November 2001): 364–72, doi: 10.1006 /pmed.2001.0901.

163 "Marijuana (pot, cannabis, weed, boo, chronic, etc.) is often used": A. Serrano, "As vets demand cannabis for PTSD, science races to unlock its secrets," *Scientific American*, January 4, 2018, www.scientificamerican.com/article/as-vets-demand-cannabis-for -ptsd-science-races-to-unlock-its-secrets/.

164 "Indeed, many people who smoke pot": National Academies of Sciences, Engineering, and Medicine, *The Health Effects of Cannabis and Cannabinoids: The Current State of Evidence and Recommendations for Research* (Washington: National Academies Press, 2017).

164 "Strains that are high in the minimally psychoactive ingredient cannabidiol (CBD)": K. Iffland and F. Grotenhermen, "An update on safety and side effects of cannabidiol: A review of clinical data and relevant animal studies," *Cannabis and Cannabinoid Research* 2, no. 1 (June 2017): 139–54, doi: 10.1089/can.2016.0034.

164 "High levels of the highly psychoactive compound delta-9-tetrahydrocannabinol (THC)": National Academies of Sciences, Engineering, and Medicine, *Health Effects of Cannabis*.

164 It's important to note that teenagers": J. Jacobus and S. F. Tapert, "Effects of cannabis on the adolescent brain," *Current Pharmaceutical Design* 20, no. 13 (2014): 2186–93.

165 "Eliminating gluten or dairy": P. Bressan and P. Kramer, "Bread and other edible agents of mental disease," *Frontiers in Human Neuroscience* 10 (March 2016): 130, doi: 10.3389/fnhum.2016.00130.

165 "Significantly decreasing highly processed food and sugar": E. Selhub, "Nutritional psychiatry: Your brain on food," *Harvard Health Publishing*, November 16, 2015, www.health.harvard.edu/blog/nutritional-psychiatry-your-brain-on-food-201511168626.

CHAPTER 11

173 "MBSR has repeatedly proven the effectiveness": *Mindfulness-Based Treatment Approaches: Clinician's Guide to Evidence Base and Applications*, 2nd ed., ed. R. A. Baer (San Diego, CA: Academic Press, 2014), 269–92, doi: 10.1016/b978–0–12–416031–6.00012–8.

174 "One study that focused on using the Body Scan": S. J. Dreeben, M. H. Mamberg, and P. Salmon, "The MBSR body scan in clinical practice," *Mindfulness* 4, no. 4 (December 2013): 394–401, doi: 10.1007/s12671–013–0212-z.

174 "A variation on the Body Scan": L. C. Van der Maas, A. Köke, M. Pont, R. J. Bosscher, J. W. R. Twisk, T. W. Janssen, and M. L. Peters, "Improving the multidisciplinary treatment of chronic pain by stimulating body awareness," *Clinical Journal of Pain* 31, no. 7 (July 2015): 660–69.

174 "*Atlas of the Human Anatomy*": F. H. Netter and S. Colacino, *Atlas of the Human Anatomy* (Summit, NJ: Ciba-Geigy Corporation, 1989).

174 "*The Anatomy Coloring Book*": W. Kapit and L. M. Elson. *The Anatomy Coloring Book* (New York: Harper & Row, 1977).

174 "listed in the Notes": "Human Body Images," sciencekids.co.nz, http://www.sciencekids.co.nz/pictures/humanbody.html; "The Human Organ Systems," lumenlearning.com, https://courses.lumenlearning.com/ap1x94x1/chapter/the-human-organ-systems/; "Human Body Diagram," bodytomy.com, https://bodytomy.com/human-body-diagram.

CHAPTER 12

184 "'They are,'" the novelist Neil Gaiman has written": N. Gaiman, *Trigger Warning: Short Fictions and Disturbances* (New York: William Morrow, 2015).

185 "As you can see, triggers shift": Kozlowska et al., "Fear and the defense cascade."

185 "We can understand this": R. M. Nesse, S. Bhatnagar, and B. Ellis, "Evolutionary origins and functions of the stress response system," in *Stress: Concepts, Cognition, Emotion, and Behavior*, ed. G. Fink (San Diego, CA: Academic Press, 2016), 95–101, doi: 10.1016 /b978–0–12–800951–2.00011-x.

186 "And to make matters even more disturbing": Sherin and Nemeroff, "Post-traumatic stress disorder."

186 "First you have to know it's happening": B. Van der Kolk, "Posttraumatic stress disorder and the nature of trauma," *Dialogues in Clinical Neuroscience* 2, no. 1 (March 2000): 7–22.

188 "As we age": J. Moye and S. J. Rouse, "Posttraumatic stress in older adults: When medical diagnoses or treatments cause traumatic stress," *Clinics in Geriatric Medicine* 30, no. 3 (August 2014): 577–89.

189 "As we breathe slowly and deeply": M. A. Russo, D. M. Santarelli, and D. O'Rourke, "The physiological effects of slow breathing in the healthy human," *Breathe* 13, no. 4 (December 2017): 298–309.

189 "Self-awareness, memory, and judgment": E. Luders, P. M. Thompson, and F. Kurth, "Larger hippocampal dimensions in meditation practitioners: Differential effects in women and men," *Frontiers in Psychology* 6 (March 2015): 186, doi: 10.3389 /fpsyg.2015.00186.

189 "Self-awareness, memory, and judgment": S. Sun, Z. Yao, J. Wei, and R. Yu, "Calm and smart? A selective review of meditation effects on decision making," *Frontiers in Psychology* 6 (July 2015): 1059.

CHAPTER 13

195 "All trauma takes a toll on our sex and love lives.": R. Yehuda, A. Lehrner, and T. Y. Rosenbaum, "PTSD and sexual dysfunction in men and women," *Journal of Sexual Medicine* 12, no. 5 (May 2015): 1107–19, doi: 10.1111/jsm.12856.

195 "When the trauma is explicitly sexual": C. Malmo and T. S. Laidlaw, "Symptoms of trauma and traumatic memory retrieval in adult survivors of childhood sexual abuse," *Journal of Trauma & Dissociation* 11, no. 1 (2010): 22–43, doi: 10.1080/15299730903318467.

195 "Survivors of sexual abuse are swamped": K. Priebe, N. Kleindienst, J. Zimmer, S. Koudela, U. Ebner-Priemer, and M. Bohus, "Frequency of intrusions and flashbacks in patients with posttraumatic stress disorder related to childhood sexual abuse: An electronic diary study," *Psychological Assessment* 25, no. 4 (December 2013): 1370–76, doi: 10.1037/a0033816.

196 "Surgery on breasts and genitals": P. Arnaboldi, C. Lucchiari, L. Santoro, C. Sangalli, A. Luini, and G. Pravettoni, "PTSD symptoms as a consequence of breast can-

cer diagnosis: Clinical implications," *SpringerPlus* 3 (July 2014): 392, doi: 10.1186/2193 -1801-3-392.

196 "Sometimes, if we've lost a lover or spouse": S. Zisook, Y. Chentsova-Dutton, and S. R. Shuchter, "PTSD following bereavement," *Annals of Clinical Psychiatry* 10, no. 4 (December 1998): 157–63.

200 "Reaching beyond the circle of complicity": R. B. Flannery Jr., "Social support and psychological trauma: A methodological review," *Journal of traumatic Stress* 3, no. 4 (October 1990): 593–611.

CHAPTER 14

209 "Thirty-five years ago": R. S. Ulrich, "View through a window may influence recovery from surgery," *Science* 224, no. 4647 (April 1984): 420–21.

209 "In the years since then": R. Parsons, L. G. Tassinary, R. S. Ulrich, M. R. Hebl, and M. Grossman-Alexander, "The view from the road: Implications for stress recovery and immunization," *Journal of Environmental Psychology* 18, no. 2 (June 1998): 113–40.

209 "Depressed people who stroll in green places": E. C. South, B. C. Hohl, M. C. Kondo, J. M. MacDonald, and C. C. Branas, "Effect of greening vacant land on mental health of community-dwelling adults: A cluster randomized trial," *JAMA Network Open* 1, no. 3 (2018): e180298, doi: 10.1001/jamanetworkopen.2018.0298.

209 "Recently, Gregory Bratman and his Stanford colleagues": G. N. Bratman, J. P. Hamilton, K. S. Hahn, G. C. Daily, and J. J. Gross, "Nature experience reduces rumination and subgenual prefrontal cortex activation," *Proceedings of the National Academy of Sciences* 112, no. 28 (July 2015): 8567–72, doi: 10.1073/pnas.1510459112.

209 "Research in England shows": Nature Nurture, "What we do," NatureNurture.org.uk, https://naturenurture.org.uk/what-we-do/.

209 "One study suggests that the *mycobacteria vaccae* organisms": D. M. Matthews and S. M. Jenks, "Ingestion of Mycobacterium vaccae decreases anxiety-related behavior and improves learning in mice," *Behavioural Processes* 96 (June 2013): 27–35, doi: 10.1016 /j.beproc.2013.02.0077.

209 "In Japan, research on *Shinrin-yoku*, 'forest bathing,'": B. J. Park, Y. Tsunetsugu, T. Kasetani, T. Kagawa, and Y. Miyazaki, "The physiological effects of Shinrin-yoku (taking in the forest atmosphere or forest bathing): Evidence from field experiments in 24 forests across Japan," *Environmental Health and Preventive Medicine* 15, no. 1 (January 2010): 18–26, doi: 10.1007/s12199–009–0086–9.

214 "The first man to walk the entire Appalachian Trail": A. Tucker, "The army veteran who became the first to hike the entire Appalachian Trail," *Smithsonian*, July 2017, www.smithsonianmag.com/smithsonian-institution/army-veteran-became-first -hike-entire-appalachian-trail-180963678/.

214 "Cheryl Strayed's account": C. Strayed, *Wild: From Lost to Found on the Pacific Crest Trail* (New York: Random House, 2012).

214 "'In wilderness,'" Thoreau observed": H. D. Thoreau, "Walking," in *Collected Essays and Poems*, vol. 124 (New York: Library of America, 2001).

CHAPTER 15

216 "they flocked to events with therapy dogs": Therapy Dogs International, "DSRD (Disaster Stress Relief Dogs)," https://www.tdi-dog.org/OurPrograms.aspx?Page =DSRD+(Disaster+Stress+Relief+Dogs).

216 "Children facing potentially fatal cancer": CRC Health, "What is equine therapy?" www.crchealth.com/types-of-therapy/what-is-equine-therapy/.

216 "For more than two hundred years": Equestrian Therapy, "History of animal assisted therapy," www.equestriantherapy.com/history-animal-assisted-therapy/.

216 "In the late nineteenth century, Florence Nightingale observed": C. Braun, "Animal-assisted therapy: Analysis of patient testimonials," *Journal of Undergraduate Nursing Scholarship* 8, no. 1 (Fall 2006).

216 "And not long afterward, stern Sigmund Freud": "Beside Freud's couch, a chow named Jofi," *Wall Street Journal*, December 21, 2010, www.wsj.com/articles/SB10001424052748 703886904576031630124087362.

216 "Several studies on healthy adults": E. P. Cherniack and A. R. Cherniack, "The benefit of pets and animal-assisted therapy to the health of older individuals," *Current Gerontology and Geriatrics Research* 2014 (2014), doi: 10.1155/2014/623203.

216 "One small study": J. S. Odendaal, "Animal-assisted therapy—magic or medicine?," *Journal of Psychosomatic Research* 49, no. 4 (October 2000): 275–80, doi: 10.1016/s0022 –3999(00)00183–5.

217 "Several years ago, Erika Friedmann and her colleagues": E. Friedmann, A. H. Katcher, J. J. Lynch, and S. A. Thomas, "Animal companions and one-year survival of patients after discharge from a coronary care unit," *Public Health Reports* 95, no. 4 (July–August 1980): 307–12.

217 "Studies also indicate": M. E. O'Haire, S. J. McKenzie, A. M. Beck, and V. Slaughter, "Social behaviors increase in children with autism in the presence of animals compared to toys," *PLoS One* 8, no. 2 (2013): e57010, doi: 10.1371/journal.pone.0057010.

217 "an article from the *New York Times*": C. Siebert, "What does a parrot know about PTSD," *New York Times*, January 28, 2016, https://www.nytimes.com/2016/01/31 /magazine/what-does-a-parrot-know-about-ptsd.html.

CHAPTER 16

222 "In 1976, Norman Cousins": N. Cousins, "Anatomy of an illness (as perceived by the patient)," *New England Journal of Medicine* 295, no. 26 (December 23, 1976): 1458–63, doi: 10.1056/nejm197612232952605.

223 "The book based on his article": N. Cousins, *Anatomy of an Illness as Perceived by the Patient: Reflections on Healing and Regeneration* (New York: W. W. Norton, 1979).

223 "improve mood in cancer patients": L. Erdman, "Laughter therapy for patients with cancer," *Journal of Psychosocial Oncology* 11, no. 4 (1994): 55–67.

223 "decrease hostility in patients in mental hospitals": M. Gelkopf, S. Kreitler, and M. Sigal, "Laughter in a psychiatric ward: Somatic, emotional, social, and clinical influences on schizophrenic patients," *Journal of Nervous and Mental Disease* 181, no. 5 (May 1993): 283–89.

223 "Laughter stimulates the dome-shaped diaphragmatic muscle": J. Yim, "Therapeutic benefits of laughter in mental health: A theoretical review," *Tohoku Journal of Experimental Medicine* 239, no. 3 (July 2016): 243–49.

224 "the 'herd level'": F. Nietzsche and T. Common, *Thus Spake Zarathustra* (Mineola, NY: Dover Publications, 1999).

227 "they are beginning to explore and make use of its power": M. Yazdani, M. Esmaeil-zadeh, S. Pahlavanzadeh, and F. Khaledi, "The effect of laughter Yoga on general health among nursing students," *Iranian Journal of Nursing and Midwifery Research* 19, no. 1 (January 2014): 36–40; D. Louie, K. Brook, and E. Frates, "The laughter prescription: A tool for lifestyle medicine," *American Journal of Lifestyle Medicine* 10, no. 4 (June 2016): 262–67.

229 "Several years ago, I was in Jordan": J. Gordon, "For Syrian refugees, a mental health emergency," *The Atlantic*, March 20, 2013, https://www.theatlantic.com/health /archive/2013/03/for-syrian-refugees-a-mental-health-emergency/274176/.

CHAPTER 17

235 "In recent years, a number of studies have shown how trauma can be transmitted": T. B. Franklin, H. Russig, I. C. Weiss, J. Gräff, N. Linder, A. Michalon, S. Vizi, and I. M. Mansuy, "Epigenetic transmission of the impact of early stress across genera-tions," *Biological Psychiatry* 68, no. 5 (September 2010): 408–15.

235 "Studies on animals": K. Gapp, A. Jawaid, P. Sarkies, J. Bohacek, P. Pelczar, J. Prados, L. Farinelli, E. Miska, and I. M. Mansuy, "Implication of sperm RNAs in transgenera-tional inheritance of the effects of early trauma in mice," *Nature Neuroscience* 17, no. 5 (May 2014): 667–69.

236 "And these changes have also been observed in the descendants": R. Yehuda, L. M. Bierer, J. Schmeidler, D. H. Aferiat, I. Breslau, and S. Dolan, "Low cortisol and risk for PTSD in adult offspring of holocaust survivors," *American Journal of Psychiatry* 157, no. 8 (August 2000): 1252–59.

237 "Genograms": M. McGoldrick, R. Gerson, and S. S. Petry, *Genograms: Assessment and Intervention* (New York: W. W. Norton, 2008).

CHAPTER 18

251 "Recent research by UCLA psychologist Shelly Taylor": S. E. Taylor, L. C. Klein, B. P. Lewis, T. L. Gruenewald, R. A. Gurung, and J. A. Updegraff, "Biobehavioral responses to stress in females: Tend-and-befriend, not fight-or-flight," *Psychological Review* 107, no. 3 (July 2000): 411–29, doi: 10.1037/0033-295X.107.3.411.

251 "The male's response is driven, as we've seen": R. Afrisham, S. Sadegh-Nejadi, O. SoliemaniFar, W. Kooti, D. Ashtary-Larky, F. Alamiri, M. Aberomand, S. Najjar-Asl, and A. Khaneh-Keshi, "Salivary testosterone levels under psychological stress and its relationship with rumination and five personality traits in medical students," *Psychia-try Investigation* 13, no. 6 (November 2016): 637–43.

251 "The female hormone estrogen and pain-relieving endorphins": T. J. Shors, J. Pickett,

G. Wood, and M. Paczynski, "Acute stress persistently enhances estrogen levels in the female rat," *Stress* 3, no. 2 (December 1999): 163–71, doi: 10.3109/10253899909001120.

252 "Over the past twenty years, we've repeatedly demonstrated": Gordon et al., "Treatment of posttraumatic stress disorder in postwar Kosovar adolescents."

252 "Students who participated in our groups": Gordon, "Mind-body skills groups for medical students," 198.

260 "Carl Jung described these meaningful but not cause-and-effect connections": C. G. Jung, *Synchronicity: An Acausal Connecting Principle (From Vol. 8. of the Collected Works of C.G. Jung)* (Princeton, NJ: Princeton Univ. Press, 2010).

CHAPTER 19

267 "Brother David Steindl-Rast": H. Walters, "Want to be happy? Be grateful: Brother David Steindl-Rast at TEDGlobal 2013," *TED Blog*, June 14, 2013, https://blog.ted.com/want-to-be-happy-be-grateful-brother-david-steindl-rast-at-tedglobal-2013/.

267 "Recent scientific studies show that these grateful people": R. A. Emmons and M. E. McCullough, "Counting blessings versus burdens: An experimental investigation of gratitude and subjective well-being in daily life," *Journal of Personality and Social Psychology* 84, no. 2 (February 2003): 377–89.

267 "Grateful people who have had one heart attack": P. J. Mills, K. Wilson, M. A. Punga, K. Chinh, C. Pruitt, B. H. Greenberg, O. Lunde, A. Wood, L. Redwine, and D. Chopra, "The role of gratitude in well-being in asymptomatic heart failure patients," *Integrative Medicine: A Clinician's Journal* 14, no. 1 (February 2015): 51.

267 "Sleep, so often interrupted after trauma": A. M. Wood, S. Joseph, J. Lloyd, and S. Atkins, "Gratitude influences sleep through the mechanism of pre-sleep cognitions," *Journal of Psychosomatic Research* 66, no. 1 (January 2009): 43–48.

268 "In fact, one Israeli study shows": Y. Israel-Cohen, F. Uzefovsky, G. Kashy-Rosenbaum, and O. Kaplan, "Gratitude and PTSD symptoms among Israeli youth exposed to missile attacks: Examining the mediation of positive and negative affect and life satisfaction," *Journal of Positive Psychology* 10, no. 2 (2015): 99–106.

270 "Robert Emmons of the University of California at Davis": Robert A. Emmons and Michael E. McCullough, *The Psychology of Gratitude* (New York: Oxford Univ. Press, 2004).

CHAPTER 20

275 "Modern science has confirmed ancient wisdom": C. vanOyen Witvliet, T. E. Ludwig, and K. L. Vander Laan, "Granting forgiveness or harboring grudges: Implications for emotion, physiology, and health," *Psychological Science* 12, no. 2 (March 2001): 117–23, doi: 10.1111/1467-9280.00320.

275 "Forgiving is therapeutic": E. Ricciardi, G. Rota, L. Sani, C. Gentili, A. Gaglianese, M. Guazzelli, and P. Pietrini, "How the brain heals emotional wounds: The functional neuroanatomy of forgiveness," *Frontiers in Human Neuroscience* 7 (2013): 839.

275 "Combat veterans who are more capable of Forgiveness": Ö. Karaırmak and

B. Güloğlu, "Forgiveness and PTSD among veterans: The mediating role of anger and negative affect," *Psychiatry Research* 219, no. 3 (November 2014): 536–42, doi: 10.1016 /j.psychres.2014.05.024.

277 "There are comprehensive, intensive programs to promote Forgiveness": International Forgiveness Institute, "How to forgive." http://www.internationalforgiveness.com /need-to-forgive.htm.

277 "Children and adults generally finish Enright's months-long programs": G. L. Reed and R. D. Enright, "The effects of forgiveness therapy on depression, anxiety, and posttraumatic stress for women after spousal emotional abuse," *Journal of Consulting and Clinical Psychology* 74, no. 5 (October 2006): 920–29, doi: 10.1037/0022–006x.74.5.920.

CHAPTER 21

290 "A 2008 study published by psychologist Joshua Smyth": J. M. Smyth and J. W. Pennebaker, "Exploring the boundary conditions of expressive writing: In search of the right recipe," *British Journal of Health Psychology* 13, no. 1 (February 2008): 1–7.

290 "Recent research on this altruistic activity": M. M. Filkowski, R. N. Cochran, and B. W. Haas, "Altruistic behavior: Mapping responses in the brain," *Neuroscience and Neuroeconomics* 5 (2016): 65–75, doi: 10.2147/NAN.S87718.

296 "Kate Wolf's": K. Wolf, *Give Yourself to Love* (Kaleidoscope Records C-3000, 1983), audio cassette.

APPENDIX: FINDING OTHER HELP

312 "In an earlier book of mine—*Unstuck*": J. S. Gordon, *Unstuck: Your Guide to the Seven-Stage Journey out of Depression* (New York: Penguin Books, 2009).

312 "The phrase he used for this relationship was 'unconditional positive regard.'": C. R. Rogers, *On Becoming a Person: A Therapist's View of Psychotherapy* (Boston: Houghton Mifflin, 1961).

316 "Cognitive-Behavioral Therapy (CBT)": N. Kar, "Cognitive behavioral therapy for the treatment of post-traumatic stress disorder: A review," *Neuropsychiatric Disease and Treatment* 7 (2011): 167–81.

316 "Developed by University of Pennsylvania psychiatrist Aaron Beck": J. S. Beck, *Cognitive Behavior Therapy: Basics and Beyond* (New York: Guilford Press, 2011).

317 "There is a significant body of research on CBT's effectiveness": P. P. Schnurr, M. J. Friedman, C. C. Engel, E. B. Foa, M. T. Shea, B. K. Chow, P. A. Resick, et al., "Cognitive behavioral therapy for posttraumatic stress disorder in women: A randomized controlled trial," *JAMA* 297, no. 8 (February 28, 2007): 820–30, doi: 10.1001 /jama.297.8.820.

317 "Trauma-Focused Cognitive Behavioral Therapy (TF-CBT)": J. A. Cohen, A. P. Mannarino, L. Berliner, and E. Deblinger, "Trauma-focused cognitive behavioral therapy for children and adolescents: An empirical update," *Journal of Interpersonal Violence* 15, no. 11 (November 2000): 1202–23.

317 "Dialectical Behavioral Therapy (DBT)": A. L. Chapman, "Dialectical behavior ther-

apy: Current indications and unique elements," *Psychiatry (Edgmont)* 3, no. 9 (September 2006): 62–68.

318 "Cognitive Processing Therapy (CPT)": K. Tran, K. Moulton, N. Santesso, and D. Rabb, *Cognitive Processing Therapy for Post-Traumatic Stress Disorder: A Systematic Review and Meta-Analysis,* CADTH Health Technology Assessment, no. 141 (Ottawa: Canadian Agency for Drugs and Technologies in Health, 2016), https://www.ncbi.nlm.nih.gov /books/NBK362346/.

318 "Acceptance and Commitment Therapy": S. C. Hayes, M. E. Levin, J. Plumb-Vilardaga, J. L. Villatte, and J. Pistorello, "Acceptance and commitment therapy and contextual behavioral science: Examining the progress of a distinctive model of behavioral and cognitive therapy," *Behavior Therapy* 44, no. 2 (June 2013): 180–98.

318 "Prolonged Exposure (PE)": E. B. Foa, E. A. Hembree, S. P. Cahill, S. A. Rauch, D. S. Riggs, N. C. Feeny, and E. Yadin, "Randomized trial of prolonged exposure for post-traumatic stress disorder with and without cognitive restructuring: Outcome at academic and community clinics," *Journal of Consulting and Clinical Psychology* 73, no. 5 (October 2005): 953–64; A. Eftekhari, L. R. Stines, and L. A. Zoellner, "Do you need to talk about it? Prolonged exposure for the treatment of chronic PTSD," *Behavior Analyst Today* 7, no. 1 (January 2006): 70–83, https://www.ncbi.nlm.nih.gov/pmc/articles /PMC2770710/.

319 "Narrative Exposure Therapy (NET)": N. Gwozdziewycz and L. Mehl-Madrona, "Meta-analysis of the use of narrative exposure therapy for the effects of trauma among refugee populations," *Permanente Journal* 17, no. 1 (Winter 2013): 70–76.

319 "Mindfulness-Based Stress Reduction (MBSR)": M. A. Polusny, C. R. Erbes, P. Thuras, A. Moran, G. J. Lamberty, R. C. Collins, J. L. Rodman, and K. O. Lim, "Mindfulness-based stress reduction for posttraumatic stress disorder among veterans: a randomized clinical trial," *Jama* 314, no. 5 (2015): 456–65; J. Boyd, R. Lanius, and M. McKinnon, "Mindfulness-based treatments for posttraumatic stress disorder: a review of the treatment literature and neurobiological evidence," *Journal of Psychiatry & Neuroscience* (2018): 7–25.

320 "can decrease anxiety": D. W. Orme-Johnson and V. A. Barnes, "Effects of the transcendental meditation technique on trait anxiety: A meta-analysis of randomized controlled trials," *Journal of Alternative and Complementary Medicine* 19 (2013): 1–12.

320 "In one randomized controlled trial": V. A. Barnes, "Transcendental meditation and treatment for post-traumatic stress disorder," *Lancet Psychiatry* 5, no. 12 (December 2018): 946–47, doi: 10.1016/S2215-0366(18)30423-1.

320 "Eye Movement Desensitization and Reprocessing (EMDR)": F. Shapiro, "The role of eye movement desensitization and reprocessing (EMDR) therapy in medicine: Addressing the psychological and physical symptoms stemming from adverse life experiences," *Permanente Journal* 18, no. 1 (Winter 2014): 71–77, doi: 10.7812/TPP/13–098.

321 "the critical role of eye movement has been challenged": M. Sack, S. Zehl, A. Otti, C. Lahmann, P. Henningsen, J. Kruse, and M. Stingl, "A Comparison of Dual Attention, Eye Movements, and Exposure Only during Eye Movement Desensitization and Reprocessing for Posttraumatic Stress Disorder: Results from a Randomized Clinical Trial," *Psychotherapy and Psychosomatics* 85, no. 6 (2016): 357–65. doi:10.1159/000447671.

321 "Interpersonal Therapy (IPT)": J. C. Markowitz, E. Petkova, Y. Neria, P. E. Van Meter, Y. Zhao, E. Hembree, K. Lovell, T. Biyanova, and R. D. Marshall, "Is exposure necessary? A randomized clinical trial of interpersonal psychotherapy for PTSD," *American Journal of Psychiatry* 172, no. 5 (May 2015): 430–40, doi: 10.1176/appi.ajp.2014.14070908.

322 "Somatic Experiencing (SE)": D. Brom, Y. Stokar, C. Lawi, V. Nuriel-Porat, Y. Ziv, K. Lerner, and G. Ross, "Somatic experiencing for posttraumatic stress disorder: A randomized controlled outcome study," *Journal of Traumatic Stress* 30, no. 3 (June 2017): 304–12.

323 "EFT": G. Craig, *The EFT Manual* (Santa Rosa, CA: Energy Psychology Press, 2011).

323 "TFT": R. Callahan and J. Callahan, *Thought Field Therapy (TFT) and Trauma: Treatment and Theory* (Nellysford, VA: Thought Field Therapy Training Center, 1996).

323 "Audun Irgens and Dawson Church": D. Church, S. Stern, E. Boath, A. Stewart, D. Feinstein, and M. Clond, "Emotional freedom techniques to treat posttraumatic stress disorder in veterans: Review of the evidence, survey of practitioners, and proposed clinical guidelines," *Permanente Journal* 21, no. 4 (Fall 2017): 27–34.

323 "Antidepressant drugs like the selective serotonin reuptake inhibitors (SSRIs)": M. E. Charney, S. N. Hellberg, E. Bui, and N. M. Simon, "Evidence-based treatment of posttraumatic stress disorder: An updated review of validated psychotherapeutic and pharmacological approaches," *Harvard Review of Psychiatry* 26, no. 3 (May–June 2018): 99–115.

323 "And these drugs have very significant side effects": James M. Ferguson, "SSRI Antidepressant Medications: Adverse Effects and Tolerability," *Primary Care Companion to the Journal of Clinical Psychiatry* 3, no. 1 (February 2001): 22–27.

324 "SAM-e plays a vital role": I. Galizia, L. Oldani, K. Macritchie, E. Amari, D. Dougall, T. N. Jones, R. W. Lam, G. J. Masei, L. N. Yatham, and A. H. Young, "S-adenosyl methionine (SAMe) for depression in adults," *Cochrane Database of Systematic Reviews*, October 10, 2016, https://www.cochranelibrary.com/cdsr/doi/10.1002/14651858.CD011286/media/CDSR/CD011286/rel0001/CD011286/CD011286.pdf.

Acknowledgments

Writing for me is solitary, mysterious. This book seemed to grow sometimes easily, sometimes with difficulty, in the dark. However, its soil and sources, the nourishment that made it possible, have been communal. This is where I thank those who have nurtured *The Transformation* and me.

First, there are my parents, Jules and Cynthia Gordon. They gave me life, invited and urged me to be a doctor, and impressed on me the power of words, even as they challenged me to deal with their trauma and the turmoil, as well the love, they brought into my life and the lives of my dear brothers, Andy and Jeff.

Next, guides on the path, especially Bill Alfred and Bob Coles, to whom I bow in this book but cannot adequately thank. Also, R. D. Laing, Lynne Dwyer, Edward Burchard, Gregory Bateson, David Cheek, Jose Rosa, and Credo Mutwa.

Then, institutions that embraced me unconditionally and welcomed all my exploration, including Harvard College and Mount

Zion Hospital. And others, that offered, along with opportunity and support, challenges that called me to find myself: Harvard Medical School, The Albert Einstein College of Medicine, The National Institute of Mental Health, and The National Institutes of Health.

I've named people in this book who over more than fifty years have helped me discover who I am. Once again, my gratitude to Sharon Curtin, great spirit, superb storyteller, my ex-wife and friend; and to Shyam Singha, healer and trickster, who shone in my life like the sun after which he is named.

There are dozens of others who appear in *The Transformation* who have been, as I've said, my teachers as well as my patients and students. All of them have been wondrously generous in sharing their stories and their lives with me and you. I am deeply grateful to them all. I have called most of them by their first names, and altered identifying details. Only they, or perhaps a partner or spouse, a parent or an intimate friend, will know who they are.

Though I have omitted many details and changed their occupations and locations, the participants in the chapter "The Healing Circle" will probably recognize one another as well as themselves. I hope that all of you feel I've been respectful and fully appreciative of your powerful, heartfelt sharing and of our experience together.

The thirty CMBM staff and our 130 international faculty are the nucleus of the healing community and the community of healers that I hoped thirty years ago to create and be a member of. In addition to those about whom I write in *The Transformation,* I want particularly to thank a number with whom I've partnered for twenty years or more: Amy Shinal, our clinical director, who tenderly and wisely mentors our faculty; Tina Fisher, who first held my DC office together and then extended her embrace to our work in Kosovo and the Middle East; Julie Staples, our tireless and scrupulous research director; Kathie Swift, the architect of our Food As Medicine program, who carefully read over and commented on my chapter on "The Trauma-Healing Diet"; Lynda Richtsmeier-Cyr, our associate clinical director; Susan Blum; Monique Class; Joel Evans; Kathy Farah; Carol Jacobs; Debra Kaplan; Jerrol Kimmel; Lora Matz; Gjorgi (Goce) Nikoloski; and Cheri Snyder.

Ten years ago, Rosemary Lombard-Murrain, my goddaughter, began work with CMBM as a skeptical but curious volunteer. "What on earth is Jim up to?" she wondered. Now she knows. She's our managing director and works closely, lovingly, with me to develop, expand, and help ensure the survival of all that we do.

CMBM's reach is increasingly worldwide. We are as much a movement for self-care and group support, for community healing and compassion, as we are a therapeutic intervention. Working and living in this larger space has given greater breadth and depth to everything I do at CMBM, to me, and to *The Transformation*.

I particularly want to thank Jamil Abdel Atti and his team, who have for the last fifteen years courageously led our program in Gaza—where we've worked with more than 170,000 children and adults; Afrim Blyta and Jusuf Ulaj, my adopted brothers, who along with Murat Butyai and the other Suhareka teachers made our foundational work in Kosovo possible; Rhonda Adessky, Naomi Baum, Danny Grossman, and Naftali Halberstadt in Israel; Linda Metayer, Regine Laroche, and Bishop Pierre André Dumas in Haiti; and Anyieth D'Awol, who is now leading the effort to bring our program to war-traumatized people in Eastern and Southern Africa.

I want to acknowledge the US staff, as adventurous as they are competent and responsible, who over the years have made this international work possible. In addition to Tina Fisher, they include Margaret Gavian, Dan Sterenchuk, Lee-Ann Gallarano, Jesse Harding, and, for the last several years, Musarrat Al-Azzeh, our wonderfully kind and skillful associate director for global trauma relief.

Thanks too to Klara Royal, who has supported all our work; Cathy

Furst and Hannah Quinn, who organize so many of our US programs with grace and efficiency; and Elizabeth Kaplan, who helps find funds for all we do.

The founding CMBM Board of Directors got us started: It included Don DeLaski, Rick deLone, William Fair, Marc Grossman, Tom Joe, Mary-Lynn Kotz, Lyn Rales, Robert Schwartz, Robert Shaye, Fera Simone, and Michael Tigar. Our current Board of Directors—Whitey Bluestein, Ann Hoopes, Mark Hyman, Dennis Jaffe, Dave Levy, Karen Saverino, and Barbara Stohlman—continues to provide guidance, encouragement, and support. A special thanks to Dave, who, attending to the call of friendship and his kinship with our mission, has done so much to raise the funds to make what we do possible.

Our Advisory Board—you'll see names and quotes from several of them on the back of this book—has always been available and encouraging.

I'm enormously grateful to the thousands of people who've supported me and CMBM. I especially want to acknowledge Don DeLaski, whose generosity and good counsel made everything possible, and his daughter Kathleen, who honors Don's legacy; Charles ("Chuck") Feeney, the founding chairman of The Atlantic Philanthropies, who saw our work in Gaza and Israel as analogous to the Irish Peace Process, which he helped facilitate, and supported us accordingly; Penny George, who with her husband Bill and The George Family Foundation have been there for and with us at critical times; Liz Salett, who has generously sustained our work in Gaza; Lisa Harris and Steve Simon, with whom we're partnering to bring population-wide healing and wellness to the people of Indianapolis; and former US Senator Tom Harkin. It was Tom who assured Bill and Hillary Clinton that I was the right one to chair the advisory council to NIH and The White House Commission on Complementary and Alternative Medicine Policy.

Many people have helped me with this book. First, my gratitude to my four executive assistants, who over the years of *The Transformation's* growth and development have worked so hard and so kindly to interpret illegible writing, transcribe drafts, offer helpful suggestions, remind me of deadlines, and organize and protect my time: Amberjade Mwekali-Tsering, Hope Rubin, Bexia Shi, and Linda Hanes. I don't know if I could have done this book without them. I do know their intelligence, support, and love have made it possible for me to do it as well as I could.

Other staff and interns have provided invaluable help with the research. Staff first: Tim Eden and Nosheen Hayatt. And the interns: David Belton II, Tiffany Chiu, Laura Farnsworth, Emily Fitzpatrick, Rachel Rubin, Seleena Saad, Harlove Singh, Monika Stedul, Kyle Tran, Sarah Woody, and Sadie Zuch.

Three other interns provided examples of commitment and intelligence, care, and kindness that I want to explicitly acknowledge. Catherine Parkhurst developed the references for "The Trauma-Healing Diet" and set a standard for all of us. Aproteem Choudhury, with great skill and patience, produced and edited the final version of the Notes that I hope will help readers of *The Transformation* to explore the scientific literature that supports it. Tatiana Znayenko-Miller worked closely with Apro and has always been there when we needed something more.

My former agent, Chris Tomasino, helped me move toward this book, and Richard Pine and Aviva Romm pointed me in the right direction.

Bonnie Solow, my new agent, worked with me—guiding, inspiring, and cheerfully, skillfully, nudging me—to make my vision a reality. Gideon Weil, my editor at HarperOne, embraced *The Transformation* with immediate warmth and graceful intelligence and has continued to shepherd it to publication. Lisa Zuniga led the copyediting and kept us moving forward.

I briefly mention my two buddies, George Blecher and Howard

(Mahadeva) Josepher, in *The Transformation*. Along with Lynne and Bill Twist and Allison Berardi, my son Gabe's mother, they've offered me homes away from home, unstinting appreciation and encouragement, and, in George's case, some clearheaded editorial guidance as well as love.

Absent friends Belle Phillips, Marshall Berman, Bob Buckley, Ragi Doggweiler, and Brenda Sowder have been present for me.

I'm grateful with every Soft Belly breath for my loving, sustaining connection to my godchildren, Rosemary's brothers, Matt and George Lombard, and Lilly-Marie Blecher, and their families, and of course, to the two children, Gabriel Gordon-Berardi and Jamie Lord, to whom *The Transformation* is dedicated.

Every day, all of you help me to remember that, as my Lakota brothers and sisters have taught me, we are all related.

Index

About the Author

James S. Gordon, MD, a Harvard-educated psychiatrist, is a world-renowned expert in using mind-body medicine to treat and prevent depression, anxiety, and chronic illness as well as psychological trauma. He is the founder and executive director of The Center for Mind-Body Medicine (CMBM) and a clinical professor in the departments of psychiatry and family medicine at Georgetown Medical School. He served as chair of the White House Commission on Complementary and Alternative Medicine Policy as well as the first chair of the Program Advisory Council of the National Institutes of Health's Office of Alternative Medicine.

Dr. Gordon has devoted almost fifty years to the exploration and practice of mind-body medicine. After graduating from Harvard Medical School and completing his psychiatric residency at the Albert Einstein College of Medicine, he was for eleven years a research psychiatrist at the National Institute of Mental Health. There he developed the first national program for runaway and homeless youth, coedited the first comprehensive studies of alternative and holistic medicine, directed the Special Study on Alternative Services for President Jimmy Carter's Commission on Mental Health, and organized a nationwide preceptorship program for medical students.

For more than twenty years, Dr. Gordon and CMBM have focused on relieving population-wide psychological trauma: in war-traumatized children and families in Bosnia, Kosovo, Israel, and Gaza and with Syrian refugees in Jordan; in US military and veterans; and in firefighters and their families in post–9/11 New York City. Dr. Gordon has also led sustainable community-wide programs of trauma healing on the Pine Ridge Indian Reservation in South Dakota; in Broward County, Florida, after the school shootings in Parkland; and following climate-change-related disasters in Louisiana (Hurricane Katrina), Haiti (the 2010 earthquake), Houston (Hurricane Harvey), Puerto Rico (Hurricanes Irma and Maria), and Sonoma, California (wildfires). In addition, Dr. Gordon and his CMBM team have created groundbreaking programs of comprehensive mind-body healing for physicians, medical students, and other health professionals and for people with cancer, depression, and other chronic illnesses.

Dr. Gordon is the author or editor of twelve previous books, including *Unstuck: Your Guide to the Seven-Stage Journey Out of Depression* (Penguin Press), *Manifesto for a New Medicine: Your Guide to Healing Partnerships and the Wise Use of Alternative Therapies* (Perseus Books), and the award-winning *Health for the Whole Person*. He has authored numerous book chapters and has published more than 130 articles in professional journals and general-interest magazines and newspapers, among them *The American Journal of Psychiatry*, *The Journal of Clinical Psychiatry*, *The Journal of Traumatic Stress*, *Traumatology*, *International Journal of Stress Man-*

agement, *Psychiatry*, *The American Family Physician*, and *BMC Medical Education*, as well as the *New York Times*, the *Washington Post*, the *Atlantic*, and the *Guardian* (US).

Dr. Gordon's and CMBM's work has been featured in the *New York Times*, the *Washington Post*, the *Atlantic*, *USA Today*, *Newsweek*, *People*, *American Medical News*, *Clinical Psychiatry News*, *Town and Country*, *Hippocrates*, *Psychology Today*, *Vegetarian Times*, *Natural Health*, *Health*, *Prevention*, and the *Psychotherapy Networker*, as well as on CBS 60 Minutes, Good Morning America, The Today Show, CNN, CBS Sunday Morning, FOX News, and National Public Radio and in his TedMed Talk on trauma.

You can follow Dr. Gordon's work around the world on www.cmbm .org and on his Twitter, Facebook, and Instagram accounts. You can contact him through the CMBM webpage. He lives in Washington, DC.